MEDIEVAL & EARLY RENAISSANCE MEDICINE

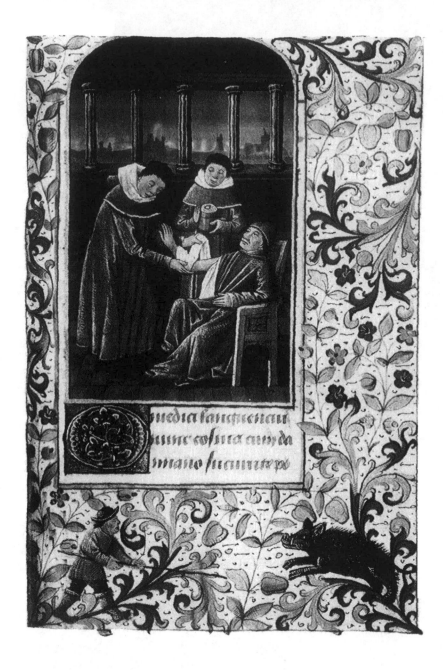

MEDIEVAL & EARLY RENAISSANCE MEDICINE

An Introduction to Knowledge and Practice

Nancy G. Siraisi

THE UNIVERSITY OF
CHICAGO PRESS
Chicago and
London

The University of Chicago Press, Chicago 60637
The University of Chicago Press, Ltd., London

12 11 10   9 8 7

Library of Congress Cataloging-in-Publication Data

Siraisi, Nancy G.
    Medieval and early Renaissance medicine : an introduction to
knowledge and practice / Nancy G. Siraisi.
        p.   cm.
    Includes bibliographical references.
    1. Medicine, Medieval.   I. Title.
R141.S546   1990   89-20368
610'.902—dc20   CIP

    ISBN 0-226-76130-4 (paper)

Frontispiece: Surgical treatment. The surgeons in this picture are actually
representations of the patron saints of medicine and surgery, Cosmas and Damian.
From a Book of Hours of the Virgin, illuminated by Jean Colombe
of Bourges about 1475. (Courtesy of Pierpont Morgan Library,
New York, MS M. 366, fol. 173ʳ.)

CONTENTS

ILLUSTRATIONS

PREFACE

The subject of this book is western European literate and technical medicine and its practitioners between about the mid-twelfth and the end of
the fifteenth century. In many respects, these centuries were part of a very
much longer period in which health conditions, attitudes to health and
disease, fundamental physiological and therapeutic concepts, and the effectiveness or ineffectiveness of medical intervention changed little. But at least
three aspects of the medicine of these centuries are of special historical
significance. In the first place, medicine has a role in the history of early
western European science and technology. As is well known, medieval
understanding of the physical universe was transformed by the twelfth- and
thirteenth-century reception of Greek science, in particular Ptolemaic astronomy and Aristotelian logic, epistemology, cosmology, and physics. The
increased knowledge of Greek medicine achieved at about the same time,
and its role in shaping medieval and Renaissance ideas about human physiology and the plant and animal kingdoms are part of the same story and no
less important.

Secondly, the history of medicine, perhaps more than that of any other
discipline or skilled occupation, illuminates broad social and cultural patterns of the period. Medicine, just as much as natural philosophy and astronomy, fully shared in the western medieval recovery of Greek, and reception
of Arabic, learning; but, unlike natural philosophy, medicine embraced
both high culture and techniques. The relation between the learned and
the technical or craft aspects of medicine was often uneasy and ambiguous
but always present. Moreover, in the complex society of the late Middle
Ages and early Renaissance, the spectrum of medical practitioners encompassed men and women, laity and clergy, learned scholastics and illiterate
herbalists; and institutions connected with medicine included both guilds
and universities. Medicine and its practitioners are part of the history of
education, of occupations and the emergence of professions, and of endeavors to manage health and disease. And—although here the historian needs
to tread with caution—attitudes, beliefs, and doctrines embedded in med-

icine may illuminate fundamental cultural assumptions about the human body, illness and wellness, the characteristics and relations of the sexes, and the stages of human life from infancy to old age.

Thirdly, the institutional, intellectual, and social characteristics taken on by medical higher education in the late Middle Ages and early Renaissance endured well into the early modern period; these characteristics formed part of the context of the advances in knowledge in the life sciences that began to accumulate in the sixteenth century. The formation of such major contributors to the creation of a new anatomy and a new physiology as Vesalius (1514–1564) and Harvey (1578–1657) took place in an environment that still owed much to the medical culture that developed in the thirteenth to fifteenth centuries.

Obviously, these three aspects do not characterize the whole of medieval and early Renaissance medicine, and this book makes no claim to survey the entire subject. The topics treated here are indicated by the chapter headings. A highly compressed chronological survey of the formation (and ancient and Islamic antecedents) of western medieval medicine is followed by chapters on practitioners and conditions of practice, medical education, physiologial and anatomical knowledge, disease and treatment, and surgeons and surgery. A brief epilogue carries the story forward to the sixteenth century. The focus is on medical practitioners—understood as including all those who made the provision of medical or surgical care, or both, their principal occupation—and on the intellectual and technical content of the medicine they studied and practiced. I hope, however, that enough is said of the social setting of medical practice, of health conditions, of the experience of patients, of the academic world of which medical learning formed a part, and of the climate of ideology and religious belief to establish a broad context for the history of medicine and its practitioners. In particular, I have tried to illuminate some of the ways in which the demand for medical care, the nature of expectations as to its results, and a shared system of medical beliefs common to practitioners and patients provided support for medicine, medical learning, and the medical profession. The medicine described in this book offered little protection against most of the factors causing human morbidity and mortality. In this respect, of course, late medieval therapies were no different from those of most other periods of history. But the ability of established forms of medical organization, knowledge, and practice to survive—despite some contemporary criticism—the crisis of the great plague epidemic of the mid-fourteenth century, and to flourish thereafter, is surely evidence that on the whole medicine adequately fulfilled contemporary expectations.

I have made no attempt to cover every topic relevant to the medical history of these centuries as understood in the widest sense. For example, Islamic medicine, a subject of great importance in its own right, is mentioned here only as an influence on the medicine of the West. Nor have I attempted to treat in any detail the history of public health or epidemiology in premodern Europe; these are the subjects of a large and increasingly sophisticated specialist literature. In particular, a systematic account of the impact of bubonic plague and other epidemic diseases upon the demography, economy, and society of the fourteenth to eighteenth centuries would take one far beyond the scope of this book and have little relevance to its central themes. Moreover, the history of medicine in this period is not closely connected with attempts to manage public health by political authorities and religious charitable foundations. The history of late medieval and early Renaissance municipal boards of health and hospitals, even though both from time to time employed medical personnel, belongs to another book.

The present state of knowledge makes it impossible to cover both intellectual and social aspects of the history of medicine in every area of medieval and early Renaissance Europe with equal thoroughness. Whereas the intellectual and technical content of medical knowledge was to a very considerable extent common throughout Europe and was shared, to a greater or lesser degree, by practitioners of many types, the social conditions of medical practice appear to have varied widely at different times and places. Moreover, excellent and comprehensive sources of information about medical ideas and knowledge are available in the shape of the numerous medieval and Renaissance medical texts, surviving in manuscript and early printed and modern editions, in Latin and in various European vernaculars, and on practical and theoretical topics. Some of these texts have, indeed, been the subject of intensive historical study, beginning in the nineteenth century. However, medical texts are essentially prescriptive; consequently, they are unreliable and inadequate sources of information about actual medical activity and its social context.

For the social history of medicine, and often for glimpses of actual practice, one must turn to other sources—to institutional and legal history and to prosopographical works of various kinds. In addition, chronicles, letter collections, saints' lives, and collections of miracles recorded at shrines or to secure a putative saint's canonization may also occasionally illuminate the experiences and attitudes of patients. Recent and ongoing studies of local archives have yielded some of the most valuable information about medical practice in different parts of Europe. At present, however, modern studies of medieval and Renaissance medical practice based on local archives are still few and scattered; additional studies of this kind, when they appear, will be important contributions to the medical history of the period.

In this book, most although by no means all of my examples come from Italy, because of the fame of its medical schools and the importance of its urban development as a social context for medical activity, and because it is the area I know best. Whatever their provenance, the examples cited are highly, although I hope not arbitrarily or inappropriately, selective. In particular, I have not attempted to convey the full range of comment on medicine to be found in medieval and Renaissance literary sources.

The expression "medieval and early Renaissance" is used here merely as a convenient way of delineating the entire span of time covered, without implying any fixed chronological boundary within it. As far as Italy is concerned, most of the period covered by this book is often called "early Renaissance"; for northern Europe in the same period, "medieval" is the term more commonly used. Moreover, the termination of the book toward the end of the fifteenth century should not be taken as meaning that 1480, or 1500, marked the end of the medicine described here, for in many respects it continued vigorously during the sixteenth and early seventeenth centuries.

My objective is to present interested readers and students of medieval, Renaissance, or medical history, or history of science with a coherent brief survey of late medieval and early Renaissance medicine as I have come to understand it. This work is not intended as a book for specialists in medieval and Renaissance medicine, to whom much of its contents should be familiar. My readings of medical and surgical texts and contemporary views on medicine and accounts of medical practice are my own, but many of these sources have also been studied by other scholars. In sketching the context of medical practice, I have benefited greatly from recent studies of the social history of medicine, of the prosopography of medical practitioners, and of vernacular medical literature. Syntheses always run the risk of being premature; I hope, however, that this one will serve as a useful introduction to the late medieval and early Renaissance medical world.

New York, New York
May 1989

ACKNOWLEDGMENTS

Much of this book was written while I was a visitor at The Institute for Advanced Study, Princeton, during the summers of 1987 and 1988. I am, as always, grateful for the ideal working conditions provided by the Institute.

I should like most warmly to thank the colleagues who read all or a section of the manuscript before publication and offered helpful comments: Jerome Bylebyl, Marcia Colish, Anthony Grafton, Robert Joy, Michael Mc-Vaugh, John Murdoch, Vivian Nutton, Dale Smith, and Noel Swerdlow. I owe a special debt of gratitude to Michael McVaugh, who has shared his profound knowledge of medieval medicine in numerous helpful suggestions and discussions. Remaining errors are, of course, my own responsibility.

Part of chapter 3 will appear in slightly different form in A History of the European Universities in Society, volume I: Universities in the Middle Ages, edited by Walter Rüegg (Cambridge, forthcoming). Thanks are due to Cambridge University Press for permission to use this material here.

Illustration credits appear in the captions to the illustrations throughout the book.

A NOTE ON NAMES

The problems of medieval nomenclature make consistency in the form of names very difficult to achieve. In this book, names of monarchs and other well known individuals appear in the form most familiar to English-speaking readers (Catherine of Siena, Petrarch, Peter the Venerable). Other personages are usually referred to in a vernacular form consonant with their region of origin or chief activity (Guglielmo da Saliceto, Ortolf von Baierland). Latin forms are occasionally used when the vernacular seems uncertain.

ONE

THE FORMATION OF WESTERN EUROPEAN MEDICINE

any institutional, social, and intellectual innovations of the twelfth to fifteenth centuries created late medieval and early Renaissance medical culture. With them, subsequent chapters will be concerned. Yet medicine's distinctive ideas and most important written sources of authoritative teaching did not originate in medieval western Europe but were drawn from Greek antiquity and the world of Islam. The reception and understanding in western Christendom of ancient medical knowledge, as of other branches of ancient science, was of course conditioned by social and cultural factors that changed over time. Hence, the emergence and character of the medical world with which this book is concerned cannot be understood without some preliminary account of the heritage of ancient medicine and its transmission to the medieval West; of the institutional, ideological and practical aspects of medicine and healing in the early Middle ages; and of the impact of the so-called twelfth-century Renaissance upon medical learning and practice in western Europe. Only the briefest sketch of this antecedent history can be given here.[1]

Ancient Medicine

Medical treatises constitute some of the oldest extant examples of Greek scientific writing; a number of the approximately sixty treatises attributed to Hippocrates date from the late fifth or early fourth century B.C. The Hippocratic collection contains important early examples of deliberate and repetitive scientific observation and of arguments for and against the worth of endeavors to base medical treatment on systematic physiological theorizing. Treatises such as the *Epidemics* show that some of the Hippocratic authors were exceptionally keen medical observers who acquired notable ability to describe the signs and course of disease in individual patients. Although the authors of the Hippocratic treatises made some use of therapeutic venesection and herbal medication and performed a restricted range of simple sur-

1

gical operations, much of their therapy consisted of the management of both health and disease by manipulation of diet. Among medical skills, they attached particular importance to accurate prognosis. Their observations and recommendations were frequently couched as brief maxims, a format that had the practical advantage of being readily memorizable.

This rational medicine and rational natural philosophy emerged at about the same time in Greece; both are rightly regarded as intellectual achievements of major importance. Yet it is necessary to clarify the meaning of rationalism in ancient medicine. Hippocratic medical authors criticized traditional beliefs and attempted to construct causal accounts of health, disease, and physiology that did not rely on magical, theological, or mythological forms of explanation. This endeavor does not, of course, imply either that the content of medicine was completely free of the influence of traditional beliefs or that rational medicine flourished in isolation from or in opposition to religious belief and, especially, religious healing. On the contrary, folkloric remedies stripped of their magical trappings, along with such popular beliefs as the superiority of right over left, found their way into medical treatises; and social factors affected, even though they did not determine, discussions of some physiological topics—for example, the role of the female in reproduction.[2]

Even more important, in Greek antiquity secular and religious forms of healing flourished side by side. Thus, the island of Cos, the birthplace of Hippocrates, became an important center of rational medicine in the fifth century; subsequently and no doubt consequently, in the fourth century it also developed as one of the main centers of the worship of the healing god and patron of physicians, Asclepius. At Cos and other similar shrines, secular and religious healing appear to have functioned in harmonious symbiosis. The god was believed to appear in dreams to supplicants who slept the night in the shrine precincts and to heal either with miraculous directness or by means of medical advice often resembling that given by human physicians. The circumstances that would lead to a patient in antiquity to prefer either religious or secular healing in a given situation are far from clear, but recourse to secular healing carried no religious stigma; and medical practitioners sometimes encouraged recourse to prayer if medicine failed or in particularly dangerous situations. One example is provided by the author of the Hippocratic treatise *Dreams*, who advised that health should be protected in ominous meteorological conditions by a change of regimen and prayer to the gods.[3]

Interaction between philosophy and medicine occurred from the earliest history of Greek science. For example, concepts shared with or derived from pre-Socratic natural philosophy (such as that of the four elements—earth, air, fire, and water) are present in some of the Hippocratic treatises, and Plato propounded physiological theories in his cosmological *Timaeus*. Aristotle's influence was especially important. In the first place, Aristotle, who was himself interested in medicine, strongly asserted a relation between medicine and natural philosophy with the remark, "But it behoves the natural scientist to obtain also a clear view of the first principles of *health* and *disease*. . . . Indeed we may say of most physical inquirers, and of those physicians who study their art more philosophically, that while the former complete their works with a disquisition on medicine, the latter start from a consideration of nature."[4] Furthermore, aspects of Aristotle's physical theory (for example, his treatment of the four elements; categorization of different kinds of motion and change; differentiation of material, formal, final, and efficient causes; and generally, biological teleology), his discussions of methods of achieving "scientific" or certain knowledge, and his techniques of argument all influenced late ancient medicine, particularly as transmitted in the writings of Galen. Moreover, in dealing with mammalian biology in his works on animals, Aristotle treated subjects of direct medical relevance, such as reproduction and physiological functions of the heart and blood. In addition, his teaching that "When the soul departs, what is left is no longer an animal, and that none of the parts remain what they were before, excepting in mere configuration"[5] perhaps helped to make the concept of dissection acceptable to some medical investigators. At any rate, Diocles, the earliest known author of a (lost) book on anatomy, may have been a pupil of Aristotle.

In Hellenistic Alexandria, anatomical knowledge was substantially increased by the investigations of Herophilus and Erasistratus (third century B.C.). Much of what is known of their work comes via the often-polemical accounts of them provided by Galen. It is clear that both Herophilus and Erasistratus engaged in extensive dissections of human cadavers—in late antiquity they were sometimes also accused of having practiced human vivisection. Among their achievements was the correct identification of the relation of the brain and the nervous system (Aristotle had believed that powers of motion and sensation originate in the heart). Yet another development of medicine in the Hellenistic period was the growth of an elaborate herbal pharmacology that found its fullest expression in a large work on materia medica by Dioscorides (first century A.D.).

As will have become apparent, Greek approaches to medicine included diverse and even contradictory tendencies. A natural result was the emergence of the so-called medical sects: rationalists (or dogmatists), empiricists, and methodists. The rationalists were those who believed that the primary task of medicine was to use reason to investigate causes of health, disease, and physiological phenomena generally and to construct physiological theories. The proliferation of such theories resulting from the work of the Alexandrian anatomists by the mid-third century B.C. engendered a reaction in the shape of the empiricist position, which held that theory is completely useless for therapeutic purposes; that the task of the medical practitioner is to treat his patients; and that his only reliable guide in so doing is experience. The third sect, the methodists, arose around the beginning of the Christian era and proposed that medical treatment could successfully be carried out on the basis of a few simple rules that could be mastered in six months; the thrust of this idea was a criticism both of the elaborate theoretical constructions of the rationalists and of the claim of the empiricists that extensive and lengthy experience was required for successful practice.

Greek medicine reached its fullest development in Galen (d. ca. A.D. 200). Galen was unquestionably one of the greatest scientists of antiquity. His contributions to anatomical knowledge—despite the limitation of his dissections to animals other than man—remained unsurpassed for nearly fourteen hundred years; and even the achievement of Vesalius, often thought of as overthrowing Galen, would have been inconceivable without Galen's foundation to build on. Galen was also a great synthesizer. His voluminous writings bring together almost the entire heritage of Greek medicine in all fields; he addressed not only anatomy but also physiology, pathology, semiotics (symptomatology), hygiene, and therapy. This terminology is not entirely anachronistic; although not Galen's own, it originated in the Hellenistic period. Moreover, as already noted with reference to Herophilus and Erasistratus, Galen's frequently polemical works are a rich, if not always reliable, source of information about the ideas and discoveries of predecessors and opponents whose books have in many cases perished.

Certainly, when he wrote commmentaries on some of the Hippocratic works, Galen remade Hippocrates, of whom he strongly approved, in his own image. Galen, who believed that the best physician is also a philosopher, tended to magnify whatever he could find in the way of philosophy or of a systematic approach to physiology in the Hippocratic works. Thus, for example, in a single passage he designated Hippocrates a philosopher (as well as a physician) and credited him with priority over Aristotle in developing a theory of qualities usually attributed to the latter.[6] Galen's own philosophical ideas were typical of late ancient eclecticism in that they contained a strongly Platonic component as well as the Aristotelian elements already noted.

The organization of physiological theory was a major concern of Galen. No single work of his can be said to present "the" Galenic system, and indeed the notion of such a system is post-Galenic. Yet, in a number of major treatises he schematized different aspects of physiological function: "faculties," "complexions," "pulses," and so on (see Chapter 4). Galen's physiological theories were to a significant extent grounded in his own anatomical work and that of his predecessors, as well as in observations made during his long and active career as a medical practitioner; they also incorporated numerous rationalizations, assumptions, and philosophical preconceptions.

On the question of the sects, Galen took a moderate position. He had no use for the methodists but tried to harmonize the views of the rationalists and the empiricists. Thus, while his works are mainly rationalist in their approach, they also contain empiricist elements. Certainly, Galen set a high value on evidence derived from personal observation and experience. In the Middle Ages and Renaissance, just as Aristotle's ideas about the relation of medicine and philosophy would influence the relation of the two disciplines and help to sustain philosophical debate within medicine, so too Galen's willingness to encompass both rational and empirical medicine would help to secure a place in medical education for works embodying both approaches.

Serious scientific investigation and writing, in medicine and related subjects as in other branches of Greek science, were the work of a very small number of individuals. Galen had no immediate successors of equal caliber. In late antiquity, medicine as a field of investigation suffered the same neglect as other scientific subjects; no significant additions to knowledge or major modifications of theory in nosology, therapy, physiology, or anatomy can be identified after Galen. Nonetheless, especially in the eastern half of the Roman empire, medical learning based on ancient and Hellenistic works continued in a relatively flourishing state. For example, schools in Alexandria in the sixth century A.D. taught a medical curriculum based on sixteen major works of Galen; and late ancient and Byzantine compilers, among them Oribasius (fourth century A.D.), Aetius of Amida (sixth century), and Paul of Aegina (seventh century), produced compendia of Galenic teaching for the use of practitioners.

In the western Roman empire, too, medicine was strongly Greek in character. Medical practitioners were frequently slaves or freedmen of Greek origin; others with an intellectual or practical interest in medicine depended on familiarity with the Greek language to read medical as well as other scientific or philosophical treatises in the original. In addition, Latin writers on medicine, of whom the most notable was the encyclopedist Celsus (first century A.D.), drew upon Greek sources in composing or compiling their own works. The cities of the western Roman empire were relatively well supplied with medical practitioners, some of whom also traveled into the countryside. In some of the larger centers, publicly salaried municipal practitioners were appointed, and medical attendants were also provided for the army. However, although Roman law regulated the liability of medical practitioners for injury to their patients, no institutionalized form of medical education or system of medical licensing developed under Roman rule, any more than it had done in Greek or Hellenistic society.

While the Roman empire was at its height during the first three centuries of the Christian era, there was little call for the translation of Greek medical works into Latin. But in late antiquity, a widening political, linguistic, and cultural gulf opened between the eastern and western parts of the Roman empire. In the Latin West, interest in medicine for practical purposes ensured the translation or adaptation of parts of the written record of Greek medical learning. What was transmitted in Latin form during this period and hence available in the early medieval West was, however, only a very slight portion of the Greek accomplishment in medicine as in other disciplines.

The translation of Greek medical works had begun by the fifth century, when Caelius Aurelianus translated a gynecological work of Soranus (first century A.D.). By the mid-sixth century, a synopsis of Oribasius' compilation and a small group of Hippocratic and Galenic writings had been translated into Latin, probably in northern Italy; the latter were apparently the subject of formal lectures, similar to those given in Alexandria, at Ravenna some time between about 550 and 570. A Latin translation of Dioscorides was also available by about that time (made in either northern Italy or North Africa).[7] Hence, although the range of Greek medical treatises available in Latin versions (at least in Italy) in the early Middle Ages was restricted, it was not negligible. In addition, in the fourth, fifth, and sixth centuries some collections of remedies were compiled in Latin: among the most important was an herbal falsely attributed to the second-century literary figure Apuleius.

From these works, readers could gain a general idea of aspects of Greek medicine: the concepts of rational and empirical medicine, the importance attached to prognosis and to management of diet and regimen, some terminology relating to diseases and symptoms, information about remedies, and a certain amount of theorizing about female reproductive physiology. Nonetheless, the Latin medical literature of the early Middle Ages represented only a few of the Greek sources and only a small proportion of their original content and conveyed only a rudimentary notion of Greek physiological theory or anatomy. In this body of writing, the main emphasis is on treatment and remedies. A few early medieval works, among them the encyclopedic *Etymologies* of Isidore of Seville (d. 636), reveal the continued presence of medicine as a branch of general learning as well as the continuity of medical ideas—but also the truncation, simplification, and sometimes the distortion those ideas had undergone.[8]

Christianity and Medicine

The rise of Christianity, and its subsequent establishment as the state religion of the Roman empire by the latter part of the fourth century, bore no exclusive and little direct responsibility for the decline of ancient medical or other science. Rather, Christianity was itself partially shaped by elements in late ancient culture that gave greater priority to rhetorical persuasion, to philosophical synthesis, to belief in the supernatural, and to various forms of magical manipulation than to the systematic investigation of nature. But the all-important influence of the Christian church in shaping the general development of the early medieval West, through the Christianization of Roman society and by carrying a modified, truncated, and transformed version of ancient Latin culture to the Germanic peoples who occupied the western empire, extended also to the particular area of medicine.

The change from classical to medieval Christian civilization affected attitudes to medical knowledge and to the relation between religious and secular healing. Christianization also gave rise to new centers of religious healing, both spiritual and physical, in the form of monasteries and the shrines of saints. And the institution of the monastery provided a new context for medical learning and some medical practice. But the emergence of Christian society of the early medieval West did not result either in the abandonment of such ancient medical knowledge as was available or in the disappearance of secular medical practitioners.

Christian ideas about medical science and about spiritual and physical healing were formed in late antiquity. To the extent that the most influential patristic writers considered anatomy, physiology, or pathology as branches of knowledge, their predominant attitude to these subjects was much the same as to most other types of information about the natural world, or to secular learning in general: modified acceptance, subordination to Christian exegetical purposes, and a rather low level of interest. Thus, for example, St. Ambrose (340–97) found it entirely appropriate to include an appreciative description of the human digestive system in his *Hexameron*, or sermons on the biblical account of the six days of creation. His immediate

7

source for the physiological material was Cicero, who had presumably drawn upon a medical author. The passage is just as characteristic in its derivativeness and its subordination of secular learning to a religious purpose as it is in its use of scientific information from non-Christian sources.[9]

However, medicine considered as healing activity rather than as a branch of learning occupied a different and more complex position in the ideas of Christians of the first six centuries A.D.[10] In the most general terms, sickness, like all the other evils afflicting human life, was conceived of as a consequence of the Fall of Man, and hence as a consequence of sin. As St. Augustine (354–430) put it,

> This very life, if life it can be called, pregnant with so many dire evils, bears witness that from its very beginning all the progeny of mankind was damned. . . . In fact, from the body itself arise so many diseases that not even the books of the doctors contain them all, and in the case of most of them, or almost all of them, the treatments and drugs themselves are painful. Thus men are rescued from a penal destruction by a penal remedy.[11]

On the question of whether disease was to be attributed to the particular sins of individuals or communities rather than to the general consequences of the Fall, different opinions were expressed. The founder of Christianity was twice recorded as refusing to ascribe injuries and disease to the sinfulness of a particular person or group rather than to that of mankind in general (Luke 13:4–5, John 9:1–3). But, unlike the author of the early Hippocratic treatise *On the Sacred Disease*, who had been at pains to deny that convulsive seizures were caused by the anger of an offended deity, Christian commentators occasionally—although by no means always—interpreted specific instances of sudden or dramatic illness as evidence of divine retribution for sin; one early example, and precedent, was set by the description of the fate of King Herod in the Acts of the Apostles (12:23). Similarly, some but not necessarily all epidemics were asserted to be the consequence of communal sin, as Pope Gregory the Great claimed of the sixth-century plague outbreaks.[12] And in all cases, for Christian theological or devotional writers it was axiomatic that the cure of the soul should take precedence over the cure of the body, and that illness might be sent or permitted by God and ought to be accepted patiently by the sufferer as a spiritual trial, test, or purification.

Such beliefs evidently did not exclude the idea that there were natural causes of disease, nor did they prohibit endeavors to restore physical health by both natural and supernatural means. Indeed, early Christianity was a healing religion as regards both soul and body. The frequency of miracles of physical healing in the Gospels could be understood as endorsing a concern for the body's well-being. But at the same time, miracles were the most striking testimony imaginable to the superior effectiveness of religious over secular healing; healing miracles were not only prominent in the Gospels, they also played a very large part in the cult of saints and shrines as it developed in the late ancient centuries. As a consequence, although secular and religious healing continued to exist side by side as they had since at least the time of Hippocrates, the relationship between them shifted as the classical world gave way to the Christian Middle Ages. St. Augustine, for instance, in recounting miracles of healing he claimed to have seen at first hand, provided emphatic and detailed accounts of the previous failure of skilled physicians to cure those subsequently healed by supernatural means.[13] Meanwhile, the physical care of the sick poor early came to be considered a characteristic manifestation of Christian charity, and, if carried out in person, of holy self-mortification on the part of the giver. One example is St. Jerome's eulogy of Fabiola (d. 399), a wealthy Roman lady whose saintly activities included founding an infirmary and caring for the sick with her own hands.[14]

The beliefs and attitudes just summarized embodied certain tensions and ambiguities. For the most part, Christian and even monastic tradition permitted, and in some respects encouraged, the preservation and study of secular medical books, a moderate concern for one's own physical health (provided the superior claims of the soul were acknowledged), and the practice of healing by members of religious communities. Thus, St. Augustine's rule for nuns (his *Letter* 211) specifically recommended consultation with a male medical practitioner by any nun who fell sick. Another influential monastic founder, Cassiodorus (d. ca. 570), assumed that the monks of the community he established in southern Italy would include men with medical learning. But a more reserved attitude to the use of medicine, especially by monks, can also be found. The enormously influential Benedictine Rule, justly famous for its moderation in regard to physical asceticism, relatively generous dietary provisions, and insistence on attentive care of sick monks in a separate infirmary, makes no mention of the possibility of consulting secular medical practitioners, although they were unquestionably present in Italy when the Rule was written (ca. 530). Indeed, the Rule's only use of the word *"medicus"* (medical practitioner) refers metaphorically to the abbot, who metes out spiritual medicine to delinquent brethren. Earlier, moreover, St. Augustine had developed the idea that Christ himself was the true physician, that is, the physician primarily of souls but also of bodies.[15]

Medicine in the Early Medieval West and the Muslim World

Whatever the concerns of ascetics and religious reformers, throughout the Middle Ages people—clergy, monks, and laity—sought physical healing by any means available. Secular medicine did not disappear in the early medieval world, although it was obviously adversely affected by the general contraction in urban life, crafts and professions, and lay literacy consequent upon the collapse of the western empire and the establishment of the Germanic successor states. In Ostrogothic Italy, King Theodoric (474/5–526) still appointed an official to supervise physicians.[16] Among a number of medical men in sixth-century Merovingian Gaul mentioned by the bishop and chronicler Gregory of Tours, one who was surely a layman was the practitioner at Poitiers who had learned how to perform castrations from surgeons at Constantinople, where eunuchs were regularly employed at the imperial court. Gregory is also a witness to the presence of Jewish medical practitioners in Merovingian Gaul. In seventh-century Visigothic Spain, secular medical practitioners apparently remained sufficiently numerous to require the reenactment of earlier legal regulations concerning medical practice.[17]

Nonetheless, as time went by, medical knowledge and healing activity tended to come more and more within the orbit of ecclesiastical communities. To the extent that it involved book learning and the transmission of Greco-Roman doctrine, medicine, like other learned disciplines, survived in western Europe between the seventh or eighth and the eleventh centuries mainly in a clerical or monastic environment. However, monks did not copy or read medical books merely as an academic exercise; Cassiodorus, in an influential work on studies appropriate for monks, recommended books by Hippocrates, Galen, and Dioscorides while linking the purpose of medical reading with charity, care, and help. Moreover, even in regions far from the cultural and climatic conditions of the late ancient Mediterranean, early medieval copying of medical books was not divorced from practical applications. For example, the *Leechbook* of Bald, a famous medical handbook written in Old English in about the early tenth century, evidently with practical use in mind, has been shown to include numerous passages selected, translated, or adapted from Latin works; similarly, the Old English translation of the so-called *Herbal of Apuleius*, presumably a monastic or clerical endeavor, shows signs of adaptation for practical use in the local environment. (Other types of treatises with no evident immediate practical application in a monastic milieu—for example, on gynecology—were, however, also copied in early medieval monastic communities.) Everywhere, the needs of their own communities, quite apart from any other considerations, were sufficient to induce western monks to acquire simple medical skills, to collect medicinal recipes, and to cultivate culinary and medicinal herbs.[18]

Clerical communities, too, were likely to be guardians of relics and shrines that represented for early medieval society the surest form of access to supernatural protection and help and that therefore attracted the sick, poor, and afflicted. Sometimes it is difficult to distinguish between physical healing and spiritual counsel and encouragement in the help offered by the clergy. One of the "miracles" attributed to St. John of Beverley (d. 721) involved his patient training of a dumb youth to speak; subsequently, the good bishop passed the patient on to a physician who prescribed an ointment for his skin disease.[19]

Religious healers and secular medical craftsmen did not always work together so harmoniously in caring for the laity in early medieval western Europe. Gregory of Tours roundly denounced the lack of confidence in the saints shown by a patient who, after being cured of blindness at the shrine of St. Martin, sought follow-up treatment from a secular—and worse, in Gregory's view—Jewish, practitioner. In reality, the most serious competitor to the healing power of the saints in the early Middle Ages was probably less the surviving tradition of ancient secular medicine than the non-Christian religious or magical folk practices and beliefs widespread in a partially or superficially Christianized society.[20]

The most important developments in medicine between the seventh and the eleventh centuries took place not in rural, thinly populated, and economically underdeveloped Christian western Europe but in the environment of the flourishing cities, developed commercial economies, and lively intellectual milieus of the Muslim societies of the Middle East and the Iberian peninsula. The Muslim conquests that began in the first half of the seventh century were followed in the eighth and ninth centuries by assimilation of Greek philosophy and science into an Islamic intellectual context. Among the Greek works translated into Arabic, often via an intermediary translation into Syriac, was much medical literature. By the ninth century, Arabic-speaking physicians had absorbed this material and begun to build on and add to it. In general, the authors of medical treatises in Arabic adopted and sometimes elaborated upon Greek philosophical and physiological systems. Where pathology and therapy were concerned, they made use of Greek materials but quite frequently added observations of their own or recommendations for treatment that drew on botanical pharmacology of oriental or Iberian origin. A characteristic but certainly not the only form of Arabic medical writing was the composition of large encyclopedic works that surveyed all aspects of the subject.[21]

Space does not permit a comprehensive list even of those among the medieval medical authors who wrote in Arabic who were subsequently most influential in western Europe. However, mention must at least be made of the leading medical encyclopedists who were to be known to the West as Rhazes (ar-Rāzī, d. 925), Haly Abbas (ʿAlī b. Al-ʿAbbās Al-Maǧūsī, fl. tenth century), and Avicenna (al-Ḥusain b. ʿAbdallāh Ibn Sīnā, d. 1037); of the author whom the West knew as Albucasis or Abulcasis (Abu l-Qāsim Ḫalaf b. ʿAbbas az-Zahrāwī, d. after 1009), who wrote a large compendium on surgery; and of the medical writing of Averroes (Ibn Rušd, d. 1198).[22] Haly Abbas, in the work known in the West in two different versions as the *Pantegni* and the *Liber regius*, and Avicenna, in the *Canon*, both strove to present ordered synopses of the whole of medical knowledge, largely but not exclusively based on Galen's teaching. Rhazes, in the work known in the West as the *Almansor*, appeared less dogmatic and more clinically oriented; his work was basically empirical in its approach and contained much information collected from his own experience. It was through these and other essentially encyclopedic or synoptic written works that Arabic medicine was to influence the medieval West. Practical aspects of Arabic medicine—for example, as regards clinical training and the development of hospitals—were of great importance within medieval Muslim society but cannot be treated here.

Although in the early Middle Ages both western Europe and the Muslim world received medical knowledge originating in Greek and Hellenistic antiquity, the extent of the material and the way it was used differed greatly between the two societies. The Arabic authors had access to many more works of Galen—in which there was a marked logical and philosophical component—as well as to much of the corpus of Greek philosophy, notably works of Aristotle unknown in the West before the twelfth century. As a result, the links between medicine and philosophy, already present in antiquity, persisted strongly among some Arabic writers. Avicenna and Averroes were philosophers of importance as well as physicians, and their philosophical views affected their medical works. Avicenna's syncretistic tendency led him to attempt to harmonize Aristotle and Galen, despite the actual opposition of their views on important physiological issues (see chapter 4). In his medical *Colliget*, by contrast, Averroes frequently adopted Aristotelian ideas and arguments. But their authors' philosophical orientation should not be allowed to obscure the fact that the Arabic medical writings were indeed medical; they were valued in Islam and later in the West for their extensive and systematic accounts of disease, symptoms, and treatment and for their collections of materia medica.

Medicine and the "Twelfth-century Renaissance"

In the rapid development of western European society that took place between about 1050 and 1225 and is often referred to as the "twelfth-century Renaissance," a population increase, economic growth, urbanization, the development of more sophisticated forms of secular and ecclesiastical government and administration, the growth of professional specialization and of occupations requiring literacy, the multiplication of schools, and the enlargement of philosophical, scientific, and technical learning were interwoven and interdependent phenomena. All had a marked impact on the study and practice of medicine.

As one might expect, increased medical activity and interest in medicine came first and no doubt helped to create the demand for a more extensive and sophisticated medical literature. Thus, Salerno, in southern Italy, probably emerged as center of medical practice in the mid-900s. By the late tenth century, the fame of Salerno had reached northern France. The Salernitan practitioners of the tenth and eleventh centuries included many clergy as well as the well-known "women of Salerno" (on women practitioners, see Chapter 2). Contemporary anecdotes about the early Salernitan practitioners, male and female, stress their skill in healing, not their book learning. In the course of the twelfth century, the medicine of Salerno appears to have become more theoretical and more oriented toward formal, academic medical education.[23] The role of late twelfth- and early thirteenth-century Salerno in shaping the curriculum of the medical faculties of medieval universities and the content of medical ideas belongs to later chapters.

Evidence of the proliferation of healers, or of sources mentioning their activities, can also be cited for both lay and clerical milieus in other parts of Europe from the early twelfth century. The complaints of contemporaries make it clear that even in monastic circles medical studies, medical practice, and reliance on medicine were taking on a somewhat secular and more specialized cast. Beginning in the 1130s, several twelfth-century church councils forbade monks and canons regular to study medicine "for the sake of temporal gain" and to leave the cloister to pursue medical studies or practice medicine elsewhere. These decrees were directed against avarice and absenteeism on the part of professed religious, not against medical knowledge or practice as such. They testify, however, to the growing appeal of specialized medical studies and paid medical practice (on later extensions and ultimate modifications of these bans, see Chapter 2).[24] Echoing similar objections, the English humanist, ecclesiastical statesman, and later bishop, John of Salisbury, complained in a work completed in 1159 of the intellectual pretensions, the technical jargon, and the avariciousness of medical practitioners who returned from studies at Salerno or Montpellier.[25] Montpellier had evidently by this time joined Salerno as a medical center of European reputation. There seems to be little or no trace of formal academic institutions at either center so early on, but at both masters were by this time instructing pupils from distant regions in book-learned as well as practical medicine.

Meanwhile, St. Bernard of Clairvaux (d. 1153) reacted strongly against the use of physical medicine and consultation of specialized medical practitioners by monk patients. He emphatically laid down a rigorist position on this issue in a letter addressed to the brethren of a monastery located in a region notorious for malaria until the twentieth century. St. Bernard wrote:

> I fully realize that you live in an unhealthy region and that many of you are sick. . . . It is not at all in keeping with your profession to seek for bodily medicines, and they are not really conducive to health. The use of common herbs, such as are used by the poor, can sometimes be tolerated, and such is our custom. But to buy special kinds of medicines, to seek out doctors and swallow their nostrums, this does not become religious.[26]

But on this issue St. Bernard's voice does not appear to have been widely heeded.

The growth of centers of medical study was in turn intimately connected with the multiplication of medical books and their accumulation, in an age in which the circulation of books was still limited, in particular places. Beginning in the late eleventh century, the body of medical writing available in Latin was greatly enlarged by translations, first from Arabic and subsequently from Greek, to include substantial parts of the corpus of Greek medical writing, especially of works attributed to Hippocrates and Galen as well as the major recent Arabic contributions. Only the most important translators and centers of translation of medical works can be noted here. Constantinus Africanus (d. 1087), a monk of Monte Cassino in southern Italy, near Salerno, translated the *Pantegni*, and much else besides, from Arabic. In the twelfth century, Gerard of Cremona and his pupils in Spain translated works of Galen, Rhazes, Albucasis and Avicenna from Arabic; Burgundio of Pisa, who travelled between Italy and Constantinople, translated works of

Galen from Greek. At about the same time, an enlarged and alphabetized version of the Latin Dioscorides became available. In these developments, of course, medicine paralleled other fields, notably logic, natural philosophy, astronomy, and geometry.[27] Medicine was fully integrated into the endeavor to secure access to the whole range of Greco-Arabic philosophy and science so characteristic of western learning between the late eleventh and early thirteenth centuries.

One must assume that, in medicine as in the other areas mentioned, the interest of scholars in securing fresh material was both cause and product of the new translations. Medical books not only held the promise of practical utility, they also contributed to the general scientific culture of the twelfth-century clerical intelligentsia. To give only two examples, Guillaume de Conches, in his *Philosophia mundi* (written about 1125), and the visionary abbess Hildegard of Bingen (d. 1179) both drew on medical material only recently made available in Latin for their descriptions of the physical universe, including human physiology.[28]

The reception of the books that began to arrive in the eleventh and twelfth centuries did not demand any drastic revolution in medical ideas or techniques. Both the medical works available in Latin in the early Middle Ages and those newly translated into that language belonged in broad terms to the same Greek medical tradition. However, the new material was so much more copious, complex, and intellectually sophisticated than most of the works available earlier that its full absorption was a slow process extending over several generations.

One effect of the expansion of Latin medical literature was greatly to enhance the theoretical, systematic, and learned elements in medicine. This tendency was further accentuated by the reception of Aristotelian logic and natural philosophy. Between the early twelfth and the early thirteenth centuries, first the advanced logical and then the natural philosophical or scientific works of Aristotle became available in Latin; in the course of the thirteenth century, the spread of Aristotelian modes of arguing, Aristotelian ideas about the nature of scientific knowledge, and Aristotelian physical science transformed European intellectual life. The impact on learned medicine was certainly very great as regards both methodology and content (see chapters 3 and 4).

Nevertheless, although the more-or-less simultaneous reception of Aristotle and of an enlarged Latin medical literature brought about an interaction of Aristotelianism and medical learning that endured from the twelfth century until the seventeenth, medicine retained its separateness from Aristotelian natural philosophy in several important respects. First and foremost, in the Hippocratic and Galenic writings medicine possessed an equally venerable scientific tradition of largely independent origin (even though Galen himself adopted some Aristotelian concepts). In addition, the reception in twelfth-century western Europe of Greek and Islamic technical astronomy and astrology fostered the development of medical astrology. Interest in medical astrology doubtless preceded its widespread application, which had to await the availability of suitable planetary tables; the actual practice of medical astrology was probably greatest in the West between the fourteenth and sixteenth centuries. Astrology linked medicine with yet other branches of knowledge distinct from Aristotelian natural philosophy.[29] Above all, medicine remained irrevocably and intimately bound to the world of crafts, "secrets" (magical or otherwise), skills, and techniques.

Thus, by the middle years of the twelfth century, the process that provided western European medicine with a rich, specialized literature, renowned centers of learning, and a flourishing tradition of practice, some at least of which was reputedly lucrative, was already well advanced. The essential groundwork for late medieval and Renaissance medical culture had already been laid.

TWO

PRACTITIONERS AND CONDITIONS OF PRACTICE

ll the most powerful *signori*, of whom there are so many in Italy, thought they would surely die if, when they fell ill, Tommaso was not their medical attendant. Because he was idolized among the Italians, he became extremely rich through large fees and enjoyed a splendid and luxurious life."[1] Tommaso del Garbo (d. 1370), the subject of this succinct contemporary summary of success in a medical career, owed at least some of his good fortune to an exceptionally favorable start. He was born into a prosperous Florentine citizen family; his father was a well-known physician, professor of medicine, and medical author; and he probably acquired his training at the University of Bologna, which at the time of his death had been for a century one of the leading centers of medical education in Europe. In light of these advantages, it is not surprising to learn that Tommaso too became a university professor, an author, and the preferred medical attendant of a wealthy and powerful clientele.

Tommaso del Garbo was a member of a medical profession in the sense of a body of recognized experts with special qualifications. Beginning in the twelfth century, there developed in western Europe a variety of ways of evaluating and attesting to the competence and legitimating the activities of medical practitioners. These were not only innovations as compared with the early Middle Ages in the West but also went well beyond the forms of legal recognition of medical practitioners in the Roman world. However, many differences separated the organization of practitioners and the concepts, let alone the application, of medical qualification and regulation of the late Middle Ages and Renaissance from those of the medical profession in a modern western society. The earliest recorded initiatives of this kind were taken by two monarchs, King Roger II of Sicily (reigned 1130–54) and his grandson, the Emperor Frederick II, who issued a law code for the Kingdom of Sicily in 1231. The kingdom was presumably the scene of a good deal of medical activity, since it included the southern Italian mainland, where Salerno was located. Whereas King Roger's statute simply ordered those who desired to practice medicine to be examined by royal officials, the Emperor Frederick II entrusted the actual conduct of licensing examinations to the "masters" of Salerno.[2]

The change in requirements between these two pieces of legislation reflected growing self-confidence and collective action among medical practitioners. As medical practitioners began to participate in both the guild and the university movements of the later Middle Ages, in many localities they formed organizations of various kinds that regulated the admission of members through examinations and other requirements; some medical corporations also obtained the legal right to approve or otherwise regulate other medical practitioners in their region. Craft guilds relating to medical practice were to be found in thirteenth-century Italy; throughout Europe they proliferated and became more specialized in the fourteenth and fifteenth centuries. For example, Florence's guild of *medici*, apothecaries, and grocers, established in 1293, had by 1314 developed into a federation of three autonomous branches; within the medical branch, university-educated physicians established their own distinct association in 1392. Barber-surgeons often belonged to the same guild as ordinary barbers, but by the fourteenth century, literate, skilled surgeons tended to form their own organizations (see chapter 6). In some Italian cities, bodies known as the College of Physicians or similar titles had been established by the late thirteenth or early fourteenth century. In university centers such as Bologna and Padua, the memberships of such medical colleges consisted of professors and leading practitioners. Elsewhere, for example at Venice, where a College of Physicians was in existence by 1316, the membership consisted of university-trained and other educated practitioners. In northern Europe, where university-educated physicians were less numerous, medical colleges were slower to appear; the College of Physicians in London was founded in 1518.[3]

Public political authorities also continued to license medical practitioners directly in the later Middle Ages and Renaissance. The practice of appointing civic medical and surgical practitioners, adopted by northern Italian cities in the early thirteenth century and subsequently by cities in other parts of Europe, notably the German lands, amounted to official endorsement by the civic government of the practitioners in question. Some kings, too, continued to concern themselves directly with medical licensing. Peter the Ceremonious of Aragon issued a number of medical licenses in the 1340s, some of them to individuals who, for one reason or another—for example, Jewish faith—would not have met with the approval of organized medical corporations. In this instance, protests on the part of "physicians and surgeons approved in medicine and surgery" subsequently induced King Peter in 1356 to reconfirm a requirement of university study and examination by a body of physicians and surgeons for medical licensing in Valencia and to rescind his own licenses previously granted to informally trained practitioners.[4]

Ecclesiastical authorities also licensed medical practitioners. From the thirteenth century, the most prestigious and thorough form of medical training was provided by university medical faculties. A university degree in medicine was everywhere recognized as a qualification to practice. But at Bologna, one of the most important centers of such training, the formal source of the license to teach, that is, the "degree," was from 1219 the Archdeacon of Bologna (the qualifying examinations were conducted by the professors, however; see chapter 3). In England, bishops routinely licensed medical and surgical practitioners during the sixteenth century.[5]

Moreover, the official motivations for requiring medical practitioners to be licensed were essentially similar to those inspiring the regulation of other crafts: maintenance of standards and provisions of legal recourse for any consumers of the craft's products or services who could show they had suffered injury through poor workmanship. Although some regulations included demands for university study on the part of candidates, the main object of licensing was to secure practitioners who were experienced and who had either documentary proof or a local reputation attesting to their honesty and competence, rather than to require any particular form of medical education as such. When the power to grant licenses was in the hands of a medical corporation, whether guild or university faculty, another function, comparable to the restrictive powers of the corporations of other trades and crafts, was to protect group interests. Medical corporations of various kinds soon acquired the power not only to license but also to prosecute the unlicensed; an early example is a well-known case in 1322, in which the Paris faculty of medicine restrained a successful woman practitioner.[6]

Hence the terms "medical profession" and "medical licensing," when used with reference to medieval and early Renaissance Europe, should not be held to imply a uniform system of medical regulation or medical qualification. By the late thirteenth or early fourteenth century, many medical practitioners possessed formal qualifications, but these could be of several different kinds: university education in medicine, membership in a guild of medical or surgical practitioners with power to examine candidates for membership, or possession of a license to practice from a public authority. All these forms of "official" qualification were fully legitimate, although university education carried the greatest prestige. Furthermore, there is every reason to suppose that many practitioners possessed none of these qualifications. In the twelfth and thirteenth centuries, licensing regulations were only just beginning to appear and applied to only a few regions; there is no way of knowing how effectively or even whether Frederick II's famous statute was enforced. Subsequently, licensing requirements became commonplace throughout Europe; however, even in important late medieval and Renaissance cities with active medical guilds, colleges, or university faculties of medicine, the regulations were often ignored, as records of prosecutions for unlicensed practice in sixteenth-century London as well as fourteenth-century Paris testify. Almost half the individuals practicing medicine in London in the last two decades of the sixteenth century did so without any form of official endorsement; it is unlikely that the regulatory net could have been wider in earlier centuries.[7] In late medieval and early Renaissance Europe numerous medical practitioners, especially but by no means exclusively those who were rural, poor, and less educated, must have been unaffected or only intermittently affected by regulation of any kind.

As the foregoing discussion implies, by the late thirteenth or early fourteenth century an informal hierarchy had come into existence. University graduates in medicine occupied the highest place, followed by other skilled medical practitioners, then by skilled surgeons, and finally by barber-surgeons and various other practitioners, among them herbalists or apothecaries. Some form of this hierarchy was to be found in most parts of western Europe, although in various regions university graduates in medicine were a rarity before the late fifteenth century; everywhere the hierarchy involved a good deal of social as well as occupational stratification. One measure of intellectual but also of social demarcation was literacy. Latin literacy was invariably possessed by university graduates and was also commanded by a good many other skilled medical and surgical practitioners. In addition, if one may judge by the appearance of a substantial technical medical literature in various European vernacular languages, by the late fourteenth and early fifteenth centuries a significant community of practitioners literate only, or primarily, in a vernacular language had come into being. The humblest empirics were unlikely to be literate at all. Only a minority of those practicing medicine resembled Tommaso del Garbo in social origin, type of training, easy geographical access to a major center of medical education, and residence in one of the most urbanized parts of Europe (let alone in the acquisition of fame, wealth, and an admiring biographer).

Yet the fluidity and inexactness of some of the terminology used to describe types of practitioners of medicine suggest that catégories were not always sharply defined. "Master" might sometimes designate a university graduate in or teacher of any subject, but it was also used as a vague general term of respect. "Doctor" always referred to a university graduate but not necessarily in medicine. Tommaso's biographer called him a *physicus* and a *medicus*. "*Medicus*" was a general term that could be applied to anyone who practiced medicine or surgery; in any particular instance, only the context gives clues to the level of knowledge or type of practice intended. "*Physicus*" (physician) in one sense implied someone who had advanced medical education and some acquaintance with natural philosophy (*physica*); but the word or its vernacular equivalent was also used more loosely to distinguish a practitioner of general internal medicine (also called "*physica*," or physic) from a surgeon. "Empiric," used by educated practitioners to refer to those whose medicine was acquired without formal education and practiced by trial and error, was more often a term of abuse than a precise description.

For Tommaso del Garbo, and unquestionably for many other practitioners, medicine was also a profession in the sense of being a money-making occupation that provided a livelihood, sometimes, as in Tommaso's case, a very good one. Medicine and law were by definition "the lucrative sciences," and medical practitioners were often accused of avarice. Chaucer's remark about the doctor of physic in the Prologue of the *Canterbury Tales* (1387–92)

> For gold in phisik is a cordial,
> Therefore he lovede gold in special.

differs only in satirical neatness, not general thrust, from many similar comments made from the twelfth century on. Nonetheless, although medicine by the thirteenth century was in many respects a commercial activity involving the selling of services, it is incorrect to suppose either that financial gain was the driving motive of all practitioners or that all practitioners grew wealthy. Some famous individuals ended their careers as rich men; one was Taddeo Alderotti (d. 1295) of Florence and Bologna, as is testified by his will as well as by anecdotal accounts. But in Florence in 1427, fewer than a third of the city's practitioners could be described as rich, and another third were clearly poor. In late fourteenth- and fifteenth-century England, those physicians and surgeons who were able to secure the patronage of members of the nobility or the royal family amassed substantial rewards in the shape of contracted annual salaries, grants of land, sinecures, gifts of money and goods, and further access to influential patrons.[8]

Wealth was loosely correlated with ranking in the medical hierarchy in the sense that learned physicians were normally a good deal better off than empirics. But the correlation was not precise. Learning carried the greatest prestige, but university professorships in medicine brought in an income (see chapter 3) considerably smaller than could be gained by outstandingly successful practice. Leading physicians combined both sources of income, but occasionally, as in Tommaso del Garbo's own case, they are said to have cut back their practice in order to free more time for study. And the most famously learned of all medieval physicians, Pietro d'Abano (d. 1316), professor of medicine and astrology at Padua and a noted author, had trouble collecting his money; when he died the Paduan civic authorities owed him three years' back salary. Furthermore, highly paid practitioners were not necessarily always drawn from the highest ranks of the medical hierarchy; a reputation for outstanding success in therapy could draw a wealthy clientele to a practitioner of any background.[9]

Moreover, one should remember that famous practitioners who are known on the basis of documentary evidence or who were alleged by contemporaries to have acquired great wealth were by definition exceptional. As will become apparent in the course of this chapter, many, perhaps most, practitioners gained only a modest or partial livelihood from medicine. Judging by the fees that fifteenth-century English practitioners charged tradesmen, clerics, and small landholders, paid medical care was beyond the reach of the poorest part of the population,[10] unless it was provided as a charity or municipal service, as was the case in Italy (see below). But abundant evidence shows that people in many walks of life consulted medical practitioners and that the great majority of patients were neither rich nor noble and could not have paid exorbitant fees. To take only one example, records of about 3,000 supposed miracles claimed by pilgrims to seven English and two French shrines between the twelfth and fifteenth centuries reveal that 90 percent of the cases involved illness, and at least 10 percent of those individuals had previously consulted medical practitioners of some kind. Sick pilgrims who did not believe themselves to be recipients of miracles were presumably much more numerous and no less likely to have sought secular medical help.[11]

Nor were all secular practitioners motivated by a desire to make money. One who was not was Guillelmus Caner, an apothecary who tried to offer his medical services without charge to the poor in mid-fourteenth-century Valencia. However, the *medici* of Valencia complained that Caner was not properly trained, even though he claimed to be "instructed in the art of medicine on account of long practice and many conversations with masters and other practitioners of medicine." In 1356, Caner turned for support to King Peter the Ceremonious of Aragon, who backed him and ordered the royal officials to allow him to practice, since he was not doing it for money.

But only a few months later the *medici*, as already noted, successfully prevailed upon the king to abrogate his own previously granted licenses.[12]

Members of the medical profession thus varied widely in training, type of formal qualification (if any), occupation, and social and economic status. Yet, despite this diversity, they shared a common medical culture in which they participated with differing degrees of intellectualization and sophistication. Hence, delineation of the general contours of medical activity in broad and nonrestrictive terms will promote an understanding of the uses to which medical knowledge was put as well as of the impact of new forms of medical knowledge as they became diffused in a variety of ways and at many different levels. Consequently, the following overview of practitioners and conditions of practice excludes only household medicine. Even this exclusion is somewhat arbitrary. Doubtless helping one's own family and helping one's neighbors for pay or as a matter of charity often shaded into each other, especially in the case of women. For example, the charities of the Roman noblewoman Francesca Bussi dei Ponziani (St. Francesca Romana, 1384–1440) included doctoring not only the members of her wealthy husband's large household but also neighbors, friends, and strangers in need.[13]

Practitioners and Their Backgrounds

There is no way of arriving at even a rough estimate of the number of people in Europe between the thirteenth and the fifteenth centuries who made the provision of physical healing a regular occupation. By no means all practitioners can have made their way into written records, and by no means all surviving records have been examined by historians from the point of view of medical prosopography. Nonetheless, it is clear that if healers in all categories are included, medical practitioners were relatively numerous; numbers were doubtless greater in some regions of the south than in the north and in urban than in rural areas. A minimum of 5,000 are known to have been active in France between the twelfth and the fifteenth centuries; when barbers who performed venesection and barber-surgeons are included, the number rises to over 7,000. About 2,000 practitioners— Christians, Jews, and Muslims—have so far been identified in an ongoing study of medicine in the Kingdom of Aragon during the fourteenth century. The single Italian region of Piedmont yields 336 names of known practitioners in the fourteenth and fifteenth centuries. In 1379, the city of Florence had about 70 established medical practitioners for a population of around 50,000. Over 1,700 practitioners have been claimed as active in England between 1340 and 1511, although more than half of this total is made up of "tonsorial barbers." These figures certainly do not include all those who practiced healing by physical means in the places named.[14]

In the two centuries of population growth that ended shortly before 1300, the numbers of medical practitioners no doubt increased with the increase in the European population as a whole. But the growth of medicine as an occupation was more than a simple reflection of demographic trends; in some regions, the medical community apparently continued to grow in size even after the general population declined dramatically in the four-teenth century (of course, allowance must be made for vagaries in the exis-tence, survival, or investigation of records). The number of known practi-tioners in France is larger for the half century following than for that preceding the demographic calamity of the Black Death; in Florence the number of practitioners was about the same in 1399 as it had been in 1338, although the population dropped by more than half during the same pe-riod.[15] The capacity to sustain a diversified medical community was a conse-quence of broad social and cultural development—primarily dissemination of written traditions of knowledge, the development of specialized crafts in urban milieus, and the spread through many levels of society of the willing-ness and ability to purchase medical help.

No general comparison is possible between the numbers engaged in medicine and in the only other comparable profession of the period, namely law. The economic and social structure of the two occupations dif-fered in ways that invalidate easy comparisons, even in the few instances where figures for the same period and place are available. In Italy, for ex-ample, in contrast to the broad economic, social, and educational range of medical and surgical practitioners, the legal profession consisted of gradu-ates in civil or canon law who constituted a clearly defined group with uniform qualifications and approximately uniform high social status. Notar-ies, whose activities were confined to drawing up contracts and wills, consti-tuted a separate and less prestigious legal occupation, with its own less de-manding training and qualifications that nonetheless always included literacy. Comparative figures for medicine and law available in Florence, where both medical and legal experts were probably more numerous than in most of the rest of Europe, are, however, suggestive. According to the chronicler Giovanni Villani, in 1338 lawyers who were guild members in Florence numbered about 80, notaries about 600, medical and surgical prac-titioners about 60, and apothecaries' shops about 100; the figure for medical and surgical practitioners has been roughly confirmed by a modern study. In the fifteenth century, the numbers in both occupations were considerably

smaller, but the balance between them had shifted slightly in favor of medicine. A study of all known, fully qualified civil and canon lawyers practicing
in Florence between 1380 and 1530 shows that in the fifteenth century the
number of lawyers who were guild members in any one year was usually
less than 25; the number of notaries in any one year in this period was about
400. In 1427 the number of medical and surgical practitioners taxed in Florence was 36 (however, occupations were by no means always reported in
the tax survey from which the last figure is drawn).[16]

Medical practitioners came from a variety of backgrounds. In northern
France and England, and doubtless elsewhere, many literate practitioners
were beneficed clergy and clergy in major orders (that is, subdeacons, deacons, or priests). Of 342 medical students or masters at French universities
before 1500 whose status can be identified, 128 were married, 13 were regular clergy (that is, monks, canons, or friars), and 201 were secular (nonmonastic) clergy. These figures include Montpellier, which had many married
laity in its medical community.[17] Although in general the importance of
monasteries as centers of medical knowledge declined from about the
twelfth century, subsequent gifts of medical books to monastery libraries
suggest continued interest in the acquisition and doubtless the use of medical information within some monastic communities (the decrees restricting
the access of monks to secular education in medicine or law did not, of
course, forbid this interest). Thus, soon after 1300 a *medicus* gave the monks
of Christ Church, Canterbury, an up-to-date collection of medical books.
Medicine did not play a large part in the intellectual life or activities of the
new orders of mendicant friars, founded in the early thirteenth century,
despite the interest in natural science of some of their most famous
thirteenth- and fourteenth-century members. Roger Bacon (d. 1292) added
medicine to his many other intellectual interests, but he was a highly unusual friar. Nonetheless, the names of a few friars who practiced medicine
are known, especially among the Dominicans (Order of Preachers); among
them was the well-known surgical author and practitioner Teodorico Borgognoni of Lucca (d. 1298).[18]

Members of the secular clergy frequently combined medical practice
with their ecclesiastical activities. The most famous such case is that of Petrus
Hispanus, who publicly taught, wrote on, and practised medicine during the
early stages of a highly successful ecclesiastical career that culminated with
his election as Pope John XXI in 1276. Secular clerics took substantial advantage of the opportunities to study medicine provided by the establishment
of medical faculties in the universities, notably at Paris, even though their
access for a time was to some extent limited by ecclesiastical regulations. In

France, at any rate, the number of practitioners who were members of the secular clergy appears to have been greatest in the fourteenth, but the number was still substantial in the fifteenth century. The combination of medical practice and priestly or ministerial activity could still be found in seventeenth-century England.[19]

Following a decree of the Fourth Lateran Council (1215) that forbade clergy in major orders to perform cautery or make surgical incisions, members of the regular and secular clergy did not normally practice surgery, although exceptions—including that of Teodorico Borgognoni, who obtained a papal dispensation to practice—can be found.[20] Throughout Europe, surgeons, barber-surgeons, and barbers usually belonged to the laity (see chapter 6 for further discussion of the hierarchy among surgical practitioners).

In Italy a sophisticated commercial economy and a wider range of secular occupations developed earlier than in the north. By the late thirteenth century, not only surgeons but probably a majority of all Italian practitioners (including university professors and students of medicine as well as others to whom the terms "*physici*" and "*medici*" might be applied) were laymen. Among lay practitioners, family status and connections played an important part in shaping medical careers. Despite the mistaken medieval belief that Avicenna, "prince of physicians," had literally been a prince, few medical practitioners came from the nobility, and by and large the social status conferred by even the most successful medical career was less than that conferred by the equivalent position in law. However, university-educated practitioners seem frequently to have come from or founded urban citizen families of substance; moreover, the practice of medicine, like other occupations, was often a family tradition. Much less is known or can be surmised about the origins of other lay practitioners, many of whom appear to have belonged to the milieu of urban guilds and crafts. It is evident that empirics usually occupied a lowly social as well as occupational position. It seems likely, too, that the practice of medicine or minor surgery was frequently combined with one or more of a variety of other petty trades or crafts, as continued to be the case in England in the sixteenth century.[21]

Medicine, like the church and the law, could offer some opportunities for improving one's social status and that of one's descendants. Taddeo Alderotti is said to have been so poor in his youth that he peddled church candles in his native Florence. He rose to become a highly esteemed professor at Bologna, a famous medical author, and a very wealthy man; his handsomely dowered daughter married into a noble family. But such a career was exceptional; Taddeo was probably able to rise in the world because he lived at a time when the medical faculty in the university of Bologna was still in its infancy, so he did not have to contend with much in the way of established tradition. The leading physicians of the medical faculty and the city of Bologna early organized themselves in a doctoral college, whose members monopolized the senior teaching positions on the medical faculty. In 1378, this body tried to exclude from membership graduates in medicine who were not Bolognese citizens by birth and the sons of native Bolognese citizens, while providing favorable terms of admission for their own sons.[22]

Women as well as men practiced medicine and surgery; as with their predecessors in the Roman empire, women's practice was limited neither to obstetrical cases nor to female patients (figure 1). For example, the names of 24 women described as surgeons in Naples between 1273 and 1410 are known, and references have been found to 15 women practitioners, most of them Jewish and none described as midwives, in Frankfurt between 1387 and 1497. In a few instances, women emerged as learned medical authors who wrote in Latin, drawing on the body of Greco-Islamic source material common to all literate medicine of the period. The most famous is Trota, or Trotula, of Salerno; her authorship—and even her existence—have long been disputed, but the most recent study places her in the twelfth century and confirms her status as an author, although postulating that she wrote a general work on medicine, not the gynecological treatise usually attributed to her. The Abbess Hildegard of Bingen, whose mystical writings not only make free use of medical ideas but also introduce her own idiosyncratic views on female physiology, may also be included in the category of women medical authors.[23]

Even in the twelfth century, however, the accomplishments of Trota and Abbess Hildegard were highly unusual. Once university faculties of medicine were established in the course of the thirteenth century, women were excluded from advanced medical education and, as a consequence, from the most prestigious and potentially lucrative variety of practice. Furthermore, it deserves to be emphasized that although women practitioners existed in many different regions of Europe between the thirteenth and the fifteenth centuries, they represent only a very small proportion of the total number of practitioners whose names are recorded—according to one estimate, about 1.5 percent in France and 1.2 percent in England.[24] It is probable that many more women may have engaged in midwifery and healing arts without leaving any trace of their activities in written records; but this in turn may imply that such women are likely to have clustered in the least prosperous sector of medical activity, or to have been part-time or intermittent practitioners.

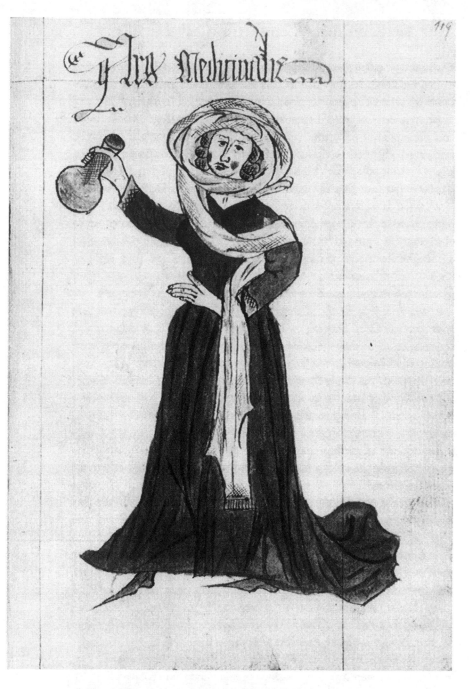

Figure 1   This imposing female figure carrying a urine flask, the universal symbol of a physician in late medieval iconography, comes from a mid-fifteenth-century German practitioner's vernacular handbook containing a treatise on *practica*, a work on bloodletting, and an herbal (all versions of Latin originals) in Middle High German. Although this figure is not a depiction of a woman practitioner but a personification of the art of medicine, the image serves as a reminder, unintended by the artist, that women's medical practice was not limited to midwifery. (Courtesy the Pierpont Morgan Library, New York, MS M. 900, Arzneibuch, South German, mid-fifteenth century, fol. 119ʳ).

Muslim (Morisco) medical practitioners were to be found in the Christian states of the Iberian peninsula. Between the ninth and the twelfth centuries, parts of Spain under Muslim rule had included notable centers of Arabic medical learning and produced some of the most famous Muslim physicians and medical authors. However, as the Iberian peninsula came under Christian rule, conditions grew progressively less favorable to the preservation of a tradition of medical high culture among Muslim practitioners. By the sixteenth century, Morisco practitioners were chiefly folk healers, with small pretension to book learning.[25]

Jewish medical practitioners were active wherever Jewish communities of any size existed, most notably in the Iberian peninsula, parts of Italy, and southern France (the linguistic region known as Occitania or Languedoc). In some places in Languedoc, more than a third of the practitioners between the twelfth and fifteenth centuries whose names are known were Jewish. In the area coterminous with modern France, the number of known Jewish practitioners was greatest between 1350 and 1450. By that time the great majority were in Provence, which did not come under the direct rule of the French monarchy until the fifteenth century (Jewish communities in Provence were augmented by refugees from the kingdom of France following the expulsion of the Jews from the kingdom in 1306 and 1322, and diminished after Provence came under the rule of the French crown). In Spain, Jewish communities, along with their medical practitioners, were transferred from Muslim to Christian rule by the progress of the Reconquista between the eleventh and the thirteenth centuries. Numerous Jewish medical practitioners flourished in the Christian Spanish kingdoms during the fourteenth century, although doubtless persecution in the second half of the fifteenth century had an adverse effect upon Jewish medical culture in the Iberian peninsula even before the expulsion of the Jews in 1492.

The strong tradition of literate, learned Jewish medicine drew on both Jewish and non-Jewish sources (figure 2). Under Muslim rule in Spain and elsewhere, Jewish physicians had come into close contact with learned Arabic medical culture and had access to the written heritage of Arabic medicine in the original language. Through this means, they too came to incorporate much of the heritage of Greek medicine into their own teaching and practice. Thus, for example, the medical writings of Maimonides (1135–1204), who spent his youth in Cordova and other parts of Spain then under Muslim rule and most of his adult life in Egypt, were written in Arabic and show extensive knowledge of Arabic versions of works of Hippocrates and Galen.[26] In the Iberian peninsula, however, the constriction of literate Arabic medical culture that followed the Reconquista reduced the likelihood

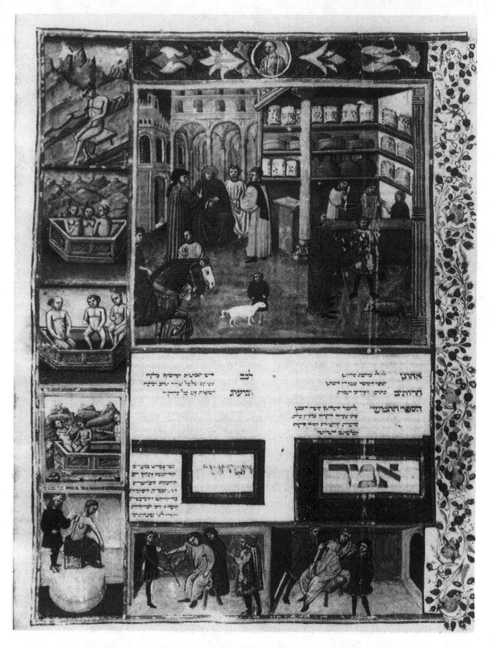

Figure 2   A page from a copy of the *Canon* of Avicenna in Hebrew, written and illuminated in Italy during the fifteenth century. The numerous manuscripts of Hebrew versions of all or part of this authoritative Arabic medical encyclopedia testify to the extent and learned character of Jewish medical practice in parts of southern Europe. The main picture appears to illustrate a cooperative arrangement of a type common in fourteenth- and fifteenth-century northern Italy between a physician and an apothecary. On the right is the apothecary's shop, with an assistant mixing a batch of medicine behind the counter. On the left, the physician holds consultations in or near the apothecary's premises. The small pictures down the left-hand edge and across the bottom of the page illustrate various forms of medical treatment, including medicinal baths. The scenes of medical activity depicted in the illustrations of this manuscript are not peculiar to the Jewish community and probably reflect the general fifteenth-century urban Italian environment. (Bologna, Biblioteca Universitaria, MS 2197, fol. 492ʳ. Reproduction authorized by the Ministero per i Beni Culturali, Italy.)

that educated Jewish medical practitioners would be able to read Arabic or have direct access to medical texts in that language. Beginning in the late twelfth century, important Arabic medical books were translated into Hebrew. For instance, there are over 100 manuscripts of Avicenna's ency-clopedic *Canon* in Hebrew translation, most of them of Spanish or Italian provenance; two separate translations were made in the late thirteenth cen-tury, and one of them was revised about 1400. By the end of the thirteenth century, information and texts were also exchanged between Jewish and Christian medical circles; in Montpellier around 1300, for example, Jewish learned practitioners, who were excluded from the university faculty of medicine, were in touch with members of the faculty, contacts that resulted in the translation of several Latin medical books into Hebrew as well as of some Hebrew medical and astronomical books into Latin. The extent of book learning doubtless varied widely among Jewish practitioners, but it is evident that their medical ideas and techniques were, like those of the Christians, permeated by the influence of Greco-Arabic medical culture.

No doubt Jewish practitioners served primarily their own communities, but they were also in great demand among Christian patients. Although both ecclesiastical and secular authorities issued decrees forbidding Jews to treat Christian patients, these decrees were frequently modified, made the subject of exemption, or ignored. The pope himself employed Jewish med-ical practitioners; six are recorded to have been in attendance during the period of the papal court's residence at Avignon. During the fourteenth and fifteenth centuries, Christian secular public authorities in Languedoc, Ara-gon, southern Italy, and Sicily habitually examined Jewish physicians and licensed them to practice. Women were to be found among licensed Jewish practitioners; for example, Floreta, who attended the Queen of Aragon for four months in 1381.[27]

The establishment of university education in medicine in the course of the thirteenth century was an institutional and cultural innovation of major significance (see chapter 3). However, between the thirteenth and the fifteenth centuries the universities trained only a minority of all medical practitioners. Of the nearly 5,000 practitioners known to have been active in France during that period, fewer than 2,000 are recorded as having studied medicine at—but not necessarily as having obtained a doctorate in medi-cine from—a university. The situation was similar in Florence, where the proximity of Bologna presumably ensured a large regional supply of university-educated practitioners. In the century following the Black Death, depending on the decade, between a third and a little over a half, of those who practiced medicine or surgery in Florence had some university education; the proportion was about the same in Piedmont in the same period. Among university-trained physicians, those who made teaching in the milieu of the faculties of medicine their main activity were yet a further minority. For example, of the almost 2,000 practitioners in France known to have attended a university, 417 are known to have been regent masters or professors.[28]

The importance of the faculties of medicine and medical professoriate lay less in their numbers than in their ability to create and maintain a medical elite and in the institutional support they offered to medical high culture. The medical training provided in universities was lengthier, more systematic, and more thorough than any obtainable elsewhere. It offered direct access to the widest range of authoritative medical information and association with other prestigious branches of learning. Ambitious prospective practitioners sought out university training, despite its duration and expense, because it enabled them to begin their careers in an advantageous position in terms of economic opportunities as well as intellectual and social status. Returning for a moment to the family of Tommaso del Garbo, we may note that his grandfather, Bono, was a skilled and respected surgeon. Bono's son Dino (d. 1327) worked with his father early in his career; like his father, he was a member of the Florentine guild that at that time included both surgeons and physicians, but Dino made the transition to the world of the universities. There he did not abandon his attachment to surgery, which he taught in a university setting (see chapter 6), but he broadened his interests to include medical theory, general therapeutics, natural philosophy, and courtly poetry. Dino's university education raised the social status of the family and opened up for Dino himself a wider intellectual universe as well as a notable medical career as professor and practitioner.[29]

The prestige of the most learned physicians was presumably supported by the widespread desire among all segments of the medical community for technical knowledge and information. As will become more fully apparent in subsequent chapters, the numerous compendia, abbreviations, recipe books, and so on that circulated in Latin or in the vernacular among ordinary medical and surgical practitioners (figure 3) usually derived many of their specific recommendations and all of their underlying theory from books and ideas first disseminated in learned milieus. In one striking instance, even a practitioner who was a fierce critic of academic medicine was unable altogether to avoid its influence in his own practice. Nicholas of Poland was a *medicus* and Dominican friar who spent the years from about 1250 to 1270 at Montpellier. As a result of his experiences there, Friar Nicholas wrote a poem denouncing the characteristic features of university med-

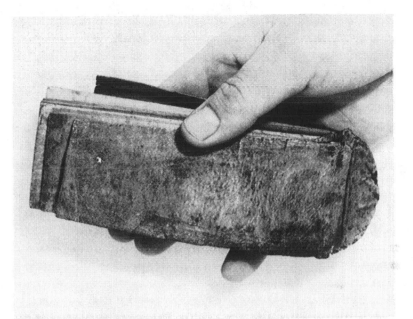

Figure 3   The portable handbook of a busy working practitioner in late fifteenth-century England. Little books of this type, designed to be hung from the belt, contained summaries and charts of essential information about such subjects as bleeding and medical astrology (see figure 27 in chapter 5). (Courtesy the Wellcome Institute Library, London, MS 40, a. 1463.)

ical training—reliance on ancient authorities, scholasticism, and rationalism. In his native Poland he tried to develop his own "natural" alternative medicine; it consisted of the idea that God had implanted special healing virtues in revolting things and led him to urge his patients to eat snakes, lizards, and frogs. The populace was horrified by these recommendations, although a local nobleman took up the new medical fad. A recent study of Nicholas suggests that the source of his ideas was essentially a religious attitude calling for acceptance of the marvelous and rejection of the search for causes; but also that the specific content of his prescriptions may have been inspired not by folk medicine but by precisely contemporary learned interest at Montpellier in the famous classical recipe theriac, the principal ingredient of which was viper's flesh.[30]

Other practitioners outside academic milieus, far from sharing Nicholas of Poland's repudiation of the learned tradition in medicine, were eager consumers of such formal medical knowledge as they could obtain. For example, Thomas Plawdon, or Plouden, a London barber-surgeon who died in

1413, commissioned the translation of a long compendium of technical and theoretical works on medicine from Latin into English. Plawdon was evidently a prosperous, literate tradesmen who could afford to spend a substantial sum of money improving his professional knowledge. Geralda Codines, a wisewoman active in the diocese of Barcelona in the late thirteenth and early fourteenth centuries, was socially and intellectually in a much humbler position. But she too sought out information derived from the learned tradition in medicine and used it to enhance her practice. She learned diagnosis by inspection of urines from a travelling *medicus* and for the next thirty years practiced this art along with conjuring away illnesses by charms. The episcopal court of the Bishop of Barcelona made repeated and apparently fruitless efforts to stop her conjuring but permitted her to continue inspecting urines, since this was a legitimate medical skill.[31]

But this very circulation of medical knowledge meant that university-educated practitioners no more had a monopoly on the command of "professional" medical information and skills hidden from the ordinary person than they had on professional legitimacy. At least for cities and towns in parts of Italy, France, and Aragon—that is, for regions within reach of the major medical university centers of Bologna, Paris, and Montpellier—it seems legitimate to say that by the early fourteenth century, practitioners in all categories competed for patients in a true "medical marketplace." Literate *medici* who were not university graduates offered therapies essentially similar to and based on the same medical concepts as those of their more highly educated colleagues. Literate surgeons had access to a substantial technical literature as well as to expertise transmitted by apprenticeship (only in Italy were a few university degrees granted in surgery). Given the considerable overlap in content between medicine and surgery in the period (see chapter 6), it is evident that trained surgeons were in many respects as well equipped as university-educated physicians to offer their services as general practitioners to prosperous and even noble or royal patients.

No doubt poor empirics and village healers did not compete with graduate physicians so much as serve a different clientele, one for whom the fees as well as the social and intellectual pretensions of university-educated physicians or other literate *medici* would have constituted an imsurmountable barrier. Yet empirics who specialized in particular procedures (itinerant eye doctors, for example) or who acquired a reputation for skill might be called upon by clients of any social standing.

One contemporary comment illustrates the overlap in some aspects of the education provided in some of the faculties of medicine and the kind of knowledge possessed by literate, skilled surgeons without university education. Writing in or shortly before 1363 and recalling the ancient medical sects described by Galen, the "surgeon and master of medicine" Guy de Chauliac asserted that those willing to undertake the care of surgical cases in his own day could be divided into five sects. The first three were the followers of different surgical authors of the twelfth and thirteenth centuries, all of whom wrote in Latin, and were divided over the technical issue of the proper treatment of wounds. Some of those among his contemporaries whom Guy placed in these three categories could have received their training in southern European universities: but other members of these same categories would have been found among literate but not university-trained surgeons. These divisions of surgical opinion are indeed something like sects in the Galenic sense of the term, although the differences Galen had in mind had philosophical foundations.

Guy's account also testifies to the continued activities of healers without any form of medical training. His fourth and fifth categories invoked social and occupational differences as well as differences of opinion. The fourth consisted of German knights who believed that God had imparted powers to words, herbs, and stones and who accordingly used incantations as well as physical care for battle wounds. In the fifth Guy placed women and the unlettered who, according to him, simply invoked God and the saints.[32] These comments are not without bias: Guy either did not know about or did not choose to recognize the undoubted presence of literate and skilled surgeons in the German lands, and his desire to emphasize the importance of Latin education for surgeons evidently led him to overlook the fact that magical remedies and Christian charms were on occasion employed by learned practitioners (see chapter 5). Yet his remarks surely constitute a realistic recognition of the diversity of available medical assistance.

There is no way of arriving at any general estimate either of patient preferences or of the actual distribution of patients among the various categories of practitioners. Geographical distribution—graduate physicians were probably a rarity in much of northern and eastern Europe before the fifteenth century, Jewish *medici* were concentrated in certain regions, and medical care was presumably much less likely to be available in the countryside than in the town—fee scales, social class, the reputations of individual practitioners, and doubtless many other unknown or imponderable factors would determine what kind of practitioner a patient consulted. The emphasis that both graduate physicians and surgeons literate in Latin placed upon their superior claims to knowledge and their frequent and unattractive expressions of hostility or contempt for "illiterates," "rustics," "old women," empirics, and Jews suggest awareness of competition. Yet these same assertions also convey the confidence of their authors that superior knowledge of authoritative traditions and texts was a socially valued commodity to which it was to their advantage to lay claim.

Occupations and Patients

Practitioners were employed in the service of both institutions and private clients. Among the latter, royalty, nobles or *signori*, and high ecclesiastics frequently sought to retain their own personal physicians and surgeons as permanent or long-term employees (in part, no doubt, because current concepts of medical care involved careful attention to diet and environment in health as well as to treatment in sickness). Ongoing studies of the records of the crown of Aragon reveal King James II as particularly lavish in his provision for personal medical care. During the spring of 1310, for example, he supplemented the services of his personal medical attendant with those of two university-educated physicians, three Jewish practitioners, and two surgeons. This ruler, who had ready access to various categories of practitioner, evidently found several equally useful.[33]

Practitioners attached to princely courts or noble households where there was less ill health (or worry about it) were likely to be asked from time to time to perform services that were not strictly medical. Since the disciplines of medicine and astrology flourished in close association, one closely related form of service was astrological prediction. Not all astrologers were *medici*, but many *medici* practiced astrology. A glimpse of the situation in the fifteenth century is provided by the French royal astrologer Symon de Phares, who around 1498 attempted to defend himself against charges of practicing illicit magical arts by writing a self-serving *Collection of the Most Famous Astrologers*. In it, he defended astrology by claiming that the art had been studied and practiced by large numbers of distinguished people, beginning with Adam. Among them he listed by name 114 astrologers who flourished between 1412 and 1495; he identified 39 of them, including himself, as physicians or surgeons.[34] In other instances, patrons demanded services of medical practitioners that could have been performed by any educated, reliable subordinate and had no particular connection with medical expertise. For example, in 1311 the Emperor Henry VII entrusted his physician, Bartolomeo da Varignana, with the responsibility of supervising the safe transport of the iron crown of Lombardy.[35]

However, full-time commitment to a single patron was probably uncommon. Practitioners normally made a living by serving a diversity of private patients (figures 4 and 5), and also, in many instances, institutions of various

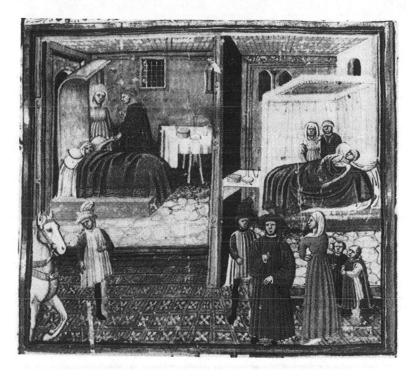

Figure 4   A physician, identified by his long robe, visits a patient and leaves
prognosis and instructions for care with the patient's family. (Bologna, Biblioteca
Universitaria, MS 2197, fifteenth century, fol. 402ʳ. Reproduction authorized
by the Ministero per i Beni Culturali, Italy.)

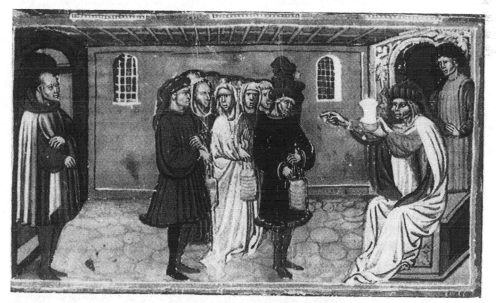

Figure 5   Consultation and examination of urines. Men and women patients
or their messengers bring flasks of urine in wicker containers to the practitioner's
premises for his expert opinion. (Bologna, Biblioteca Universitaria, MS 2197,
fifteenth century, fol. 7ʳ. Reproduction authorized by the Minstero
per i Beni Culturali, Italy.)

kinds.[36] The following examples of types of medical practice and patients, drawn from the late thirteenth- and fourteenth-century Italian scene, probably reveal a wider availability of and reliance upon paid medical care from lay practitioners who made medicine their sole or principal occupation than was the case in all but a few areas of northern Europe during the same period.

Even professors of medicine in the universities, who made teaching and writing a major focus of their activities, simultaneously engaged in extensive private practice. Taddeo Alderotti's patients included both men and women (he practiced gynecology but not obstetrics); ranged socially from a blacksmith to the Doge of Venice, although the wealthier classes predominated; varied in age from adolescence to the sixties; and resided all over northern Italy. He also provided consultations by letter for other practitioners who wanted advice about their patients. For the most part, the more elite the physician, the more general the practice. Specialization in particular kinds of care—eye conditions, hernia, midwifery (the last practiced only by women)—was a mark of low status.

Among the most important institutional employers were the towns themselves. In Italy, urban governments early came to regard the supervision of public health as part of their duty; to this end, during the fourteenth and fifteenth centuries, the rulers or governing bodies of various cities issued sanitary regulations, instituted provisions for quarantine in times of plague, and appointed boards of health. These institutions were civil magistracies in which medical practitioners played little part, filling at most an advisory role. In the early thirteenth century, however, as already noted, some municipal governments in Italy began regularly to hire both medical and surgical practitioners (*medici condotti*) to care for their citizens. By the mid-fifteenth century, *medici condotti* were to be found in cities and towns, large and small, throughout Italy. Large cities employed several practitioners at a time; for instance, between 1333 and 1377, Venice employed an average of about 7 *medici* and about 10 surgeons every year. Over the course of the fourteenth and fifteenth centuries, 138 practitioners (63 of them university trained) were employed by public authorities in Piedmont. Duties and salaries varied widely but commonly included the obligations of residing in the city and of treating the poor gratis.[37] Municipalities also hired medical and surgical practitioners for particular tasks—for example, to report on the cause of death or injury in disputed cases or to advise administrative boards of health when these were formed.

In the fourteenth and fifteenth centuries, pious foundations and religious institutions, including houses of monks and nuns concerned to provide regular medical attendance for their own members, also retained the services of paid medical practitioners. In Florence, *medici* were engaged by various charitable confraternities that included service to the sick among their objectives. Moreover, while most of the institutions termed "hospitals" in this period provided chiefly food, shelter, and prayer to the indigent, aged, and pilgrims as well as to the sick, a few gave a measure of medical care and some paid medical practitioners a retainer for regular attendance. A famous but untypically large and medicalized example is the hospital of Santa Maria Nuova in Florence. Founded in the 1280s, it had 300 beds in the late fifteenth century and by 1500 employed nine medical practitioners.[38]

The large size, substantial wealth (even after the demographic and economic contraction of the fourteenth century), and sophisticated administrative structures of great cities such as Florence and Venice doubtless facilitated the demand for and supply of paid medical care. But by the early fourteenth century, essentially similar provisions could also be found in considerably smaller centers in Italy. For example, the records of a papal commission of inquiry in 1318–19 into the sanctity and miracles attributed to Chiara of Montefalco (d. 1308) incidentally reveal the extensive availability and use of paid secular medical care in Spoleto and the surrounding region.[39]

Chiara was a member of a community of nuns with connections to both the Franciscans and the Augustinian Hermits. Her reputation for sanctity and the supposed discovery of symbols of Christ's passion in her heart and gallbladder at the time of her death led to the development of a cult and the attribution to her of numerous posthumous miracles, most of them involving physical healing. Almost all the witnesses who testified before the papal commission enthusiastically endorsed her sanctity; many believed that they or members of their families had been beneficiaries of healing miracles. A lone dissenter, Friar Tommaso Bono OFM, adduced Chiara's suspicious friendships with heretics, the good food she ate, and the fact that she was attended by the best doctors (*optimi medici*). Friar Tommaso obviously regarded Chiara's use of medical attendants as incompatible with ascetic sanctity, although not necessarily as wrong in itself. His evidence was explained away by Chiara's natural brother Francesco, also a Franciscan friar. Friar Francesco asserted that she cared nothing for her own bodily health, but that he himself had summoned to attend her "a most excellent *medicus*, by name Master Mercato of Gubbio, one of the best practitioners in the whole of Italy." Master Mercato "by means of most certain signs that he knew from the subtlety and height of his command of the art of medicine" diagnosed that she was suffering from urinary obstruction "owing to the extremely tight closure of her virginity." The certain signs were evidently not based on

direct physical examination, since Chiara's modesty forbade her even to apply any medication herself for her condition, whatever it may have been.[40]

When Chiara lay dying, she was attended not by Master Mercato but by
Simone da Spello, the *medico condotto* of the little town of Montafalco. He
appears to have been neither particularly gifted in prognosis nor particularly
sympathetic to his patients. The night before Chiara died, Simone told Friar
Francesco that she was completely recovered except for "elevations and
carrying away of the mind" which were injuring her greatly. Simone da
Spello was clearly not impressed by Chiara's devotional outpourings. The
nuns knew better and told Francesco to stay if he wanted to see his sister
alive. Next morning, when Simone returned, Chiara was dead. Because she
was sitting erect, the *medicus* did not realize death had taken place until he
attempted to find a pulse. Accordingly, he began his visit by scolding the
grief-stricken Friar Francesco for weeping "like the women."[41]

The nuns of Montefalco did not defer to their medical attendant or
show any great reliance on his expertise. Before she died, Chiara told her
sisters in religion that she had Christ in her heart. Being literal-minded
women, they promptly cut open her body after death and were gratified—
although not at all surprised—to find formations inside the heart that they
took to be symbols of the passion. They then asked Simone to open up her
gallbladder, and "they put it in his hand." On his refusal, "because he did not
feel himself worthy, as he said," the sisters dissected that, too.[42] It is quite
likely that experience of the farmyard and butchery had given them as
much familiarity with and rough understanding of gross anatomy as a small-
town medical practitioner possessed.

The commissioners routinely asked witnesses attesting healing miracles
whether medical attention previously had been sought for the patient.
There is nothing to suggest that the clerical commissioners asked this question because they regarded a first choice of secular means of healing as a
sign of lack of faith. Rather, as products of a society that by this time took
the availability and use of secular medicine for granted, they seem to have
wanted testimony that medical practitioners had diagnosed the extent and
severity of prior disease because it constituted particularly telling evidence
that a miracle had in fact subsequently occurred. The replies to the question
reveal the presence of a number of practitioners in Spoleto and the surrounding region during the decade 1308–18 and much demand for their
services. No doubt some were empirics, but Master Niccolo, *physicus*, Master
Giovanni, *physicus*, and Master Filippo, a surgeon, all of Spoleto, sound as if
they had received academic or other formal training.[43]

By no means all who sought healing from Chiara had made previous efforts to obtain treatment by physical means; and some had medicated themselves or their children or gone to medicinal baths. The large minority who had sought out a medical practitioner cannot be identified with any particular social class. No doubt ability to pay played a part in the decision to secure medical treatment beyond self-help. *Medici condotti* did not necessarily provide free services for noncitizens or transients. Some time in the first decade of the fifteenth century, when St. Francesca Romana came upon a homeless man lying in the streets of Rome with a gaping, maggotty wound in his arm, her reaction was to ask him, "Poor man, why don't you go for treatment and get cured?" His answer was, "I haven't any money."[44]

The main impression left by the clients of Chiara of Montefalco who stated that they had used practitioners is of a strong demand for any service that offered the help of physical relief. For example, those who consulted practitioners at all frequently consulted more than one. Women seem very often to have initiated the search for medical treatment for themselves or their children, although this perception may be skewed by the fact that women were frequent supplicants at Chiara's shrine and therefore make up a large number of the witnesses questioned by the inquisitors. A striking feature of the testimony is the readiness with which practitioners were called to attend babies and small children; evidently high infant mortality did not breed resignation or acceptance in these parents.

Indeed, the medical needs and hopes of the witnesses, many of them parents of sick children, make sad reading. One woman consulted "many *medici*" for her uterine prolapse, and three were summoned to examine the swelling on a baby's eyelid. A boy was taken from Spoleto to Gubbio to see a "famous *medicus*" for his hernia, and *medici*, in the plural, despaired of the health of six-year-old Napoleone, who had suffered from fever for 15 days on end without eating anything. When a woman whose face was so disfigured by a "a kind of leprosy" that the other women would not give her the kiss of peace in church told her brother that she felt better after praying to Chiara, he retorted, "You said the same thing the times you were treated by a *medicus*, and every time your infirmity came back." Her neighbor heard Vannuctia Angelicti crying for many, many days from the pain in her right breast and weeping again when the *medici* said the only remedy was the knife. Lady Alegra's husband, Bertoldo Massarecto, was so distressed by her stomach pains, which were much worse than the labor pains she had had in bearing her seven children, that he consulted numerous *medici* on her behalf, including the emperor's own (the emperor in question was presumably

Henry VII, whose Italian expedition took place during these years; perhaps the practitioner was Bartolomeo da Varignana).[45]

Expectations and Critiques

The demand for medical care at all social levels was fueled by the overwhelming health needs of a society characterized by low life expectancy, high infant mortality, high morbidity, and, among the poor, widespread malnutrition, inadequate housing, and urban overcrowding.[46] Of course, readiness to seek out and pay medical practitioners implies not only medical need but also acceptance of the validity of current medical knowledge and forms of practice. The development of the late medieval and Renaissance medical profession (in the most inclusive sense of the term) is inexplicable unless one recognizes that the knowledge claims of practitioners were generally accepted and their various activities were broadly consistent with current social expectations of medicine. The privileged place of learned physicians in the medical hierarchy reflected both the general social prestige of learning of all kinds and the value set on access to the most detailed sources of medical information. As for practical results of therapy, medieval and Renaissance practitioners and patients alike knew that successful cures depended on the knowledge and skill of the practitioner, but also on factors beyond his control: ultimately the will of God and, more immediately, the healing power of nature,[47] external conditions, and the patient's willingness or ability to follow medical instructions. Unfavorable outcomes were on occasion blamed on the ineptitude of individual practitioners;[48] but the existence of such accusations is in itself evidence that practitioners were normally thought of as competent and that it was considered possible to distinguish competence from incompetence. Hence, bad or inconclusive results of medical treatment would be no more likely to be destructive of general confidence than an individual's failure to obtain a miracle would be likely to shake confidence in the healing power of saints' shrines. And practitioners and patients also knew that many conditions were beyond the powers of medicine to heal. But recognition that the powers of medicine are limited is not incompatible with the belief, whether or not well founded, that it may be useful in some circumstances.

Thus, not even the mid-fourteenth-century calamity of the Black Death, when disease in the face of which the medical community was totally helpless killed perhaps one third of the population of Europe was sufficient to produce a general or lasting loss of confidence in established medical theory, education, and practice. That crisis produced some bitter comments, such as the remark of a Florentine chronicler, à propos of the behavior of his city's medical practitioners during the first great plague outbreak: "Some of them, for the sake of making a profit, visited patients and gave their explanations, but they showed by their deaths that their art was feigned."[49] But the inability of medical practitioners to explain or arrest the course of an epidemic of unfamiliar type and unprecedented virulence certainly did not have the effect of invalidating the entire complex structure of medical knowledge and its underlying physiological theories or of diminishing the actual or presumed usefulness of medical attention in many of the ordinary vicissitudes of life. Medicine as a profession seemed less attractive to members of prosperous Florentine families in the second than in the first half of the fourteenth century, but "new men" from lesser families or the surrounding countryside flocked to take their place.[50] Throughout Europe, continued recruitment of practitioners during the second half of the fourteenth and the fifteenth centuries testifies to continued demand for medical services of the same type as those available before the plague. Leading university-trained physicians and professors of medicine of that period enjoyed fame and intellectual prestige just as great as that of their predecessors around 1300. More important, the institutions and content of academic education in medicine, the central role of texts of Greek and medieval Islamic origin as the ultimate source of most medical and surgical information and ideas, and the conditions of medical and surgical practice—all survived the Black Death essentially unchanged.

The criticisms of medical practitioners that were frequently voiced usually sprang less from dissatisfaction with medicine's limited effectiveness than from religious tradition, with its powerful themes linking healing with religious charity and miraculous intervention, and its assertion of the priority of the healing of the soul over the healing of the body. But by the thirteenth century, ideals as well as realities were undergoing modification. In general, while traditional religious ideas about medicine and physical healing continued to find expression, ecclesiastical authorities moved toward the acceptance of the use of specialized medical care as a social norm and the endeavor to regulate it in the interests of the Christian community.

As mentioned earlier, the first ecclesiastical response to the growth of commercial medical practice and nonmonastic centers of medical learning had been to try and prevent the participation of monks. The most important such prohibition was a decree of the Council of Tours (1163) that was subsequently included in various canon law collections. In the early thirteenth century, the impulse was still to control by prohibition; indeed, the prohibition was considerably expanded by a papal decree of 1219 that forbade secular clergy in responsible positions—priests, deacons, and holders of benefices—to absent themselves from their ecclesiastical duties in order to study medicine or law. In 1298, the restrictions on absence for purposes of medical studies for all categories of clergy, including monks, were modified into the reasonable requirement that permission of superiors be obtained.[51] And numerous documents requesting benefices for or conferring benefices upon medical masters and students preserved in the records of the Portuguese University (Coimbra-Lisbon), to choose only one example, show that in the fourteenth and fifteenth centuries this method of financing medical teaching and studies was taken for granted by medical masters and students, university officials, and the papacy.[52] Medicine, of course, was only one of many fields in which ecclesiastical benefices held in absentia were used to support intellectual, professional, or administrative activities, a practice that was widespread in the fourteenth and fifteenth centuries.

The church also sought to regulate medical practice from the standpoint of the welfare—chiefly, naturally, the spiritual welfare—of the patient (figure 6). Rightly or wrongly, ecclesiastical authorities were suspicious that medical practitioners put patients' physical health before their spiritual well-being, and their own fees before either, a belief also voiced by moralists and satirists (figure 7). The Fourth Lateran Council (1215) obliged physicians to insist that patients summon a confessor before any other treatment and strictly forbade the use of any medical treatment by "sinful means" (for example, prescriptions to eat meat on fast days or engage in sexual intercourse outside of marriage). Also in the late twelfth and early thirteenth centuries, canon lawyers and theologians confronted new social realities in discussions of the legitimacy of taking fees for transmitting knowledge; they came to a consensus that moderate fees or salaries to meet the needs of the physician, like those of the lawyer or teacher of secular subjects, were licit, although there was supposedly an obligation to provide good service in return and to treat the poor for nothing.[53]

The life of St. Francesca Romana reveals something of the attitude of a deeply religious person in the fifteenth century to the use of medicine. Francesca was personally an ascetic of such austerity that she wore a hair shirt to the marriage bed. Repelled by marital sexual relations—she had been forced into an arranged marriage at the age of eleven—and by upper-class social life, she developed a passionate concern for the poor and especially the sick. As a result, although she repudiated all use of medicine for herself, she expended her energies in securing it for others, and she evidently devoted thought to securing the right kind of medicine for each case. She herself practiced healing, usually by prayer and touch alone but

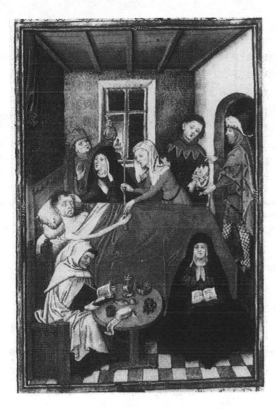

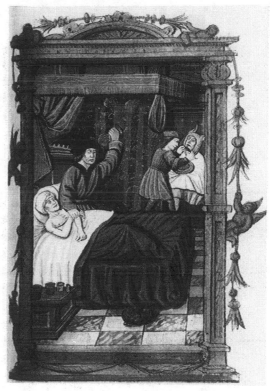

Figure 6   In this deathbed scene from a Book of Hours illustrated in the Low Countries about 1440, both the patient's soul and his body are objects of concern. However, the inclusion of this illustration in a prayer-book and its specific representation of a dying patient dictate the evident subordination of prognosis and physical care, in the shape of the medical practitioner shown with his urine flask at the far left and the woman stroking the sick man's forehead, to religious consolation and preparation for the soul's departure, personified by the praying religious in the foreground. (Courtesy the Pierpont Morgan Library, New York, MS M. 917, Hours of Catherine of Cleves, p. 180.)

Figure 7   A sickbed scene from the section on medicine of a satire on "the abuses of the world" written and illustrated at Rouen for King James IV of Scotland in about 1510. The young and healthy-looking patient, lying in a bed that looks considerably more luxurious than that depicted in figure 6, is attended solely by a medical practitioner; religion literally does not enter the picture. An array of containers for medicines stands on the bedside table. The abuses of medicine on the part of practitioners denounced in the accompanying text include corrupt financial arrangements with apothecaries, lack of sufficient training, and consequent ignorance; practitioners prescribe medicines by chance and learn on their patients. Those who rush into practice without enough knowledge of medical "art" or "science" are compared with the young barber in the background of the picture who, although a mere apprentice, started to offer his services as soon as he had learned to give a shave. Patients who abuse medicine are those who place too much value on preserving their youth and good looks or who think that their wealth will enable them to cheat death. (Courtesy the Pierpont Morgan Library, New York, MS M. 42, Pierre Gringore, *Les abus du monde*, fol. 55.)

sometimes by also employing ointments or liquids. She also told a woman who consulted her about a dumb child that it would be better to take the little girl to a *medicus*, by whom she meant a male Christian practitioner with some form of medical training; Francesca firmly warned anyone who consulted her away from women who used charms or spells and away from Jewish physicians.[54]

The depth of Francesca Bussi's religiosity and of her social concern was as unusual in her own society as in any other. But Christian traditions concerning medicine and healing continued to provide ammunition for literary or rhetorical critiques of the medical profession. These traditions made medical practitioners—especially university-educated physicians with claims to philosophical learning as well as medical expertise—particularly susceptible to charges that they pursued for money subjects that should be studied for the sake of either charity or pure knowledge; hence Dante's contrast of Taddeo Alderotti's pursuit of medical knowledge for worldly gain with the purer motives of St. Dominic (*Paradiso* 12.82–84).

To be sure, not all criticisms originated from religious belief or feeling. The poet and humanist Petrarch (d. 1374) denigrated medical practitioners for religious and moral failings; but he also scorned their intellectual pretensions and claimed to find their practical activities squalid. He jeered that one practitioner owed his pallor not to philosophical studies, as he maintained, but to contact with the excreta of sick bodies. Petrarch's comments stand in striking contrast to the view implied in the biography of his contemporary, the Dominican tertiary and ecstatic mystic St. Catherine of Siena (d. 1380). The life of this most celebrated of the numerous holy women associated with the mendicant orders in fourteenth-century Italy was written by her confessor and fellow-Dominican, Raimondo of Capua. He evidently believed Catherine's willingness to have physical contact with the excreta of the revoltingly sick to be a mark of sanctity. In a lengthy chapter devoted to recounting in detail the cases of three sick women nursed by Catherine, Raimondo held up for particular admiration Catherine's acts of self-mortification in first kissing, and on another occasion drinking pus from, the cancerous sore on one of these patients. These feats were of course designed to have therapeutic effects on Catherine's soul rather than on the sick women. Catherine's patients did not necessarily appreciate having their suffering used as an opportunity for her spiritual edification; at any rate at one time or another each of the three took a dislike to her.

Petrarch's and Catherine's or Raimondo's reactions to the realities of illness represent extreme responses in which there is a strong rhetorical or dramatic element. Endorsement of their respective attitudes could be found in philosophical tradition and in ascetic (perhaps especially mendi-cant) spirituality. Yet neither attitude was sufficiently generally or pro-foundly held to discourage entry into the medical profession or the wide-spread search for physical healing by any means available, whether secular or religious.[55]

Nor was Petrarch's attitude necessarily typical of humanist intellectuals. In the view of another early humanist writer, Filippo Villani, author of a set of lives of notable Florentines including the account of Tommaso del Garbo quoted at the beginning of this chapter, medicine took its place among the disciplines supposedly restored to life by the efforts of modern Italians. This claim ignored historical continuities, not to mention the contributions of Islam, various translators, Salerno, and Montpellier, but it initiated a literary tradition in which the development of medicine was treated as a source of pride. In subsequent collective biographies of distinguished men written in Italy during the fourteenth and fifteenth centuries, physicians were fre-quently included, and the aspect of medical accomplishment that was most often stressed was medical learning. The model physician described in most of these biographical and bibliographical sketches was a medical author and university professor who also attended patients.[56]

As the foregoing account makes clear, such men formed only one com-ponent in the multifarious community of medical practitioners. The au-thors of collective biographies, however, were correct in perceiving that learned physicians (and, one would add, learned surgeons) had an impor-tance disproportionate to their numbers in shaping and transmitting the culture of medicine and in preserving medicine's place among the presti-gious branches of knowledge. Even though relatively few practitioners par-ticipated fully in the high culture of medicine, the extensive medical and surgical activity described in this chapter was fostered, directly or indirectly, by intellectual and educational developments as well as by economic capac-ity and social needs.

THREE

MEDICAL EDUCATION

n innovation in medical education with profound and lasting consequences took place in western Europe in the
twelfth and thirteenth centuries. As a result of developments in medical pedagogy that began in twelfth-century
Salerno and of the subsequent rise of universities,* medi-
cine became one of the small range of subjects taught in a university setting
during the Middle Ages and Renaissance. The distinct type of professional
and intellectual formation thus initiated shaped Europe's medical elite until
well into the early modern period. The institutional organization of university faculties of medicine, parts of the actual curriculum, and the claims to
social and intellectual primacy of university-trained physicians within the
hierarchy of practitioners all exhibited much continuity between the thirteenth and the seventeenth, and in some respects and some places, between
even the thirteenth and the eighteenth centuries. Moreover, although
medieval and early modern universities enrolled only a minority of all medical practitioners, university curricula systematized the transmission and reinforced the authority of a body of medical books, concepts, and techniques that provided the basis for medical practices and beliefs broadly
disseminated throughout society. University records, taken in conjunction
with the pedagogical writings of professors, are thus a rich source of information about the training of an elite and about the intellectual basis of
medical ideas.

Faculties of medicine were included in almost all universities established
before 1500.[1] But the distribution of universities throughout Europe was
chronologically and geographically very uneven, and, as we shall see, their

*Throughout this book, the word "university" is used, except where otherwise
noted, in the modern sense, to mean an entire academic community and its constit-
uent institutions. In a medieval and Renaissance context the more technically correct term is *"studium generale," "universitas"* being reserved for a self-governing association of students or masters in a particular discipline or disciplines within a *studium
generale.*

medical faculties varied widely in size, influence, and prestige. The medieval university movement took place in two distinct stages. The oldest universities, in France, England, Italy, and the Iberian peninsula, appeared in the late twelfth and the thirteenth centuries. Although their development was legitimated, regulated, and encouraged by religious and local and regional political authorities, almost all of them came into being more or less spontaneously, and their origins involved some degree of autonomous self-assertion by scholars or masters. Fundamental to the successful establishment of medicine as a discipline in these oldest universities, as it was to the university movement in general, was the general economic, demographic, and urban growth of western Europe in the same period. More specifically, university education in medicine first emerged in the context of a recent multiplication of schools providing Latin literacy, the early stages of the impact of Aristotelian logic and philosophy on ideas and pedagogy, a new availability of many medical textbooks in Latin, and the appearance of new forms of authentication of medical practitioners. The creative process of development, selection, and adaptation of basic methods and materials for the university curriculum in medicine thus extended from about the late twelfth to the early fourteenth century.

The second stage of the university movement occurred at a time when teaching methods and materials in Latin academic medicine were already well established. The foundation of universities in the German lands and central Europe began with the charter granted to the University of Prague by the Emperor Charles IV in 1348 and continued until after 1500. The main motivating force behind these foundations was usually the will of the secular ruler and his perception of the needs of the state. Meanwhile, the process whereby Italian universities were brought under the control of the Renaissance state had already begun in the fourteenth century.

Despite the great institutional, professional, and intellectual importance of the medical faculties of the medieval and Renaissance universities, the content of the discipline studied and taught in them was neither their creation nor ever their exclusive property. Because medicine was at once a system of explanation and a set of techniques, the acquisition of medical expertise was both an intellectual enterprise and a process of gaining skills. The intellectual enterprise was, as has already been indicated, grounded in the medicine, the logic, the natural philosophy, and the astrology of antiquity and the Islamic world. Its pursuit normally involved acquaintance with books, although for less-educated practitioners this acquaintance might be slight; evidently, oral transmission of ideas emanating from the learned tradition also took place. The skills came by way of some combination of formal or informal apprenticeship to an older practitioner, personal experience, hearsay, and folklore. Both forms of learning could and did go on inside and also outside the university setting. Hence, throughout the twelfth to fifteenth centuries (and for long thereafter), the task of acquiring medical expertise was pursued in a variety of contexts and at widely varying levels of formal organization, intellectualization, and sophistication. Medical education was formally acquired in the university classroom or informally through private study or shared experience. In some settings Latin literacy was a prerequisite; in others, literacy in a vernacular sufficed; and in still others literacy was doubtless not involved at all.

Varieties of Medical Education

Because ancient Greek and medieval Islamic medicine, in both its explanatory and its technical aspects, constituted the most advanced medical knowledge available, its study was necessarily a major component in advanced medical education (figure 8.) And because in western Europe the most direct access to Greco-Islamic medicine was through the medium of such texts as had been translated into Latin, higher medical education was necessarily book learned and Latinate (figure 9). Only a handful of translators and Jewish physicians had access to material in languages other than Latin or western European vernaculars. Graduates of (and dropouts from) university faculties of medicine were assuredly equipped with Latin medical learning; in addition, they were supposedly able, at least ideally, to enrich their medicine with rational arguments and knowledge of general physical science gained through the study of liberal arts and natural philosophy.

But Latin literacy was not, of course, confined to the universities. Latin medical books could be and were copied, studied, compiled, and composed in other environments. In the twelfth century, monastic libraries built up medical holdings that served to train monk-practitioners and were also an important source of ideas about human physical nature for theological and philosophical writers (see chapter 4 and figure 15 in that chapter). In the following centuries the numerous clergy who practiced medicine were unquestionably literate in Latin, but most of them must have gained their medical as well as their other learning in a religious rather than in a university context. For example, in the 1340s and 1350s, Berthold Blumentrost, who had himself probably studied arts and medicine at the universities of Paris and Bologna, respectively, taught in a house of canons in Würzburg. The medical works he composed there included a set of questions on the section of embryology in Avicenna's *Canon* that showed he had fully absorbed, and

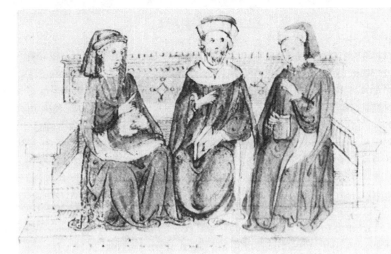

Figure 8   Three medical authorities in discussion, as envisioned by an artist in
Lombardy around 1400. The figures probably represent Hippocrates (late fifth–early
fourth century B.C.), Dioscorides (first century A.D.), and Sextus Placitus (fifth century A.D.?), although the copyist appears to have confused the last name with that
of Plato. The manuscript in which this picture is found consists chiefly of a collection of Latin books on remedies compiled in late antiquity; it includes an herbal
incorporating translated portions of Dioscorides' work on materia medica, the herbal attributed to Apuleius, and Sextus Placitus's treatise on medications obtained
from animals. (Courtesy Yale Medical Library, MS 18, fol. 3ᵛ.)

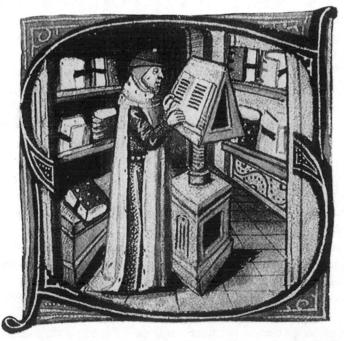

Figure 9   A learned physician in his study, from a collection of works of Galen
copied in the Low Countries or northern France around 1460. (Sächsische Landesbibliothek, Dresden, MS Db 93, fol. 407ᵛ; courtesy Sächsische Landesbibliothek and
Vivian Nutton.)

presumably passed on to his students, the philosophical approach to medicine inculcated in some university courses. However, the most important new educational institutions of the thirteenth century other than the universities, namely the *studia* of the friar orders, seldom seem to have provided much opportunity for medical study, for their libraries were usually specialized collections of works in theology and philosophy and contained few medical books. But proximity to a major center of secular university medical education might affect the libraries and interests of friars, as may have occurred when the university professor of medicine Taddeo Alderotti willed his medical textbooks to the Franciscan friars of Bologna.[2]

Furthermore, in the thirteenth and fourteenth centuries, major textbooks of surgery written in Latin and based on ancient and Islamic teaching were composed by surgeons who were unconnected or only loosely connected with university faculties. Surgery, indeed, is especially notable for the way in which it bridged learned and technical traditions, the academic world and the world of crafts (see chapter 6). In fifteenth-century Padua, and no doubt in other secular urban milieus of the same period, Latin as well as Italian medical and astrological works were studied by surgical and other practitioners who did not have university training as well as by literate citizens in other occupations.[3]

In the late fourteenth and the fifteenth centuries, books on medicine and surgery in vernacular languages surely played a significant part in the training of many lay practitioners outside academic and religious milieus (see figure 17 in chapter 4). Doubtless, too, the audience for vernacular medical books included some readers from outside the medical profession (see figures 25, 26, 28, and 32 in chapter 5). Practitioners who used vernacular medical books for study and reference learned to participate in essentially the same system of medical ideas as their Latinate colleagues, since most vernacular writings on medicine drew in one way or another on Latin texts. The extent to which the study of vernacular medical books was likely to be accompanied by formal instruction or guidance from a teacher is unclear. It seems highly likely, however, that apprenticeship to a practitioner would involve gaining some acquaintance with any books he or she might have owned.

Growth in the variety, scope, and depth of medical writing in vernacular languages can be illustrated with examples drawn from the English scene. Although there are some important early medieval medical texts in Old English from the Anglo-Saxon period, only a few recipes for remedies survive in Middle English from the twelfth and thirteenth centuries. Anglo-Norman (French) medical writings of that period also consist largely of recipes or other brief practical texts. One example is a medical poem, found in a thirteenth-century manuscript, that provides summary versified remedies for the treatment of conditions ranging from worms to sleeplessness. In the fourteenth and fifteenth centuries, collections of remedies and other simple texts were produced in quantity in Middle English. Often, a number of treatises were assembled into a manuscript book covering various aspects of medicine, so that the owner had a general work of reference at his or her command. By the end of the fifteenth century, however, translations or adaptations of medical textbooks from Latin into English included a number of lengthy, complex, and sophisticated works. By that time, according to one expert, English was as important a language as Latin in medical book production in England. The works selected for translation were usually of relatively recent date and practical in focus; for example, treatises on surgery, bloodletting, and gynecology composed or compiled in Latin between the twelfth and the fourteenth centuries were translated into English in the late fourteenth or early fifteenth century. Nonetheless, these works were themselves heavily indebted to the medicine of antiquity and of medieval Islam, and they included much theoretical and explanatory material. The translators of medical and surgical books accepted a difficult assignment, since they were often faced with technical Latin terms for which there was no existing vernacular equivalent. Their inventive solutions to this problem helped to create vernacular technical vocabularies, just as those who had earlier translated from Greek and Arabic into Latin had helped to enlarge the Latin technical vocabulary. By the fifteenth century, practitioners who owned technical books on medicine and surgery in English ranged from graduate physicians who could also read Latin to the London barber-surgeon mentioned in chapter 2.[4]

A similar story could be told of the expansion of technical writing on medicine in other vernacular languages over the same period. In the German lands, where the late foundation and small size of university faculties of medicine meant that university-trained physicians were a rarity before the fifteenth century, the dissemination of medical books in the vernacular took on a special importance. For example, perhaps as early as 1280, Ortolf von Baierland (Bavaria), a practitioner in Würzburg, put together in German a comprehensive handbook of medicine in 167 chapters. It transmitted some account of physiological theory as well as information about diseases and remedies and drew on standard Latin or translated Greek and Arabic authors—Constantinus Africanus, Hippocrates (the *Aphorisms*), and Avicenna. In the course of the fourteenth and fifteenth centuries, Ortolf's work became one of the most widely disseminated medical textbooks in

Germany and central Europe; it was translated, wholly or in part, into a variety of languages, Latin among them, and in one form or another it survives in numerous manuscripts and early editions.[5]

Written materials emanating, directly or at one or more removes, from the world of Latin formal education were clearly important in the broad dissemination of concepts of medical explanation. The role of the written word is more obscure when it comes to the actual acquisition of therapeutic techniques. Most of the forms of intervention known to medieval medicine had been described by Greek medical authors and their Islamic amplifiers and interpreters; works embodying this information were, of course, prominent among those studied in and outside the universities, in Latin and the vernaculars. No doubt such books played a part, perhaps a major part, in disseminating information about techniques and perhaps also in promoting some techniques and discouraging the use of others. But the real relation between ancient descriptions of therapeutic techniques, their subsequent Islamic and western elaborations and interpretations in learned books, and actual medieval and early Renaissance practice remains highly problematic (see chapters 5 and 6).

Yet it is obvious that, just as the influence of Latin academic medical learning was by no means confined to the universities, so too the ability to put techniques into practice and to vary them as local, temporal, and individual circumstances demanded could only have been acquired through the observation of experienced older colleagues at work and through "hands-on" experience that was essentially common to practitioners in all categories. To the extent that licensing regulations or requirements of guild membership involved examinations or the imposition of rules based on norms developed in the learned medical milieu, they may have helped to standardize practice. For example, a decree issued in 1332 by King Alfonso of Aragon followed the advice of technical manuals on phlebotomy in forbidding barber-surgeons in Valencia to practice bloodletting in the heat of summer (the dog days) except "when evidently necessary or by advice of the *medici*."[6] Despite the range of contexts and levels in which and at which a practitioner might acquire the knowledge and skill he or she needed, there seems to have been much broad similarity in the concepts and techniques transmitted in most of the milieus of which we have any knowledge.

It was, however, in the universities that the most sophisticated, systematic, and prestigious form of medical education was imparted. Juridical and institutional features distinguished universities from all other schools: the presence of legally recognized, self-governing academic associations with the power to determine their own membership; a papal bull recognizing the university as a *studium generale;* some form of official recognition from secular political authorities: and fixed curricular arrangements and academic exercises. Above all, only the universities recognized the various stages of academic progress of bachelors and masters, and only in the university could the doctorate be earned. This highest degree usually was granted by an official empowered by ecclesiastical authority after the candidate had satisfied faculty examiners as to his competence. In medicine as in other subjects, the doctorate took the form of a license to teach in any university whatsoever (*licencia ubique docendi*). Thus, although the doctorate in medicine was always accepted as a qualification to practice medicine, its absence never implied that a *medicus* was unqualified to practice.

Origins, Distribution, and Relative Importance of University Faculties of Medicine

Despite the presence of faculties of medicine in most universities, major centers of academic medical education were always few in number. In terms of the chronological and geographical distribution of such centers, the salient facts are the early emergence and early decline of Salerno (the late eleventh through the early thirteenth centuries) and the subsequent predominance of just three centers: Bologna, Montpellier, and Paris. A fourth center, Padua, the home of medical studies since the thirteenth century, increased in size and importance in the course of the fifteenth century.[7] Mention may also be made of Ferrara, which, although small, became a center of intellectual influence in medicine during the last thirty years of the fifteenth century. The leading position of these medical schools—as measured by reputation among contemporaries, ability to attract students from far away, output of medical writings, presence of numerous or famous teachers, and, where known, numbers of graduates with medical degrees— was not challenged in the period before 1500. Additional universities of medieval foundation attained more than local renown for medical teaching in the course of the sixteenth century, but they were not major centers for the study of medicine at an earlier date. This description applies as much to Salamanca, an important university since the thirteenth century, as to the regional education center of Tübingen, still small, struggling, and recently founded when the fifteenth century ended.[8]

The differences between the various faculties of medicine lay more in size, reputation, and institutional position than in curriculum. The common heritage of Greek and Islamic medical learning and Aristotelian natural philosophy ensured a good deal of curricular uniformity throughout Europe, but the intellectual as well as the professional and collegial ambience of the various medical faculties varied widely. In all these respects, the experience of the 4 otherwise-obscure doctors of medicine who taught at Poitiers in the fifteenth century must have been very different from that of the more than 125 professors (including a number of well-known medical authors) and promoters of candidates for medical degrees at Padua during the same period.[9]

Yet developments in even the less-celebrated faculties of medicine probably had a local or regional impact on the medical profession. Oxford may serve as an example. Despite the fame of the university in other respects, the medical faculty at Oxford was small and on the whole undistinguished. For the entire fourteenth century, the names of only 40 medical masters and students are known; all of them appear to have been beneficed clergy or members of religious orders, and for many of them medicine was decidedly subordinate to other intellectual interests or career activities. The only two medical authors, John of Gaddesden and Simon Bredon, were both associated with Merton College, to which Bredon left a respectable collection of medical books. Merton was one of several Oxford residential colleges that from time to time had one or two medical students or masters among its members, perhaps to treat the other fellows. In the course of the fourteenth century, the faculty of medicine secured the right to license medical practice in Oxford, which at that time was only a small provincial town.

In the fifteenth century, although the faculty increased only modestly in size (54 masters and students), some Oxford-educated physicians began to be active in a wider medical context. At least three were laymen; a higher proportion appear to have made medical practice their main activity, although this impression may be an accident of record survival; and some had connections with the Cambridge University faculty of medicine, which was also small, or with the world of medical practice in London, a much larger and more important city than Oxford. In the 1420s, English university-educated physicians petitioned King Henry V to restrict any right to practice physic to university-educated physicians licensed by (not necessarily educated at) the English universities. Soon afterwards, graduate physicians united with London surgeons in short-lived joint association that sought the right to regulate medical and surgical practice in London. However, no lasting results came of these efforts. Although by this time physicians trained in English universities clearly aspired to dominance within the medical profession in England, they were unable to achieve this result, largely because their numbers were too small, and the university medical faculties were too weak and located too far from the wealth and professional opportunities of

London. But it is probable that Oxford and Cambridge university medicine, not to mention the presence in England of foreign medical graduates from universities abroad, had an indirect influence on English medical practice, since medical masters and students were among the most likely owners of Latin medical books from which vernacular medical collections might be compiled.[10]

In the newer universities of Germany and central Europe, too, medicine was normally the smallest faculty. Such influence as the professors of medicine had often derived more from the support of the local prince or from their position as leading practitioners and substantial citizens in the town than from the place of medicine in the university community. Between the founding of the University of Prague in 1348 and the Reformation, some 250,000 individuals frequented these institutions; during the first decade of the sixteenth century, about 6,000 students per year attended universities in the German lands. But only a very small number studied medicine. For example, at Cologne between 1395 and 1445, 500 students—more than 65 percent of the total—matriculated in the faculty of arts; civil and canon law together accounted for 143 students, or almost 19 percent. By contrast, the 8 students of medicine amounted to only 1 percent of the total. Among those who did study medicine in German universities, many also went to Italy for at least part of their medical education.[11]

Investigation of the social and professional context of the small faculties of medicine, and the careers and backgrounds of those who studied and taught in them, will add considerably to our knowledge of the diverse social and institutional history of medicine in different parts of Europe during the late Middle Ages and Renaissance. Knowledge of this aspect of university education in medicine is still scattered and incomplete, although a number of valuable local studies have appeared.[12] But understanding of the goals, methodology, accomplishments, and limitations of university medical teaching is best gained from consideration of the most successful schools.

Between the late eleventh and the early thirteenth centuries, Salerno, long famous as a center of medical expertise and medical practice, developed into an extremely influential center of medical education where important characteristics of academic medical teaching took shape. In one sense, however, Salerno does not belong in a discussion of the principal medieval university faculties of medicine; formal university organization was not introduced at Salerno until the second half of the thirteenth century, after the end of the period of its predominance as a center of medical education.

The introduction of an academic and book-oriented emphasis in Salernitan medicine was the result of a confluence of factors. Access to some of the medical writings in Latin available in Italy during the early Middle Ages no doubt played a part. In addition, the geographical situation and early medieval history of the southern part of the Italian peninsula provided opportunities for intellectual contact with both the Greek- and Arabic-speaking worlds. Among the Salernitan clergy, Archbishop Alfano (d. 1085) translated a treatise with physiological content from the Greek.[13] Extremely important was the presence nearby of the celebrated Benedictine monastery of Monte Cassino, where Constantinus Africanus was a monk. As noted in chapter 1, Constantinus' *Pantegni* and other translations provided the first access in western Europe to a substantial corpus of medical literature derived from Arabic sources.

In addition to writing various guides to medical practice, twelfth- and early thirteenth-century Salernitan authors brought together a collection (subsequently known as the *articella*) of short treatises conveying the rudiments of Hippocratic and Galenic medicine to serve as a basic curriculum, and they established the practice of teaching by commentary on these texts. The collection as first compiled in the twelfth century (later other texts were added) consisted of two Hippocratic treatises, the *Aphorisms* and the *Prognostics*; a brief Galenic treatise known under various titles (*Ars medica, Ars parva, Tegni,* or *Microtechne*); an Arabic introduction to Galenic medicine known to the Latins as the *Isagoge* of Johannitius; and short tracts on the main diagnostic tools of the medieval physician, namely pulse and urine. The association of medicine with natural philosophy was also emphasized at Salerno; Salernitan masters were among the earliest Latin writers to reflect some knowledge of Aristotle's writings on physical science, and the well-known "Salernitan questions" mingled medical and general scientific topics.[14]

Historians at various times have posited Salernitan, Iberian Muslim, and Jewish influences as sources of the early development of medicine at Montpellier.[15] The career of Gilles de Corbeil (ca. 1140 to ca. 1224) provides one example of personal contact between Salernitan academic medicine and the schools of Montpellier. He was born in northern France, studied in Salerno, spent some time in Montpellier (where he became involved in acrimonious controversy with the Montpellier masters) and at the end of his life taught medicine and served as a royal physician in Paris.[16] In general, however, evidence of knowledge of Salernitan and Arab medicine among Montpellier masters must be ascribed to their study of written works. And although intellectual contacts between Jewish and Christian medical scholars and practitioners at Montpellier undoubtedly took place, there as elsewhere

Jews were excluded from teaching in the faculty of medicine once it took institutional shape.

Montpellier had become known as a center of medical activity by about the middle of the twelfth century. Medical teaching was being carried on there before the century's end. Medical masters and students at Montpellier were already organized into a university in 1220, when they were the recipients of a set of statutes granted by the papal legate. The earliest surviving written exposition of a medical textbook by a Montpellier master appears to be a commentary by Henry of Winchester (fl. 1239–40). A papal bull of 1289 recognized Montpellier as a center of education where a license conveying the *ius ubique docendi* might be obtained in canon and civil law, in arts, and in medicine.[17]

Medicine emerged as a discipline at Paris in approximately the same period as at Montpellier. A list of medical books read at Paris has been ascribed to Alexander Nequam, who studied there from about 1175 until about 1182. The oldest traces of medical teaching date from 1213; statutes listing books to be studied by candidates for a Parisian license in medicine were issued between 1270 and 1274.[18]

In northern Italy, Parma was the home of an early and important medical school before the development of formal university organization for the teaching of medicine. The surgeon Roger Frugard was teaching and practicing at Parma before 1180 (see chapter 6). A handbook on medication has been attributed to Roger's colleague, Guido of Arezzo the younger. In this, the author confidently put forward his own recipes and methods; pointed out his own differences of opinion with "the ancients;" criticized the *medici* of his own day for arrogance, ignorance, and lack of concern for the poor; and scornfully dismissed the "arid" medical teaching of both Salerno and Montpellier. The author of this work, who even if he was not in fact Guido of Arezzo (fl. ca. 1170 or 1180), certainly wrote no later than about 1230, preferred instead the *Canon* of Avicenna.[19] Thus he was among the pioneers in introducing a medical textbook that would be widely used for several hundred years.

But within a generation, Bologna had superseded Parma as northern Italy's main center of medical learning. Roger Frugard's pupil, Rolando or Rolandino (see chapter 6), an influential teacher in his own right, moved to Bologna, where the presence of a number of physicians, surgeons, and medical students is documented during the first two decades of the thirteenth century. In the 1260s and 1270s, notable Latin treatises on surgery were written by surgeons who had previously been trained by apprenticeship at Bologna or had practiced there (see chapter 6). The organization of medical masters and students into academic corporations had probably taken place by the 1260s. The first recorded public *laurea* (degree) in medicine, following examination by a group of masters, was awarded in 1268. Tax and other privileges were extended to medical masters and students by the city government between 1274 and 1288.[20] There developed a fairly constant circulation of medical faculty among Bologna, Padua, and other less-celebrated centers of medical learning that multiplied in northern Italy from about the mid-thirteenth century, so that it is probably unwise to attribute ideas exclusively to any one of these schools.

The strong development of philosophical and Aristotelian aspects (already present to a lesser extent, as we have seen, in the medicine of Salerno) in northern Italian academic medicine was stimulated by a general growth of philosophical studies in Italian schools; however, in the nascent faculties of medicine such interests may also have been fostered by influences from Paris as well as Salerno. Petrus Hispanus, a major writer on logic as well as medical author, studied at Paris and subsequently taught medicine in Siena from 1245 to 1250. The almost equally celebrated Pietro d'Abano returned about 1306 to teach medicine, philosophy, and astrology at Padua after some years at Paris. What is perhaps more important, Pietro incorporated the fruits of his Parisian study and, apparently, teaching of those subjects into his *Conciliator of the Differences of the Philosophers and, Especially, the Physicians*,[21] a work that retained an influence in the Italian schools for centuries.

The organization of the faculty of medicine differed at Paris, Montpellier, and Bologna. At Paris, the faculty of medicine consisted of a group of teaching masters. At Montpellier, the separate university (this time used in the narrower medieval sense of an academic corporation pertaining to a particular discipline or cluster of disciplines) of medicine in the thirteenth century seems to have included both professors and students.[22] The arrangements at Bologna, and similarly at Padua and other southern European centers, consisted of a doctoral college and a student university, each of which conjoined arts and medicine. As already noted, the doctoral college was an association that included both senior professors and medicine and physicians practicing in the town; membership was restricted in number and by 1378 limited to Bolognese citizens. By contrast, the university of arts and medicine was an association of students who were not of Bolognese origin.

Regardless of the differences in their internal organization, the medical professoriates of Paris, Bologna, and Montpellier all represented the summit of the medical profession. Although their social origins and acquired status were as a rule more modest than those of lawyers of equivalent achievement or professors of theology, senior professors of medicine in the great centers of medical education were citizens of substance. Their incomes came primarily from practice (particularly the patronage of wealthy individuals) and to a lesser extent from student fees, but also from public sources, including in some cases ecclesiastical benefices.

In Italy, where medical teaching in the universities was an occupation in which married laymen predominated, a few publicly salaried medical professorships were provided at an early date. At Bologna a professor of medicine was on the public payroll in 1305, and a professor of medical *practica* was receiving a municipal salary in 1324. At Cologne and the other universities of Germany and central Europe, founded in the second half of the fourteenth and in the fifteenth centuries, salaries for medical professors as for those in other areas were provided at the time of or very soon after foundation.[23]

In medicine, as in other faculties, the provision of salaried professional chairs by local municipalities or territorial rulers strengthened both the ties of the professors to outside authorities and the control of those authorities over the academic community. At Bologna the medical professoriate was an integral part of the same citizen class that, at different times, either controlled a communal government or retained much influence at the lower levels of signorial administration. As just noted, the senior teaching positions in medicine were reserved for Bolognese citizens, a privilege jealously guarded by the college of medical doctors. From 1378, non-Bolognese graduates in medicine at Bologna were obliged to swear not to attempt to lecture in the morning hours when the principal or "ordinary" lectures were given. In universities in regions under the rule of territorial princes, ties between an academic faculty of medicine and a princely court often developed; a physician who was in personal attendance on a ruler might also occupy a professorial chair. Princely patronage was, for example, a major factor in the development of the University of Ferrara as a center of medical teaching the late fifteenth and early sixteenth centuries, and the provision of a medical teacher for the University of Aberdeen in the early sixteenth century was possible only when the position was combined with that of royal physician.[24]

The principal medical faculties occupied positions of importance in the public sphere as well as within the academic community. They were used by public authorities—royal, noble, ecclesiastical, or municipal—as guarantors of medical standards, sources of medical information, and a reservoir of reliable practitioners. Thus, at Paris, Montpellier, and elsewhere, the faculty of medicine acquired the right and responsibility to examine and license all medical practitioners in the city. At Bologna, where a surgeon was already maintained on the municipal payroll in 1214, the public provision of medical or surgical treatment for the citizens antedated the appearance of academic medical corporations. But shortly after a formally organized faculty of medicine appeared, professors of medicine were being called upon to provide expert medicolegal opinions for the civic authorities; by the first decade of the fourteenth century, the public services asked of these professors on occasion included the performance of autopsies. The most famous example of a request by a governmental authority for the expert opinion of a medical faculty is doubtless the solicitation of a report on the causes of the Black Death from the Paris faculty by King Philip VI in 1348.[25]

Medical students at each of the major centers of medical education came from all over Europe as well as from the surrounding region. For example, of the university men active in the diocese of Liège before 1350, those known to have studied medicine and whose place of study is known all went to Paris, Bologna, or Montpellier.[26] Moreover, the establishment of universities in the German lands in the fourteenth and fifteenth centuries did not diminish the ability of Bologna and Padua to attract German medical students in significant numbers. If anything, the foundation of German and eastern European universities may have widened the pool from which the Italian medical schools drew. Ambitious medical students could now complete the necessary preliminaries in liberal arts and the first part of their medical studies locally (and inexpensively) and then cross the Alps to a more prestigious institution for the final stages of their medical education and possibly graduation. At Padua, for much of the fifteenth century, scholars from northern Europe earned 30 to 40 percent of all the degrees awarded in all disciplines.[27]

Practitioners trained at the most prestigious universities for medicine found positions all over Europe. Master Pancius of Lucca (d. 1340) will serve as an example. In this homeland, Pancius was modestly successful. Probably educated in medicine at Bologna, as a young man he became personal physician there to his compatriot the bishop, Dominican friar, and surgical writer Teodorico Borgognoni of Lucca. He also took some part in academic medical debate, since one of his opinions was subsequently quoted by Gentile da Foligno (d. 1348), a well-known medical author. In England, however, Pancius was able to translate this respectable but hardly distinguished record into a richly rewarded position as household physician, general factotum, and moneylender to King Edward II and King Edward III,[28] a position he held from 1317 until his death.

In the fifteenth century, faculties of medicine in the new universities of the German lands and central Europe provided teaching opportunities in their homelands for northern European graduates of Paris and especially of the Italian schools. For example, the medical faculty of the University of Erfurt had 37 known members between its foundation in 1392 and 1521, all of whom were of German origin. It is not known where 5 of them received their degrees. Of the remainder, 5 received the doctorate in medicine at Erfurt and 8 received their doctorates at other northern universities; 3 studied at Paris; and 16 received medical degrees from Italian universities, with Padua and Ferrara by far the most popular.[29]

The total number of those who taught and studied medicine at Paris, Bologna, Montpellier, Padua, and in lesser faculties of medicine between the thirteenth and the fifteenth centuries cannot be recovered. As a rule, only indirect or anecdotal evidence is available for the thirteenth and the first part of the fourteenth centuries. For the following period, extensive matriculation records survive for some universities in northern Europe but not for the major centers of medical education. Moreover, although it is clear that the size of various medical faculties was from time to time affected by general demographic trends, by local or regional political or epidemiological crises, or by the drawing power of a famous teacher, the effect of these factors and their interaction on either numbers or quality was seldom simple or obvious. One can, however, arrive at some idea of the relative size of the student body in these medical faculties at different times, as compared with one another and with other faculties in the same center. Thus of 1,681 practitioners in France before 1500 whose university affiliations are known, 1,008 went to Paris, 376 to Montpellier, and 297 elsewhere. In France, the number of university medical students seems to have peaked in the second half of the fourteenth and first half of the fifteenth centuries. Evidently neither the Black Death nor the Hundred Years' War discouraged ambitious students from embarking on academic medical training.[30]

At Bologna, between 1419 and 1434, 65 degrees in medicine and 1 in surgery were awarded; these figures cannot necessarily be extrapolated to other periods of Bologna's medieval and early Renaissance history. By contrast, Turin (founded in 1404) granted only 13 medical degrees between 1426 and 1462, while in the entire period from its foundation in 1477 until 1534, the University of Tübingen granted 35 doctorates in medicine.[31] These figures, of course, imply that even at the famous medical school of Bologna, at any rate in the 1420s and 1430s, the number of medical masters and students present at any one time was not large. Yet it is not easy to estimate the ratio between the number of medical degrees and the size of student medical population in any given time and place. A full medical course lasted four to five years; but it is also necessary to allow for those—and they were many—who either abandoned their studies before graduation or studied at one university and graduated from another. Furthermore, students or teachers in other faculties might have a secondary interest in medicine. Hence, as far as students are concerned, a multiplier of at least 10 for each degree awarded is reasonable.

The largest community of medical students and professors in Europe before 1500, and one probably unprecedented in size, may have been that in mid-fifteenth-century Padua. At Padua, the number of medical degrees awarded rose from four in 1407 to eight in 1434, to nine (two of these being in surgery) in 1450. If the multiplier suggested in a previous paragraph is used, the award of eight or nine degrees in medicine in a given year may imply a medical student body approaching 100. This estimate may be roughly confirmed by the facts that in 1457 the total number of students in all faculties at Padua is known to have been 800 and that in 1450, when 9 medical and surgical degrees were awarded, the total number of degrees was 93.[32]

While the names of many teaching masters are known, it is often difficult to arrive at the size of a group actually teaching medicine in any one place in any given year. For example, at Bologna in the late fourteenth century, the college of doctors of arts and medicine was limited to 15 Bolognese citizens, some but not all of whom were senior professors of medicine in the university. There was also a smaller handful of publicly salaried teaching positions in medical subjects, the holders of which were not necessarily all citizens. To these overlapping but otherwise more-or-less determinate categories must probably be added an indeterminate number who taught briefly or informally and whose activities may have left little record. Fairly full information exists for Padua regarding the number of faculty holding salaried chairs during the fifteenth century. The number fluctuated from time to time, but over the century as a whole it tended to increase. In 1436, Padua had a salaried medical teaching faculty of 16: 7 professors, 2 ordinary (senior) and 5 extraordinary (junior), taught medical theory; 4 professors, 2 ordinary and 2 extraordinary, taught practical medicine; and there were 5 professors of surgery, a number increased from 1 in the previous year. Medical students would probably also have attended some of the lectures of the 3 professors of astrology and 5 professors of natural philosophy.[33]

Light of a different kind is thrown on the relative positions of the major centers of university medical education if one attempts to compare not numbers of degrees or of students but contributions to medical learning. Collectively, the contribution of the faculties of medicine to the written output of late medieval medicine was disproportionately large, since university-educated physicians, and, in particular, professors of medicine, were naturally far more likely than other medical or surgical practitioners to write books. Among the faculties, Paris appears to have trained more practitioners than Montpellier, although this may be an impression created by the accidents of documentary survival. But, as far as is known, Montpellier was the affiliation of a larger number of medical authors than Paris. And medical writers associated with the northern Italian universities, collectively considered, outnumbered authors from Montpellier, especially if one uses as a measure commentaries on the Hippocratic works most widely studied in the universities, namely, the *Aphorisms*, *Prognostics*, and *On Regimen in Acute Diseases*. Moreover, Montpellier authors were most productive of these commentaries in about the half-century turning on the year 1300, whereas the output by Italian medical writers continued into the later fourteenth and the fifteenth centuries.[34]

The Relation of Medicine with Other Academic Disciplines

In the medieval university system, medicine was one of three higher faculties, the others being law (canon and civil) and theology, the study of all of which, at least in principle, followed training in liberal arts. Not all three higher faculties were present in all universities; for example, Bologna and Padua lacked theological faculties until the 1360s, and even thereafter theological teaching was largely in the hands of members of local religious communities. By contrast, Paris was, as is well known, famous for its faculty of theology, but civil law was not taught there. Relations among the higher faculties varied in different places. As already noted, medicine was usually the smallest and weakest of the faculties in universities in the German lands and central Europe. In the northern Italian schools, law was usually the most prestigious and powerful disciplinary community, with medicine an ambitious and competitive second. As a result, at Bologna and Padua the rivalry of the two professional disciplines sometimes manifested itself in unedifying squabbles over such matters as precedence in academic processions. At Paris and Oxford, the presence of faculties of theology made the practice of obtaining a combined medical and theological training relatively common.[35]

By far the most important relation with another faculty was that with the faculty of arts. In institutional terms, this relation was very different in different parts of Europe, both because the respective strengths of arts and medical faculties varied and because of differences in institutional arrangements. The joining of arts and medicine in the academic corporations of Italian universities has already been noted. Although the arts faculties of Bologna and Padua were strong for much the fourteenth and fifteenth centuries, the needs and interests of the medical professoriate and students usually predominated in these organizations. By contrast, the newer northern universities enrolled numerous arts students, relatively few of whom pursued higher degrees or had any connection with the higher faculties.

But the main importance of the relation of arts to medicine was not institutional but intellectual. In the medieval universities, all students began and many ended their academic careers in the arts faculty. The content of the arts curriculum was neither static nor everywhere the same between the thirteenth and the fifteenth centuries. But it can be broadly described as providing prolonged and intensive training in logic, exercised in disputation (formal debate); a grounding varying in thoroughness from time to time and place to place in natural philosophy—that is, chiefly in Aristotle's writings on scientific methodology and physical science; and a rather cursory overview of arithmetic and introductory geometry, astronomy, and music theory. In addition, the arts course both assumed the student's initial command of basic Latin literacy and served continually to reinforce his grasp of philosophical and scientific vocabulary and techniques of argument in that language. Among the principal medical schools, not only Paris but also Bologna and Padua flourished as centers of advanced teaching in arts and philosophy.

The full assimilation of Aristotelian logic and natural philosophy, subjects that came to dominate the arts curriculum, is the central fact of the intellectual history of western Europe in the thirteenth century and in one way or another affected ideas and pedagogy in almost all disciplines. The scholastic method of inquiry associated with the introduction of Aristotelian logic provided a new tool for analyzing texts on many subjects, medicine among them. And for medicine, the reception of Aristotelian natural philosophy was especially important, because in some areas the subject matter of the two disciplines overlapped. Indeed, as has already been noted, in the twelfth century *medici* were among the pioneers in introducing Aristotelian ideas into western Europe.

Venerable truisms, repeated by university medical writers, asserted that all the liberal arts and natural philosophy were necessary for medicine.[36] This belief, as well as institutional history and convenience, underlay the arrangements linking arts and medicine in a single university and a single doctoral college at Bologna, Padua, and elsewhere. At Montpellier, the expectation that a medical student should be competent in arts was made explicit by provisions in the statutes of 1240 and the papal bull of 1309 to the effect that students already proficient in arts could complete their medical studies in a shorter period than those lacking such preparation.[37]

Some parts of the medieval university arts course did indeed constitute a highly practical preparation for the kind of medical education provided in the universities. As Pietro d'Abano put it, certain disciplines were especially necessary adjuncts to medicine: "Logic, since it is the condiment of all the sciences, just as salt is of food; natural philosophy, since it shows the principles of everything; and astrology since it is directive of judgments."[38] Pietro's estimate of the importance of the study of logic and natural philosophy is readily understandable. Command of logic provided the would-be medical student with the major tool of medieval scientific inquiry. University-trained medical authors such as Pietro himself habitually used Aristotelian logic to isolate arguments in medical texts for analysis and criticism. The study of natural philosophy, primarily in works of Aristotle, the chief ancient authority on the subject, provided a grounding in what may be described as general physical science and also equipped students with a knowledge of philosophical and scientific Latin.

Less obvious, perhaps, is the role of elementary astronomical instruction. Officially prescribed university instruction in astronomy usually took place at an extremely modest level; often it amounted to little more than lectures on the elementary and largely qualitative cosmological treatise entitled *On the Sphere* by John of Sacrobosco and on a greatly simplified textbook of Ptolemaic planetary theory. Despite the widespread general interest in matters astrological during the late Middle Ages, no doubt many university students rested content with this elementary survey. Between astrology and medicine, however, strong ties existed. The heavenly bodies were universally believed to influence human as well as all other sublunar bodies: the good physician was supposed always to take astral influences—on the patient at conception and at crises of life and of health or illness, on medications, and on parts of the body—into account. Both medicine and astrology involved prognosis, and both had to account for the discrepancy between apparently certain theory and uncertain results. And, as previously remarked, medical and astrological practice were often combined in a prosperous career, especially in the service of princes. Prospective medical students were thus especially likely to pursue astrological and hence also astronomical studies beyond the elementary level, to study more advanced expositions of the subject privately, or with a tutor, and to acquire familiarity with appropriate tables, ephemerides, astronomical instruments, and other aids to actual astronomical computation for astrological purposes. Indeed, in at least one instance the introductory course on Sacrobosco's cosmological treatise had a good deal of astrological content: the lectures given at Bologna in the early 1320s by the astrologer Cecco d'Ascoli were prefaced by a justification of the value of astrology for medical studies.[39] (Cecco d'Ascoli's subsequent death at the stake, possibly for his astrological determinism, may have caused a temporary diminution of interest in astrology among medical students at the University of Bologna.)

Some measure of astrological competence was indeed one of the marks separating an educated practitioner from an empiric. Nonetheless, the level of training varied widely. Both the writings of *medici* and the general history of astronomy and astrology in western Europe suggest that emphasis on astrology in the education of intending *medici* may have increased as time went on. Medical-astrological culture was particularly strongly developed in fourteenth- and fifteenth-century Italian universities, most notably at Padua. There, in a milieu suffused with astrological belief, a few learned physicians unquestionably gained full mastery of contemporary cosmological theories as well as command of a good deal of technical Ptolemaic planetary theory. These men wrote treatises on astronomical or astrological subjects, adapted sets of tables, and designed astronomical instruments such as the famous planetary clock made by Giovanni Dondi of Padua (d. 1370). Many more university-educated physicians were able to employ astrological techniques without necessarily fully grasping the underlying astronomical theory. They learned to use astronomical tables to draw up general forecasts for the coming year or to cast the horoscopes of princely employers, a level of astrological competence that appears to have been common in the late fourteenth and fifteenth centuries. Practitioners outside the university milieu were of course equally convinced of the validity and medical relevance of astrology, but they would be likely to receive their cosmological and astrological information in simplified form and to acquire little or no expertise in technical astrology or in mathematical astronomy for themselves. It was presumably for such practitioners that medical-astrological charts in the form of volvelles (superimposed disks of parchment that could be rotated to show different combinations of data) or little folding books to hang from the belt were prepared (see figure 3).[40]

There can be no doubt that leading Latin medical writers of the thirteenth to fifteenth centuries were indeed the products of extensive training in logic and natural philosophy, and increasingly as time went on, in astrology as well. A few of them—Pietro d'Abano himself is an especially celebrated example—had a command of these subjects equal to that of any of their colleagues in other faculties, along with a pronounced interest in philosophical questions. Many others whose treatment of philosophical issues was abbreviated or routine nonetheless displayed in their writings extensive familiarity with Aristotle's books on natural science and a competence in handling syllogistic arguments.

When one turns to the teaching careers of medical masters in the major schools, a similar picture emerges. Of 14 doctors involved in drawing up a set of statutes for the medical branch of the Bologna College of Doctors of Arts and Medicine in 1378, 7 are recorded as having degrees in philosophy as well as medicine, and 5 are known to have taught logic and natural philosophy as well as medicine. Indeed, a common career pattern in the Italian schools was to teach arts while studying medicine, that is to say, to finance graduate studies by teaching undergraduates. Furthermore, it is evident that a substantial proportion of the graduates in medicine from Italian universities also obtained degrees in arts. Thus, of the 65 medical graduates at Bologna between 1419 and 1434, 31 already had degrees in arts at the time of their graduation in medicine, and 2 more took arts and medical degrees simultaneously. Among northern professors of medicine, Bartholomeus of Bruges (d. 1356), who taught at Paris and Montpellier, also held degrees in, and wrote on, both arts and medicine.[41]

Individuals did not always or even customarily obtain their arts and medical degrees from the same university; on the contrary, students often moved from one place to another. Furthermore, in those universities that had conjoint corporations of arts and medicine, courses of study in arts and medicine remained separate. Bologna in the early fourteenth century and Padua in the fifteenth century were significant centers of philosophical teaching in their own right, apart from any connection with medicine. But the medical and the arts faculties in these centers evidently supported one another in terms of attracting and providing for students and teachers.

The education in arts acquired by university-trained physicians did not always concentrate exclusively upon subjects and approaches considered most useful adjuncts to medicine. In particular, although Italian Renaissance humanism (most simply defined as a new attention to the style, language, and original meaning of ancient books) began to have an impact upon medicine itself only in the last two decades of the fifteenth century, long before then individual Italian professors of medicine were taking an interest in literary humanism. Two noteworthy examples are the friendship and correspondence between Giovanni Dondi, the professor of medicine at Padua already mentioned as the designer of a complex astronomical clock, and Petrarch; and the career of Michele Savonarola (d. after 1466), who moved with apparent ease not only between the world of literary humanism and an academic environment but also between ordinary medical practice among the mothers and children of Ferrara and one of the most lavish of early Renaissance princely courts. Savonarola probably studied Latin literary subjects as a private pupil of the humanist Giovanni Conversini da Ravenna. He graduated in arts and medicine at the university of Padua; subsequently he became a professor of medicine first at Padua and later at Ferrara, where he combined his teaching with the position of court physician to successive rulers of that city. Savonarola's intellectual range is revealed in his works, which included Latin treatises on medical practice, one of the earliest books on pediatrics in Italian (addressed to women), a humanistic Latin encomium of the city of Padua, and a courtier's praise of his patron and patient, the despot of Ferrara Borso d'Este.[42]

Savonarola's cultivation and attainments reveal a medical culture that was by no means narrowly professional. Membership in the elite group among university-trained physicians who occupied senior professorial chairs at leading centers of learning, wrote extensive Latin medical works, or served at major princely courts implied a broad education with substantial preparation in liberal arts. But doubtless many university-trained practitioners studied arts or philosophy only to the minimum extent necessary for medical professional purposes and retained no interest in those subjects once their education was finished.

The Medical Curriculum and Teaching Methods

By the time the first medical faculties were established in the universities, material could be selected for teaching and study from an abundant Latin medical literature of Greek and Arabic origin. In addition, the reception of the eleventh- and twelfth-century translations stimulated the production of Latin medical writing, much of it the work of university masters or professors. Genres included works directly interpretive of the Greek and Arabic sources (commentaries, compendia, glossaries, and so on) and medical treatises drawing extensively on their content. Unquestionably these endeavors made possible a fuller knowledge of ancient medical and physiological concepts and introduced a larger and more refined technical vocabulary. However, it should be emphasized both that masters and students in the universities before the late fifteenth century could still obtain only a partial idea of ancient medicine, and that only a portion of the Greco-Islamic material that had been translated into Latin was in regular use in the university curriculum.

Thus, by the end of the twelfth century more than forty treatises passing under the name of Hippocrates and a considerably larger body of material attributed to Galen existed in Latin translation. But although these works included treatises attributed to Hippocrates in antiquity and a number of authentic books by Galen, the medieval Latin Hippocrates and Galen were incomplete, especially as regards Galen's major anatomical treatises. His lengthy physiological and anatomical treatise *On the Usefulness of the Parts of the Body*[43] was translated into Latin in the early fourteenth century, but it was too long and too difficult for use as a university textbook in its entirety, and a short compendium based on the work was already in existence. Possibly as a result, *On the Usefulness of the Parts* was known to few physicians before the sixteenth century. Galen's practical and detailed dissection manual, *On Anatomical Procedures*, was not translated into Latin until the sixteenth century. The teaching of the ancient authors was also contaminated by spuria, such as an allegedly Hippocratic work on medical astrology. Only in the late fifteenth century did the endeavors of humanists open a new phase of study and translation of Greek texts that significantly extended knowledge of ancient medicine.

Judging by the small number of manuscripts in which some works survive, one must conclude that only a few of the most learned professors could have been familiar at first hand with more than a portion of the Latin medical literature in existence. Furthermore, students grasped ancient medical ideas only partially through direct consultation of the longer treatises of ancient authors; a large role was also played by highly abbreviated or aphoristic treatises, by compendia, and by the mediation of the Arabic medical encyclopedias. Lists of books officially assigned for medical lectures at Montpellier in 1309 and 1340 and at Bologna in 1405 (the Bologna statutes probably formalize arrangements made in the late thirteenth century) show a curriculum of courses on works in the *articella* collection, which continued to supply the pedagogical need for brief statements of fundamental concepts; on up to a dozen or more longer works of Galen; and on selections from Arabic writers, notably Avicenna.[44] The cycle of lectures does not appear to have been arranged in order of ascending difficulty, but certain books nonetheless functioned as basic texts. These were the brief Galenic compendium known as the *Tegni*, *Microtechne*, or *Ars parva*; the Hippocratic *Aphorisms*; and sections of Avicenna's encyclopedic *Canon*. The parts of the *Canon* regularly used as textbooks for university lectures contained a synopsis of physiology (Book 1, Part 1), a treatise on fevers (Book 4, Part 1), principles of disease and treatment (Book 1, Part 4) and diseases from head to toe (Book 3). The writings of Rhazes on diseases also frequently served as the basis of lectures. The exposition of the Ars, the Aphorisms, and the Canon was hence a major task of late medieval medical masters, as a large body of surviving commentaries on these works bears witness.

Statutory lists of books and lectures tell only part of the story of academic medical education. Professors' commentaries on assigned texts (based on their lectures) show that there was considerable room for variation and personal opinion in the way the standard works were interpreted. The prescribed public lectures (figure 10) and other exercises were supplemented by "extraordinary" lectures on works chosen by the master and by private teaching and study. Moreover, antedating and surviving the formation of relatively impersonal and sometimes mutually adversarial academic corporations of medical teachers and students was another kind of relationship, that between an individual practitioner and a younger socius, who was his master's pupil, assistant, apprentice, and potential successor. At Bologna, before medical teaching was provided in the university, the surgeon Ugo of Lucca (fl. 1214) passed on his skill to a select, closed circle of younger relatives or apprentices. At Montpellier, the oldest regulations referring to a medical university (1220) required each student to choose a master and penalized attempts to lure a scholar away from his master.[45] Academic medicine probably always retained elements of craft training and personal apprenticeship.

The length of the medical course varied. At Montpellier, statutes of 1240 provided that the status of bachelor of medicine could be attained by a student not already proficient in arts after three and a half years of study and six months of practice outside Montpellier; the papal bull of 1309 fixed the entire course of study at six years for students not previously proficient in arts (five years for those who were), and extended the practicum to eight months, or two summers. At Bologna, the statutes of the University of Arts and Medicine issued in 1405 provided for three years each of philosophy and astronomy-astrology and four years each of medicine and (medical) practica, that is, lectures on books about particulars of disease and treatment (figures 11 and 12).[46] All these subjects are treated under a single rubric of the statutes, all presumably being regarded as pertaining to medical students. No doubt at least some of the courses in different subjects could be taken concurrently. In medicine as in other disciplines, the requirements for graduation were hearing lectures on prescribed books, participation in disputation, and success in oral examination.

The curriculum was geared toward training practitioners, for practice was the acknowledged goal of university medical education. All university teachers of medicine trained students who would practice, and most professors were also practitioners themselves, often successful and highly rewarded ones. It is doubtless true that the practice of some leading professors of medicine was largely consultative and that those university-trained physicians who could afford to do so tended to delegate some forms of physical intervention to assistants. As one might expect, attitudes to practice among individual university professors varied: Tommaso del Garbo, according to his biographer, regarded the demands of practice as a burden that distracted him from study. It is recorded of Gentile da Foligno, an exceptionally prolific medical author who commented on almost the whole of Avicenna's *Canon* (which is about one million words long), that he died in 1348 during the great plague epidemic "from too constant attendance on the sick."[47] But for lay physicians, including university professors, practice of some kind was an economic necessity, since it was their most lucrative source of legitimate income (there are some indications that professors of medicine and law in thirteenth-century Bologna occasionally added to their income by lending money at interest to students, a practice illicit by thirteenth-century standards and reprehensible by twentieth-century ones[48]). The frank admission of Taddeo Alderotti, one of the most celebrated medical professors of Bologna, that he had temporarily suspended writing commentaries in favor of lucrative practice merely made explicit the main source of the substantial wealth revealed by his will. Moreover, medical writings produced in the ambience of the universities devoted much attention to topics related to medical practice: regimen, symptoms, disease, and remedies.

Furthermore, university education in practical medicine involved not merely the study of texts and attendance at lectures about diseases, remedies, and so on but also such requirements and opportunities as a period spent in actual practice before graduation (as already noted, such practice was obligatory at Montpellier from 1240), the study of collections of *consilia* describing individual cases, and attendance upon a senior professor and practitioner when he visited patients (figure 12). As is well known, medieval university medical students also attended anatomical demonstrations on the human cadaver. Public dissections were instituted at Bologna by 1316 and made statutory at Montpellier in 1340 (see chapter 4).

Nevertheless, university medical education relied primarily on the study and exposition of authoritative texts. Hence, lectures on the texts and disputations, or formal academic debates, about problems of textual interpretation or the reconciliation of conflicting opinions were as central to instruction in medicine as they were in other academic disciplines. Both courses in theory (that is, philosophy of medicine and principles of physiology and pathology) and courses in *practica* (that is, the study of specifics of diagnosis and treatment) into which university curricula in medicine came

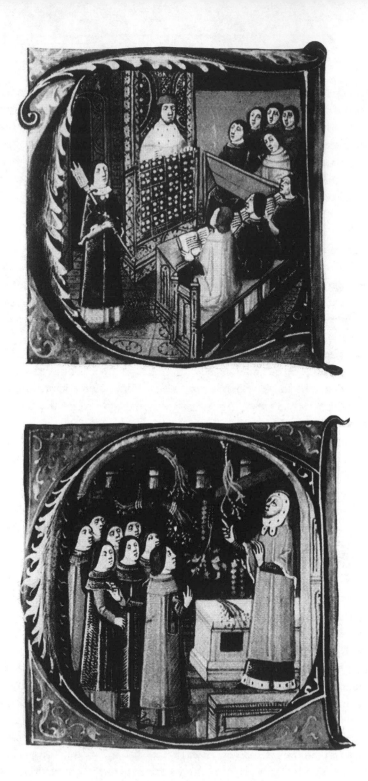

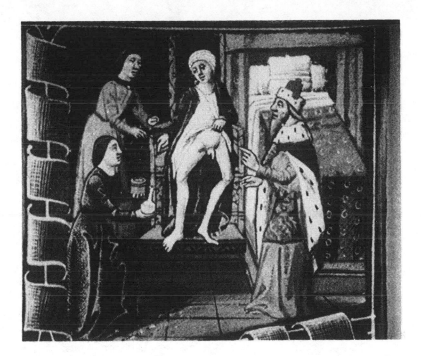

Figure 12   Practical teaching at the patient's bedside. A richly dressed physician (intended to represent Hippocrates) gives instruction to students or assistants in the recognition and treatment of a swelling probably intended to represent a plague bubo. The scene is suggestive of the supervised practice often listed among the requirements for graduation in medicine from medieval universities. The picture illustrates the Hippocratic *Epidemics* and is thus a reminder both of the way in which "new" diseases such as plague were interpreted in the light of Hippocratic-Galenic understanding and of the practical usefulness attributed to the study of ancient medical texts. (Sächsische Landesbibliothek, Dresden, MS Db 93, ca. 1460, fol. 458^r; courtesy Sächsische Landesbibliothek and Vivian Nutton.)

Figure 10 (Opposite, top)   A university lecture on medicine. (Sächsische Landesbibliothek, Dresden, MS Db 93, ca. 1460, fol. 503^v; courtesy Sächsische Landesbibliothek and Vivian Nutton.)

Figure 11 (Opposite, bottom)   A medical lecture on *practica*, in this case on herbs and their uses, with a demonstration of dried specimens. The miniatures in this volume of Galen's collected works illustrate the subject matter of each of the various treatises included; the lecturer is Galen himself, depicted as the source of medical teaching. Hence the scenes of medical education include both realistic and symbolic or imaginative elements. Figures 9 and 10 appear to be realistic representations of fifteenth-century medical study and lecturing. Other illustrations obviously cannot be taken literally. For example, in one accompanying a treatise on the elements, the lecturer is placed outdoors in a garden setting and is surrounded by earth, air, and water, and various animals; and in another, he points out to students a standing naked pregnant woman (fols. 443^r and 295^v, both reproduced in E. C. van Leersum and W. Martin, *Miniaturen der lateinischen Galenos-Handschrift der Kgl. Oeffentl. Bibliothek in Dresden Db 92–93* [Leiden, 1910]). The scene shown here may well be realistic but is not necessarily so. (Sächsische Landesbibliothek, Dresden, MS Db 93, ca. 1460, fol. 397^r; courtesy Sächsische Landesbibliothek and Vivian Nutton.)

to be divided were taught in this way, a method often termed "scholastic." In university lectures, medical books on essentially practical topics were treated to full scholastic analysis. Questions on which opinions differed were isolated, the views of authorities were listed and distinguished, objections to each were raised and solved in turn, and so on. An example may be seen in Dino del Garbo's exposition, written between 1311 and 1319 while he was lecturing at Bologna and elsewhere, of a portion of Avicenna's *Canon* dealing with methods of therapy.[49]

Intellectual criteria established in the thirteenth century, with the reception in western European schools of Aristotle's theory of knowledge, ensured that such exposition supported the claim of medicine to be one of the higher branches of learning. Scholastic method was believed to fulfill Aristotle's requirements for the achievement of certain knowledge (*scientia*); according to the first book of the *Posterior Analytics*, this type of knowledge could only be attained in disciplines that began from accepted first principles and proceeded by way of rational argument to demonstrate universally valid conclusions. Academically educated physicians wanted at least some aspects of medicine to qualify as *scientia*, although they readily admitted that much of it was more like the kind of knowledge termed "*ars*"—a word used in different contexts for both crafts and liberal arts but always with implications of skill and ordered knowledge rather than of reasoning toward universal truths. Given that medicine was a discipline involving both the study of received texts and knowledge of the natural world, the introduction of scholastic method had both advantages and disadvantages. It fostered critical comparison of statements in supposedly authoritative texts (even though the goal was usually reconciliation) and developed habits of rational analysis. But it also encouraged excessive expenditure of ingenuity in elaborating intricate arguments about textual interpretation; and it focused attention on issues to which observation was largely irrelevant.

The characteristics just indicated probably did not vary much from one of the principal centers of medical education to another. For example, a recent examination of the use of and attitudes toward sections of the *Canon* of Avicenna as medical textbooks at Paris and Montpellier in the thirteenth and early fourteenth centuries has shown that there appears to be little basis for the idea that the teaching of Montpellier was more "practical" or more "Hippocratic" than that of Paris. Moreover, some important developments in medical teaching were not confined to any one school but affected the major centers at about the same time. Thus, in the decades before and after

1300, an expansion of interest in the direct study of works of Galen occurred at both Bologna and Montpellier.[50]

By the early fourteenth century, the medical faculties of Paris, Bologna, and Montpellier were at the height of the first stage of their development. Very shortly thereafter, the flourishing medical faculties were confronted by the medical calamity of the great plague epidemic. At Bologna, for example, plague in conjunction with regional political and economic problems made the mid-fourteenth century a period of serious, if temporary, difficulty for the university. But the system of medical education provided in the academic medical faculties was so securely established that it recovered with the general recovery from crisis. Some of the most celebrated Italian and French scholastic medical commentators—Giacomo da Forlì (d. 1414), Ugo Benzi (d. 1439), and Jacques Despars (d. 1458)[51]—belong to the late fourteenth and the early fifteenth centuries. The vitality of fifteenth-century university medicine is evident from a number of important new developments. Padua rose to the position of prominence it would retain throughout the sixteenth century; fifteenth-century Padua was noted for some celebrated professors of practical medicine and for a distinguished tradition of philosophical teaching, regarded as highly relevant to medicine. Connections established between the young medical faculties in German-speaking regions and the flourishing medical schools at Padua and Ferrara in the fifteenth century were subsequently to prove an important channel for the transmission of innovative ideas in medicine from Italy to Germany. And by the turn of the fifteenth and sixteenth centuries, at Ferrara, Paris, Montpellier, and elsewhere, humanistically educated medical professors who aspired to a fuller and more accurate knowledge of Greek medicine than was provided by the medieval textbooks were beginning to stir up lively debate over the curriculum. University education in medicine was a durable but by no means a static institution, one that would continue to show new life in the sixteenth century.

FOUR
PHYSIOLOGICAL AND ANATOMICAL KNOWLEDGE

he subject matter of medicine included the study of the organization and functioning of the human body. As the famous opening definition of the *Canon* of Avicenna ran, "Medicine is the science by which the dispositions of the human body are known so that whatever is necessary is removed or healed by it, in order that health should be preserved or, if absent, recovered."[1] These words of Avicenna attach a value to formal and systematic knowledge about the body that is also implicit in the considerable output of western medieval writing on physiological theory, the smaller amount on anatomical description, and the occasional practice of some dissection for instructional purposes.

Moreover, writers on medicine fostered the idea that the study of the human body was a dignified and worthwhile scientific undertaking. The most famous medieval treatise on dissection, the *Anatomy* of Mondino de' Liuzzi (d. 1326), is introduced by a paean of praise to the superiority of man (that is, humankind) to all other animals. Man, according to Mondino, is distinguished by his upright stature, his intellect, his power of judgment, and his tool-making abilities. The implication of the passage is that the body of so noble a creature is a subject specially meriting study. Other authors emphasized the superiority of the kind of intellectual activity that learning about the human body involved. For example, in comparing medicine and law, a favorite rhetorical theme in fourteenth- and fifteenth-century Italy, Bartolomeo Fazio, or Facio (d. 1457) defended the nobility of medicine on the grounds that it involved knowledge of the causes of things in nature. He demanded rhetorically: "What could be more ingenious than to grasp through reason the composition, structure, order, and the very causes of the diseases, of our bodies?[2]

The topic of this chapter is, accordingly, the understanding of the human body acquired by those trained in medicine or surgery. What is described is the level of knowledge of those who obtained advanced instruction and direct exposure to major texts in Latin; less highly educated practitioners shared the same basic concepts, but in much simpler form and without either the seductive distractions of scholastic elaboration or the advantages of scholastic rationality.

Physiology and anatomy were neither independent disciplines in their own right nor wholly subordinated to medicine. In particular, physiological knowledge was as much a part of natural philosophy as of medicine, the study of the subject being equally valid under either discipline. Furthermore, theologians who included discussions of physical human nature in their works did not merely draw on physiological information but made their own contributions to physiological debate, as we learn, among other possible examples, from the treatise on embryology by Aegidius Romanus (d. 1316). In many respects, treatments of physiological subject matter in medical, in natural philosophical, and in theological works written during the thirteenth to fifteenth centuries are apt to resemble one another closely. The same standard question topics; the same scholastic apparatus of arguments, objections, and solutions; and many of the same citations of authorities often crop up in all three.[3]

Yet, despite these shared attributes, medical explanations of physiology were also characterized by emphases, goals, and approaches peculiar to the discipline of medicine. Moreover, although passages of anatomical description occur in philosophical works—a notable example being the treatment of human anatomy by Albertus Magnus (d. 1280) in his works on animals—anatomy was chiefly of interest to *medici* and surgeons. Furthermore, the *medici* themselves considered their understanding of the human body to be of a kind distinct from that obtained through natural philosophy; although their claims mixed rhetoric with reality, they contained a measure of truth.

First and foremost, medical authors repeatedly asserted that the salient characteristic of medical understanding of the body was an ultimately practical aim. Physiological theory provided a general conceptual underpinning for explanations of illness and prescriptions for treatment. Both were, for example, frequently couched in terms derived from the theory of *complexio*, or temperament, that is, of the role played by the balance of the elementary qualities of hot, wet, cold, and dry in the body. A much more specific kind of usefulness of knowledge of the body for therapy was suggested by Galen's *On the Affected Parts* (also known as *On the Internal Parts*), a treatise on pathology introduced for study at Montpellier and Bologna in the late thirteenth century. Readers of this work encountered the idea that study of anatomy would enable the physician to locate and identify diseases in the hidden internal organs of living patients. In the words of an abbreviated version of the book by Arnald of Villanova (d. 1311), who was a leading medical figure at Montpellier during the 1290s, the wise *medicus* "ought to be informed about the nature of every one of the internal organs by anatomy, whether it is cartilaginous or fleshy, etc. . . . to know the afflictions of the hidden parts it is necessary to have knowledge of their action and purpose and anatomy."[4] The ideal of practical diagnostic application of detailed anatomical knowledge held up in this passage is echoed in the opening chapter of one of the principal works on surgery written in the fourteenth century, Guy de Chauliac's *Inventarium*, commonly known as the *Great Surgery* (1363); but it was not an ideal that could often have been realized.

In reality, the goal of physiological or anatomical study was, in many instances, a better understanding of texts. In the context of the intellectual life of the thirteenth to the fifteenth centuries, that goal was, of course, entirely valid. The milieu of university faculties of medicine in which medical study of physiology was for the most part pursued also contributed certain characteristics. Physiological knowledge constituted only one part of medical theory, which was in turn only one branch of the university medical curriculum. Expositions of physiology thus constitute only a small proportion of the total output of late medieval medical writing, by far the largest part of which is concerned with disease and treatment. Extended accounts of physiological topics by medical writers are mostly to be found in learned Latin commentaries on general introductory works (notably, the first part of the first book of the *Canon* of Avicenna) and hence fall within the most scholastic and bookish genre of medical discourse. Most of these expositions therefore show few if any signs either of therapeutic concern or of readiness to modify theory on the basis of evidence drawn from clinical experience. Academic medical writers tended to stress the links between physiological theory and natural philosophy. Contemporary intellectual and associated social values fostered their propensity to treat physiological topics in a scholastic, philosophically oriented fashion; the ability to do so was a skill that both made individual reputations and also helped to secure for medicine a position of respect. Some of the most renowned fourteenth- and fifteenth-century *medici* earned at least part of their reputations by their ability to contribute from a physiological standpoint to discussions of contemporary philosophical interest.

By about the mid-thirteenth century, a second salient feature of the medical treatment of physiological topics was recognized. It became a medical commonplace that a series of differences over specific physiological issues separated "the philosophers and the physicians," differences that were to provide the theme and the title for one of the most celebrated of Latin medical books, Pietro d'Abano's *Conciliator of Differences*. The differences were real enough, being those between the physiological doctrines of Aristotle, the master of the philosophers, and those of Galen and his followers. Both Avicenna and Averroes had discussed these differences and thus helped to focus the attention of Latin authors upon them.[5] Medical writers identified themselves as the heirs and exponents of a primarily Galenic physiological tradition. Adherence to a learned tradition expressed in a body of authoritative medical writings constituted a guarantee of the separate identity of rational inquiry about the human body by *medici* as an authentic intellectual enterprise, distinct from natural philosophy. Moreover, in general Galenic medicine provided a more richly detailed account of the human body than Aristotelian natural philosophy, and one that in many particulars was likely to be confirmed by the experience of practitioners. On the other hand, the philosophical authority of Aristotle was as powerful for *medici* as for scholars in any other discipline. The situation was further complicated by the fact that Galen himself had had eclectic philosophical interests, drawing upon both Plato and Aristotle, and that philosophical concepts underlay many of his physiological formulations. Hence, the elucidation, discussion, and, where possible, reconciliation of differences between the Aristotelian and the Galenic points of view on various physiological topics soon became and long remained a central preoccupation (figure 13).

But, like medicine's ultimately practical goal, the differences between the philosophers and the physicians did not lead to any radical or unambiguous separation of the medical from the philosophical approach to physiology. Differences between Aristotle and Galen over such subjects as the role of the female parent in conception could not be resolved by the only available form of observation, namely, gross anatomy. And even in instances where sense evidence appeared to support the Galenic position, the Aristotelian view was not thereby disproved, since it did not necessarily depend on such evidence. Injuries to the brain and spinal cord resulting in paralysis were much discussed in surgical writings (see chapter 6) and certainly provided experiential confirmation of the connection Galen proposed between the nerves of motion and sense and the brain and spinal cord, whereas no such claim could be made on behalf of Aristotle's ascription of dominion over motion and sensation to the heart. But the usual solution was to introduce a conceptual hierarchy in which the heart ruled the brain in some ultimate or philosophical sense and the brain ruled the nervous system directly. Learned medical men, like philosophers, hence had little incentive to abandon discussion and speculation in favor of any other form of investigation. Although medical writers were more likely to take a Galenic than an Aristotelian position on particular physiological issues, learned opinion was certainly not divided into monolithic philosophical and medical blocs with adherence to one position or another determined solely by disciplinary allegiance. Moreover, despite their endless discussions of specific differences between the two physiological traditions, academically educated physicians continued, to a greater or lesser extent, to share with philosophers a familiarity with both philosophical and medical source texts, a bent toward conciliation or harmonization of conflicting authorities, and a generally Aristotelian epistemology and method of inquiry.

The practice of dissection, undertaken as a form of medical and surgical instruction (see below), seems a much more clearly distinctive characteristic of the medical approach to knowledge of the human body than either a supposed commitment to an ultimately practical goal or the differences between Aristotelian and Galenic physiological doctrines. Yet the academic environment in which the dissection of the human cadaver was regularized integrated the occasional presentation of the body itself as the object of study with frequent and habitual attention to learned texts on the subject. Nonetheless, the origins of human dissection are obviously also connected with the growth of surgical activities and skills and have been linked with the development of autopsy for legal purposes, with its demand for specific information about appearances in individual cadavers.

Figure 13 (Opposite)   The sense organs and localization in the brain of the so-called internal senses, or powers of the mind, as depicted in a late fifteenth-century Latin manuscript (written in Germany) of works of Aristotle and others on logic and natural philosophy. The five small circles within the brain represent ventricles that are supposedly the sites, reading from left to right, of common sense (a power bringing together the input of the senses), imagination, fantasy, cogitative power (not the same thing as reason), and memory. The division of mental activity into distinct processes which were allocated among specific sites within the brain was a medieval concept that derived from Galenic ideas about brain function. A fourfold scheme was frequently used; the fivefold division seen here seems to have been introduced by Avicenna in his commentary on Aristotle's *On the Soul*. By using this image the writer of the manuscript was bringing ideas ultimately originating in a medical tradition to bear on Aristotle's teaching. Thus, the drawing depicts the power of sensation as linked to the brain, as Galenists held; but the label to the first ventricle refers to Aristotle's location of the powers of sensation in the heart. In this way, the picture and legend are located in the context of the discussions of the differences "between the philosophers and the physicians." (Courtesy the Wellcome Institute Library, London, MS 55, fol. 93ʳ.)

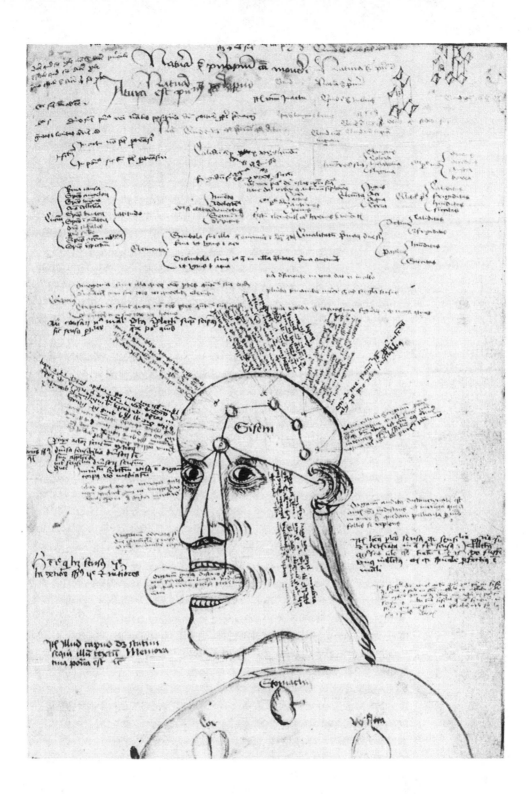

Sources and Methodology

The principal sources of information were, of course, books. The most influential books all transmitted a physiological and anatomical teaching that was in its main outlines Galenic. As already noted, the more learned physicians also drew on Aristotle's works on natural philosophy and made some use of his biological works. Knowledge of Galen's physiological theories was, however, fuller than acquaintance with his achievements in anatomy. By around 1300, some of Galen's fundamental expositions of physiology were being intensively studied in Latin translation at Montpellier, Paris, Bologna, and probably elsewhere. For example, *On Complexions* provided an account of the theory of temperament, and *On the Natural Faculties* explained nutrition, growth, and reproduction. For Galen's physiological anatomy, recourse could be had to the compendium that presented an abbreviated (and distorted and simplified) version of *On the Usefulness of the Parts of the Body*.[6] The physiology and anatomy transmitted in Galen's own works were supplemented by the versions of his teachings found in the various encyclopedias, summaries, commentaries, and pseudo-Galenic treatises of medieval origin. In particular, the organization and presentation of physiological and anatomical topics in basic textbooks—notably the *Isagoge* of Johannitius and sections of the *Canon* of Avicenna—strongly influenced the medical approach to the study of function and structure.[7]

In the *Canon*, for example, Avicenna provided his readers with a summary account of physiology and some aspects of anatomy in the first section of the work. This account occurs in close proximity to philosophical generalizations about the nature of medical knowledge and the assertion that medicine is divided into theory and practice. Furthermore, the physiological subject matter opens with a brief account of the four elements (earth, water, air, and fire), components of the human body as of all other material substances. The treatments of element theory found in Avicenna's and various other medical works often served medieval and Renaissance Latin commentators as an invitation to expatiate upon topics remote from medicine in general and physiology in particular; their discussions ranged from tangential philosophical problems, such as that of the fate of the elements in mixed bodies, to the completely unrelated subjects of tides and comets. The other topics included in this first part of the *Canon* all deal exclusively with physiological function, except for an anatomical section on bones, muscles, nerves, veins, and arteries (termed "simple" members). But for the anatomy of other organs classified as "composite" parts (for example, ear, eye, liver, spleen), the reader must turn to Book 3, which deals, in a head-to-toe arrangement, with diseases peculiar to different parts of the body and with their treatment; each section opens with a brief chapter on the anatomy of the organ under discussion.[8]

Avicenna's arrangement thus joins physiological with philosophical generalities and yields no unified treatment of anatomy, either as a subject in its own right or in relation to physiological function. Moreover, although the first part of Book 1 and Book 3 were both used as university textbooks, they belonged to different parts of the medical curriculum. And Latin commentators on the *Canon* reduced the significance of the anatomical content by their usual practice of omitting from consideration the chapters on bones, muscles, nerves, veins, and arteries in Book 1. Furthermore, although most of the *Canon* deals with practical topics relating to disease and treatment, the physiological summary in Book 1 is handled in a deliberately abstract and generalizing way. For instance, the teaching of Avicenna's chapters on complexion, or temperament, is very similar in its essentials to that in Galen's *On Complexions*. But Galen wrote in the context of his own clinical experience, in which, for example, his encounters with many patients taught him that no general or universal difference between the temperamental heat of children and that of adolescents can be discerned by touch; and Galen was concerned to refute specific views held by other physicians. By contrast, the summary in the *Canon* appears primarily intended to formulate the underlying theory into a set of clearly organized basic principles, or rules.[9]

An arrangement that gave much greater prominence and unity to anatomy than did the *Canon* was, however, to be found in a number of other well-known and influential general works. Thus, the *Pantegni* adopted the division of bodily parts into simple and composite but treated them in two consecutive sections near the beginning of the work. The treatise on pathology, diagnosis, and therapy by Rhazes, known as the ninth book of the *Almansor*, begins with a section of systematic anatomical description; so (after a preface) does the *Colliget*, Averroes' survey of medicine. Among works originating in the West, similar introductory sections on anatomy are to be found in some general books on surgery, notably those by the two leading fourteenth-century surgical authors, Henri de Mondeville (d. ca. 1320) and Guy de Chauliac. The content of these sections was, of course, drawn from earlier texts. Henri de Mondeville explicitly stated that anatomical chapters at the beginning of his *Surgery* (originally a separate set of anatomy lectures he had given at Montpellier) were based on the anatomical material in the *Canon* of Avicenna but were recast and abbreviated in the more convenient form of a coherent introductory summary.[10] Awareness of the value of a preliminary grasp of anatomy in studying medical subjects may have come most naturally to surgeons but was not confined to them. Gentile da Foligno complained of the practice of omitting the anatomical sections from lectures on the first section of the *Canon* of Avicenna, and averred that knowledge of anatomy was as essential a first step in medicine as a knowledge of the alphabet was in reading.[11]

Among the sources and methodology for knowledge of the body must be counted the study of the body itself as a physical object. In the examples just given, "anatomy" refers to written descriptions, most of them embedded in general texts. But in twelfth-century Salerno the actual practice of dissection was initiated for the first time since antiquity, along with the production of accompanying brief anatomical manuals.[12] The animal used for dissection was the pig (chosen for the allegedly close resemblance of its interior organs to those of human beings, especially in the female).[13] A well-known decree of Frederick II, dated about 1241, which ordered the study of "the anatomy of human bodies" by candidates for a license to practice surgery in the Kingdom of Naples, probably assumed that this requirement would be fulfilled through the study of texts and dissection of animals. Interest in anatomy as a distinct branch of study had spread to northern Europe by about 1225, when a manual of anatomy was probably compiled in Paris. Naturally, the anatomical manuals, whether or not they were intended to accompany dissection, drew information and theories from existing textbooks.[14]

Dissection of human bodies appears to have begun by the end of the thirteenth century. At Bologna and elsewhere, dissection of humans seems first to have occurred in the course of autopsies for legal purposes. This activity was soon followed by the introduction of dissection of the human cadaver as part of medical and surgical education. The term "anatomy" acquired the sense of the exercise consisting of the dissection of an individual human body according to prescribed rules. The *Anatomy* of Mondino de' Liuzzi, written in 1316, was designed by its author, a professor of practical medicine at Bologna, as a handbook to accompany such a dissection (figure 14). Since Mondino referred openly in his text to the use of the cadavers of executed criminals, it is to be presumed that the local public authorities provided them, as was certainly the case later. Some unofficial dissection also went on; in 1319 a group of medical students at Bologna who took steps to secure their own cadaver were prosecuted for sacrilegious grave robbery.[15] Dissection was probably introduced at Montpellier at around the same period; the provision for it in the Montpellier University statutes issued in 1340 has already been mentioned. In Venice, a decree of the Great Council dated

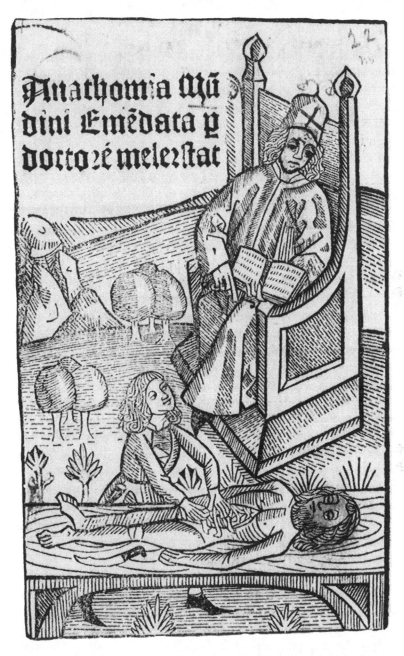

Figure 14   Dissection scene from the title page of an early printed edition (ca. 1493) of Mondino de' Liuzzi's *Anatomy*. The outdoor setting is not necessarily unrealistic; dissections were sometimes performed outdoors in the fourteenth and fifteenth centuries. However, the purpose of the illustration is not to show a realistic dissection but to provide a standard (imaginary) author portrait of Mondino (d. 1326) and to encapsulate the subject matter of his book; hence, the picture cannot be read as evidence for the view that lecturers on anatomy invariably deputed actual dissection to assistants. (Courtesy the New York Academy of Medicine Library.)

1368 obliged the College of Surgeons to conduct at least one annual dissection; in 1370 the city's *medici* were ordered to contribute to the costs on the
grounds that attendance at a dissection was important for them as well as
for the surgeons. Annual anatomies (that is, dissections) became part of the
formal academic curriculum at both Bologna and Padua. The practice is referred to as already established in a set of university statutes from Bologna
dated 1405; a year earlier, the first public anatomy in Vienna was conducted
by a professor from Padua. Statutes of the arts and medicine branch of the
University of Padua, dating from 1465, refer to the annual anatomy as a well-
established practice. The earliest anatomies for university students took
place privately in the houses of professors or students; by the late fifteenth
century, a temporary theater was being constructed for each annual anatomy at Padua.[16]

The reintroduction of human dissection on a regular basis, presumably
for the first time since early in the Hellenistic period, is a deservedly famous
episode in the histories of both anatomy and medical education. It is also
evidence of a striking commitment on the part of some *medici* to first-hand
sense experience, as well as theoretical understanding, of the human body's
inward parts. It seems likely that the institution of human dissection in the
medical schools was inspired by the intensification of direct study of the
works of Galen that took place at both Bologna and Montpellier in the late
thirteenth century. Even though the full range of Galen's anatomical activity
and teaching was not known, the Galenic works that were studied contained numerous allusions to knowledge gained through dissection and ex-
hortations to practice it. And Guy de Chauliac was presumably not alone in
believing that Galen had dissected human beings as well as animals.[17] Con-
ceivably, studies of late medieval attitudes to the human body from an an-
thropological perspective, which have recently begun to interest some historians, may throw some additional light on broader cultural reasons for the
emergence of interest in human dissection.

But although the innovation was of the first importance for the future
development of anatomical science, its immediate impact on knowledge
was necessarily limited. The reasons were not those given in many popular
accounts: the Church did not issue blanket prohibitions against dissection in
medical schools as such, nor did medieval lecturers on anatomy invariably
delegate the actual work of dissection to assistants. Nevertheless, other social, technical, and intellectual constraints did affect the practice of dissection.

Thus, late thirteenth- and early fourteenth-century ecclesiastical prohibitions against boiling or dismembering bodies, primarily intended to re-

strain excesses in burial practices and the cult of relics, may have discouraged some anatomical activity, especially in France.[18] In an age with no means of preserving cadavers, dissections could take place only in the winter ("before the end of February" at Padua), and there was a strong incentive to complete them rapidly. The practice of human dissection was established at only a few centers of medical training in the fourteenth or fifteenth century, and at those centers it was infrequent; the Paduan university statute just referred to provided for the dissection of one male and one female cadaver per year. Even in these favored localities, and allowing for supplementary private dissections, the opportunities for medical practitioners, professors, or students to attend, much less participate in, dissections of the human cadaver cannot have been numerous before the late fifteenth century. And the time any individual was able to spend performing or attending dissections could seldom have been sufficient for the assimilation of much detail. As for medical and indeed surgical practitioners outside a few major centers, it seems likely that the great majority of them were never instructed by means of dissection, either as observers or as participants. Of course working surgeons, however trained, must have learned at least some anatomy from direct encounters with the human body in the course of their practice.

But probably the most important reason why dissection remained infrequent before the end of the fifteenth century was that, as far as general understanding of physiological anatomy was concerned, the dissected cadaver seemed to add relatively little to the information available from other sources. Appearances in dissection were unlikely either to throw general doubt on or to greatly clarify preexisting physiological theories and anatomical descriptions; the study of gross anatomy offered no immediately useful contribution to the debates over various problems of interest to learned physicians, as for example, the difference of opinion between Aristotle and Galen as to whether and in what sense the heart could be described as the ruling organ of the body.

The objective of the dissections conducted as part of medical or surgical training in the fourteenth and fifteenth centuries was not investigation but instruction. In this context, dissection seldom functioned as a means of controlling or correcting the written word and certainly not as an independent research tool. Indeed, to the limitations mentioned above may perhaps be added a certain philosophical unwillingness to criticize supposedly general or universal principles on the basis of particulars seen in individual cases. Rather, the practice of dissection served primarily as a visual aid to the understanding of physiological and anatomical doctrines found in texts.

The real usefulness of dissection as an exercise in medieval medical education was perhaps not altogether dissimilar from that of other forms of illustration. "Trees" and "wheels" designed to represent the theory of temperament, stylized pictures of plants, drawings diagramming bodily systems, and endeavors to illustrate anatomy lessons with pictures had in common the aim of helping the reader to grasp organizing schemes rather than that of naturalistic depiction.[19] Most medieval anatomical illustrations were lacking in detail and were not intended to be representative or naturalistic. Illustrative material about anatomy in medical works was primarily schematic and mnemonic. For example, the pictures formerly known as the "five-figure series," showing the arteries, veins, muscles, nerves, and bones, versions of which are found in both Islamic and Western manuscripts, served as diagrams to help the reader understand and memorize Galenic physiological-anatomical concepts (figure 15).[20] Two surgeons active in France in the first half of the fourteenth century, Henri de Mondeville and Guido de Vigevano (fl. ca. 1340), tried to develop new types of anatomical illustration to use in teaching; Guido specifically announced his intention to use pictures as a substitute for dissection. But the actual pictures produced were not very anatomically informative.[21] By the first half of the fifteenth century, however, a few instances of relatively naturalistic anatomical illustration were beginning to appear (figures 16 and 17). Dissection itself provided a general map of the body to accompany the books; at best, books and body helped to explain each other.

Moreover, the sequence in which dissection was carried out and the method of exposition was organized and understood in the light of the written, learned tradition. Mondino de' Liuzzi incorporated the conceptual division between simple and composite members into his anatomical practice. He asserted that anatomical dissection of the simple members was an entirely separate undertaking, requiring a differently prepared body than that needed for dissection of the organic or composite parts. Guy de Chauliac described the teaching format for anatomical dissection devised by Mondino de' Liuzzi and adopted by his student, and Guy's own master, Niccolo Bertruccio (d. 1347), as based on a Galenic classification of bodily parts and following an expository pattern modeled on a commentary on Galen's *On the Sects*—a treatise justifying the combination of rationalism and empiricism in medicine. Master Bertruccio pointed out nine things about each body part he discussed, among them its shape, location, relation to other parts, and also its temperament, or complexion, the diseases to which it was subject, and their cure.[22]

The fact that dissections were carried out in the light of a textual tradition does not necessarily imply that the working anatomist expected habitually to be able to match details in a precise, written description with appearances in the cadaver. Even in the fullest authoritative texts available, actual descriptions of individual organs in a good many cases were brief, not very detailed, and interwoven with nondescriptive material. For example, the entire chapter "On the anatomy of the kidneys" in Avicenna's *Canon* rightly impresses the reader as much more informative than the curt statement on the same subject in the early twelfth-century Salernitan *Anatomy of a Pig*, which asserts only that "urine with the four humors is transmitted to the kidneys. The kidneys are oblong hollow organs situated at the upper part of the loins." Some of the extra information provided in the *Canon* is indeed anatomical in the strict sense. Avicenna included a number of details about the shape, structure, situation, and consistency of the kidneys, but the descriptive material is a scattered and subordinate ingredient in a chapter the main thrust of which is to describe the purpose and functioning of the kidneys. The situation was probably conducive to a large measure of tolerance for deviations between textual descriptions and physical appearances.[23]

Thus, special explanation is scarcely needed for the well-known fact that Mondino's *Anatomy*, while undoubtedly based in part on its author's own dissections of the human cadaver—which impressed his contemporaries as numerous—repeats a number of erroneous descriptions from textual authorities. Some of the errors were originally made by Galen and derived from the application of information drawn from his dissections of animals to human beings, or from the requirements of his physiological system. Into this category fall the assertions that a *rete mirabile* ("marvelous net") of vessels is found at the base of the human brain and that a small amount of blood can cross directly from one side of the heart to the other through supposed pores. Other errors arose from misinterpretations of Galen or from efforts to combine the teachings of Galen and Aristotle. For example, Mondino followed Avicenna, who followed Aristotle in asserting that the heart had three ventricles, whereas Galen had clearly and correctly stated that there were two.[24]

Moreover, a theory that was satisfactory for philosophical, astrological, or numerological reasons was unlikely to be displaced, however difficult it might be to demonstrate it visually in dissection. A striking example is provided by the concept of the seven-celled uterus. Galen maintained that the human womb had two cavities, in which he was followed by the major Arabic medical writers. The idea that there were seven divisions, three warmer ones on the right engendering males, three colder ones on the left engendering females, and a seventh, in the middle, producing a hermaph-

Figure 15 (Above and opposite)   A set of the anatomical drawings sometimes known as the five-figure series. Drawings of this type, with accompanying brief, explanatory text, are found in a number of both Persian and Latin manuscripts; in some versions there are as many as nine figures. Pictures and text provide anatomical teaching that is Galenic in its essentials, although greately compressed and simplified. They may derive at several removes from a tradition of diagrammatic representation of anatomy originating in Hellenistic Alexandria. The copy illustrated here was the work of a Benedictine monk at the Bavarian abbey of Prüfening in the mid-twelfth century. Each figure diagrams a different physiological system. The left-hand page shows arteries (right) and veins (left). The right-hand page shows bones (top left), muscles (bottom left), and nerves (top right). (Courtesy Bayerische Staatsbibliothek, Munich, CLM 13002, twelfth century, fols. 2ᵛ–3ʳ.)

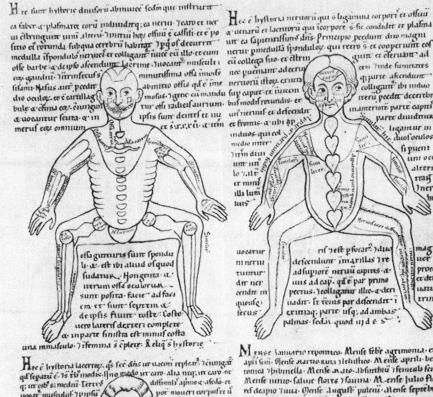

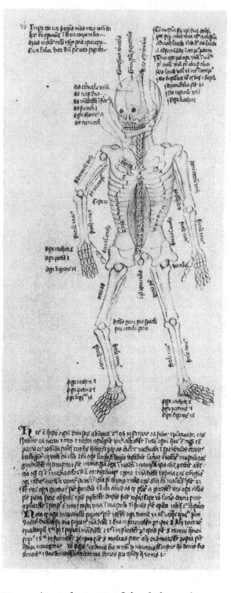

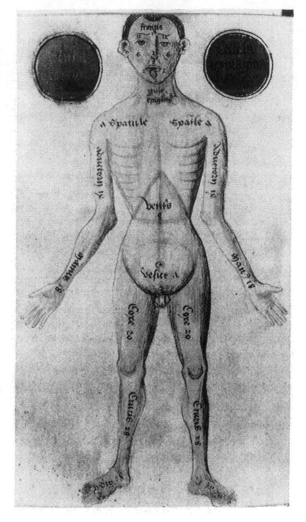

Figure 16   A depiction of the skeleton drawn about 1420 in Germany with considerably more naturalism and depiction of detail than that in the bone picture of the five-figure series in figure 15. The conventional squatting posture has been abandoned, labels name a number of individual bones, and ribs and vertebrae are numbered. The picture illustrates a pseudo-Galenic treatise. (Courtsey the Wellcome Institute Library, London, MS 49 [Wellcome Apocalypse], fol. 37ʳ.)

Figure 17   The body and its parts, ventral (above) and dorsal (opposite) views, as seen by the illustrator of a manuscript containing two brief works on anatomy, namely, one of the Salernitan treatises on the dissection of a pig and a short treatise claimed to be by Galen. The Latin originals of these treatises date from the twelfth and thirteenth centuries. In this manuscript, written in the mid-fifteenth century, the text is in English, although Latin terminology has been retained for the body parts in the illustrations. Proportions here are fairly naturalistic; some internal organs as well as visible body parts are labeled. (Courtesy the Wellcome Institute Library, London, MS 290, fols. 49ᵛ–50ʳ.)

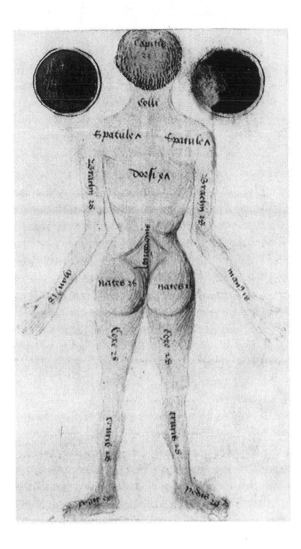

rodite, may have resulted from a systemization in Byzantine medicine of various separate ancient ideas bearing upon multiple births and sex differentiation; these were the perceived mystic qualities of the number seven, the importance of right and left, and the effects of warmth and cold on generation. The theory became known in the West during the twelfth century and was further disseminated by a treatise, falsely attributed to Galen, titled *On Sperm*, which began to circulate in Latin translation some time during the thirteenth century. As is well known, the seven-celled uterus was also accepted by Mondino de' Liuzzi and was asserted as fact by numerous other medical and nonmedical writers in Latin and in various vernaculars. Hence, the idea of the seven-celled uterus gained rather than lost in popularity just at the time when increased interest in dissection, including the dissection of human beings, was appearing.[25] However, some learned physicians, among them Pietro d'Abano, continued to follow the Arabs closely on this issue and to describe a bipartite uterus.[26]

Yet, despite all the difficulties, the practice of dissection evidently did allow some surgeons and anatomists to recognize specific differences between authoritative textual accounts and appearances in the cadaver. One such instance, brought to light in a recent study of medieval medical approaches to sexuality, concerns the hesitation or outright scepticism with which two surgeons, Guglielmo of Saliceto (fl. 1270s) and Henri de Mondeville, and two learned physicians with experience of dissection, Mondino de' Liuzzi and Gentile da Foligno, greeted the assertion in Avicenna's *Canon* that there are three separate passages in the penis, one for urine, one for semen, and one for a third substance. The two surgeons expressed their doubts; Mondino omitted any description of one of the supposed channels, and Gentile specifically mentioned the contrary evidence of dissection.[27] Of course, it is possible that some of these authors may have known of each other's work; their descriptions of the anatomy of the penis remained imprecise; and no major tenet of Galenic physiology was affected, whether or not Avicenna's account was accepted.

Mondino's textbook continued to accompany demonstrations on the cadaver until the early part of the sixteenth century, but changes that eventually contributed to the advances in anatomical knowledge, techniques, and illustration in the age of Vesalius had already begun in the latter part of the fifteenth century. To trace these changes is beyond the scope of this book, and they will only briefly be mentioned here. Developments of undoubted importance for the future of anatomy were increased writing on the subject and more frequent actual dissections by medical faculty, attention to the full range of works of Galen in Greek by medical humanists, and the invention of printing.

Connections are also often suggested between the development of Italian Renaissance art and Renaissance anatomy, although here the evidence is ambiguous. Changes in artistic style and values unquestionably made the study of anatomy a subject of interest to artists. The belief that artists should know anatomy had already been expressed between the 1430s and the 1450s in the influential writings of Leon Battista Alberti and Lorenzo Ghiberti. Their views were a natural concomitant of the concept, especially stressed by Alberti, that the depiction of the idealized human body in its proper proportions was a major task of sculpture and painting. Ghiberti seems to have had in mind the study of anatomy as taught in the schools, since he referred to anatomy as part of the study of medicine, wrote of the desirability of "seeing" an anatomy and drew on Avicenna. Alberti advised artists to study the body itself directly and closely:

> So one must observe a certain conformity with regard to the members, and in this it will help, when painting living creatures, first to sketch the bones, for, as they bend very little indeed, they always occupy a certain determined position. Then add the sinews and muscles, and finally clothe the bones and muscles with flesh and skin. . . . As Nature clearly and openly reveals all these proportions, so that zealous painter will find great profit in investigating them in nature for himself.[28]

Later in the century, as is well known, some artists carried their investigation of anatomy to the point of engaging in dissection for themselves; it has recently been argued that Pollaiuolo (ca. 1431–98) was the first to do this, but the most famous case is that of Leonardo da Vinci, who performed a number of dissections and made anatomical drawings over a period of some thirty years, beginning about 1487.[29] Masterly though Leonardo's drawings are, they should not be regarded as either a totally new departure in anatomy or as a strong influence on the development of anatomical studies. Although these drawings record much careful observation, their visual persuasiveness cannot always be equated with anatomical accuracy in depicting human organs (figures 18, 19, and 20); further, they remained in private notebooks. Nevertheless, in a broader sense, trends in fifteenth-century art may have contributed to the subsequent development of improved techniques of anatomical illustration and also helped to create a new climate of visual attentiveness to the skeletal and surface anatomy of the human body.

Major Concepts

Medieval anatomical and physical ideas were, by and large, inherited from ancient medicine. It is not appropriate to look for radical conceptual changes or large increments of new knowledge in the work of *medici* who—despite their willingness to criticize respected authorities on specific points—perceived their task in regard to anatomy and physiology as one of understanding, interpreting, and passing on an existing tradition of learning. Indeed, certain basic physiological concepts and associated therapeutic methods—notably humoral theory and the practice of bloodletting to get rid of bad humors—had a continuous life extending from Greek antiquity into the nineteenth century.

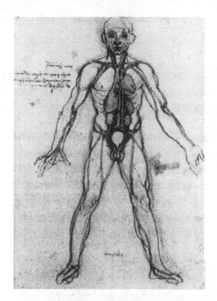

Figure 18 Leonardo da Vinci, drawing of a male anatomical figure depicting veins, arteries, and principal internal organs, probably dating from the 1490s (R. L. 12597R). The internal anatomy is probably based on Mondino and Avicenna in conjunction with some dissection of animals. (Courtesy Windsor Castle, Royal Library. © 1988, Her Majesty Queen Elizabeth II.)

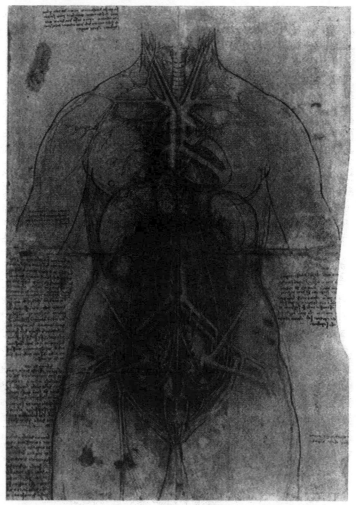

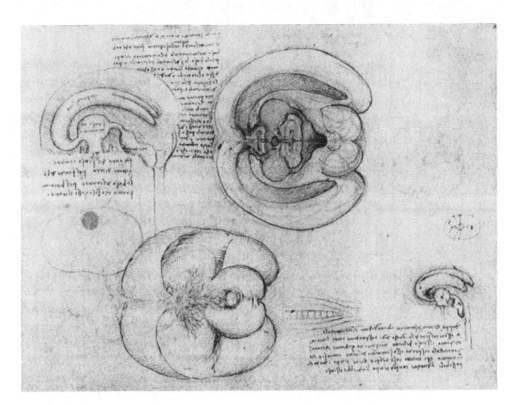

Figure 20   Leonardo da Vinci, drawings of the brain (of an ox?) (ca. 1509–1510) injected with wax to preserve the shape of the ventricles (R. L. 19127R). Leonardo attached importance to ascertaining the shape of the ventricles correctly because, as the labeling of the drawings shows, he shared the standard beliefs about the localization of mental faculties within the brain. The method of wax injection, which came into general use among anatomists only in the seventeenth century, was his own invention. The lettering on the drawing gives a description, in mirror writing, of the procedure of injection. Counterclockwise from the left, the three large drawings show the lateral view of the cerebral ventricles; the base of the brain with the retiform plexus, or rete mirabile—believed to be present in human beings, actually present in the ox—in which the spirits were supposedly refined for transmission to the brain; and a transverse section. The shape of the ventricles was actually somewhat distorted by the wax. Compare these drawings with the presentation of essentially similar theories about the localization of mental activity in figure 13. (Courtesy Windsor Castle, Royal Library. © 1988, Her Majesty Queen Elizabeth II.)

Figure 19 (Opposite)   Leonardo da Vinci, drawing of a female anatomical figure (ca. 1510?) (R. L. 12281R). This drawing shows much evidence of direct observation; however, most of the anatomical details are based on dissections of animals. (See Charles D. O'Malley and J. B. de C. M. Saunders, *Leonardo da Vinci on the Human Body* [reprinted New York, 1982, originally published 1952], 456.) The drawing also shows more detailed knowledge of Galenic anatomical and physiological theory than the earlier drawing shown in figure 18, for example, in the representation here of a two-chambered heart (the auricles not being regarded, or depicted, as part of the heart). (Courtesy Windsor Castle, Royal Library, © 1988, Her Majesty Queen Elizabeth II.)

The predominance of Galen's ideas over those of other ancient medical authors further ensured broad areas of general agreement, especially after the late twelfth century. For example, it has recently been suggested that the account of the female reproductive system given by the first-century physician Soranus, known in a Latin version to twelfth-century Salernitan *medici*, had less influence thereafter, being largely replaced by the different, Galenic descriptions in the works of Haly Abbas and Avicenna.[30] In the later Middle Ages, the multiplicity of texts of various chronological, geographical, and linguistic origins, together with scholastic ingenuity in elaborating interpretation and occasional original contributions, guaranteed diversity; nevertheless, most of the variations were in detail only.

Thirteenth- to fifteenth-century Latin writing about physiology falls into two distinct phases. Until about 1300, medical writers tackled the task of absorbing the newly translated technical literature; they elaborated physiological and pathological narrative, identified major themes, and enlarged the technical Latin vocabulary.[31] The themes and vocabulary of physiological discourse established in this period remained much the same until the sixteenth century. The contributions of fourteenth- and fifteenth-century learned physicians to physiological theory were more likely to consist of highly abstract discussions of topics overlapping physiology, logic, and natural philosophy. One example is provided by the controversies about the nature and action of heat among Giovanni Marliani (d. 1483), who taught medicine at Pavia and Milan, and his contemporaries in both medicine and philosophy. Because of their interest in changes in the human body that took place as health gave way to sickness and vice versa and in how the body changed or was changed by food and medicines, respectively, academic physicians also interested themselves in late medieval philosophical debates concerning the composition of bodies and changes in their qualities. They joined in discussions of the state of the elements in mixed bodies and the intension and remission of forms and inquired whether there was a "latitude" (that is, a gradual intension or remission) of health.[32]

A comprehensive account of Galenic physiology, which was well understood by some learned physicians in western Europe by the fourteenth century, together with a systematic review of its Islamic and Western medieval modifications and of medieval anatomy, would extend far beyond the scope of this book. The following paragraphs merely describe some basic concepts in fairly standard form, with little attention to variations and refinements. This necessary simplification may make the whole complex of ideas appear more static, unified, and coherent than was in fact the case. The texts from which the examples were drawn were all used, and some were composed, in western European medical schools between 1200 and 1450.

Basic constituents of the human body, like deadly sins and cardinal virtues, formed part of a conventional set. This was the list of "things natural," which were, in turn, one of a group of three categories: the naturals, the non-naturals, and the contra-naturals. As the explanation of the three categories in the elementary textbook of medicine known as the *Isagoge* of Johannitius made clear, the contra-naturals, or things against nature, were pathological conditions of all kinds. The non-naturals were a mixture of physiological, psychological, and environmental conditions held to affect health: air, exercise and rest, sleep and waking, food and drink, repletion and excretion, and the "accidents of the soul," or passions and emotions. The list of six factors affecting health was drawn from Galen, as was the terminology and concept of non-naturals, although these appeared in different works.[33] The set of non-naturals often served the practical purpose of providing a series of headings under which recommendations for regimen could be compiled.

The list of things natural differed slightly in terminology and number of subdivisions in different versions; it usually included elements, complexions (sometimes divided into *commixtiones* and complexions), humors, members, virtues, operations, and *spiritus*. The things natural thus joined together alleged material components imperceptible to sense (the elements of earth, air, fire, and water in the human body, and *spiritus*, which was supposedly a substance manufactured in the heart from inspired air and transmitted through the body via the arteries); physically perceptible bodily parts (humors, that is, body fluids; and members, that is, parts of the body); and activities or functions (virtues and operations). This list will serve here merely to introduce three main organizing concepts: complexion, the humors, and systems assigning relations between bodily parts and functions.

Complexion

The term "complexio" was, from the twelfth century, the Latin commonly used for the Greek *crasis*, or temperament, that is to say, the balance of the qualities of hot, wet, cold, and dry resulting from the mixture of the elements in the human body.[34] Since it served as a fundamental concept, not only in physiology but also in pathology and therapy, complexion theory provided important support for the idea that medicine constituted a unified and rational body of knowledge. The general theory, already quite fully developed in the works of Galen, underwent considerable further elaboration during the Middle Ages. Some scholastic physicians gave discussions of the subject a highly abstract and philosophical turn; they argued, for example, over whether complexion constituted a fifth quality distinct from the primary four and whether it was to be identified with "form" or "substantial form" in medieval Aristotelian philosophical usage.

Doubtless such recondite questions were of slight or no interest to most medical practitioners. For them, complexion theory functioned as a system of explanation providing the rational link between disease and therapy; sickness occurred when the balance of qualities in an individual was upset; the physician might restore nature's balance by prescribing medications in which the qualities were matched inversely to the patient's disordered complexion. These pathological and therapeutic aspects of complexion will be discussed more fully in chapter 5; they depended upon the underlying biological or physiological idea that all corporeal living things are complexionate, each plant or animal species having its own characteristic complexion.

Among human beings, furthermore, each person was endowed with his or her own innate complexion; this was an essential identifying characteristic acquired at the moment of conception and in some way persisting throughout life. In this sense, complexion was a fundamental organizing principle of each individual human organism considered as a whole. Thus, a particular person might be characterized as having a hot complexion relative to other human beings, and this characterization would apply to him or her throughout life.

In addition, the complexion of human beings varied according to conditions of life and external circumstances. It was affected by the passage of time; heat and moisture in youth gave way to coldness and dryness in old age. It differed according to sex; most authors considered women as a group to be colder and moister in complexion than men as a group, though an individually exceptional woman or man might have a complexion hotter or colder than a member of the opposite sex. Complexion also varied among different peoples or geographical regions; Scythians, who lived in a cold climate, were supposed to be colder and moister in complexion than Ethiopians, who lived under the hot sun.

Again, each organ of the human body was considered to have its own predominant complexional quality. The heart was always hot, or at any rate hotter than the brain; the brain was always cold, or at any rate colder than the heart; and so on. Medical textbooks provided four long lists of bodily parts arranged in order of hotness, dryness, wetness, and coldness, respectively.

In principle, complexion—normal and abnormal—was supposed to be a physically perceptible quality that could be discerned by touch. It was never an absolute but always a relative quality, one that had to be ascertained by comparison with the norm for the species or individual or bodily part in question. The ideal complexion, ensuring perfect health and functioning, was temperate, that is, well balanced. However, what constituted a good complexion would vary with the species or, among human beings, with the race or the individual; presumably a perfectly healthy Ethiopian would have a hotter complexion than a perfectly healthy Scythian. Among species, human beings were the most temperate; in the human being, the palm of the hand was the most temperate part of the body. A perfectly temperate complexion was an ideal that could be approached but probably never reached.

Complexion theory usefully accounted for psychological and social as well as physiological characteristics or stereotypes. The cold and moist complexion attributed to women explained timidity as well as menstruation.[35] The theory also drew upon or reinforced observations or truisms common to medicine and other disciplines, as the following examples may briefly show. The difference in complexion between the Scythians and Ethiopians discussed in Galen's *On Complexions* also occurs as an example of the effect of the climates of different latitudes on their inhabitants in Ptolemy's (fl. mid-second century A.D.) work on astrology, the *Tetrabiblos* (known in its medieval Latin versions as the *Quadripartitum*). And long before either Ptolemy or Galen, a Hippocratic writer had similarly compared Egyptians and Libyans with the Scythians.[36] Again, the idea that complexional heat and moisture decrease with age is a theme in Galen's writings on the subject of complexion. However, even earlier Aristotle had taken up the subject of heat and moisture in living animal bodies, introducing the idea that in some animals the innate heat consumes the body's moisture over the lifespan and suggesting the metaphor of a flame consuming fuel. Galen himself knew and alluded to these remarks of Aristotle. By the time the topic of changes in complexion due to aging and their outcome in natural death was taken up by thirteenth-century authors, a whole cluster of elaborations and interweavings of the Galenic and Aristotelian ideas was also available from various intermediate writers, notably Avicenna.[37] In the physiology of complexion, as in other branches of medieval learning, such echoes and repetitions from one work to another, one author to another, and one discipline to another were often taken as providing corroboration and confirmation from independent sources.

The fundamentally simple nature of the ideas of complexion, its apparent confirmation not only by a wide range of authorities but by facts of sense experience (heat and moisture are characteristics of living mammals, shriveling does take place in old age), the comprehensiveness of the concept, its flexibility, and its potential for elaboration doubtless all explain the attraction of complexion theory. Nevertheless, obvious difficulties with the theory did not go unnoticed.

Gentile da Foligno, for example, expressed dissatisfaction with the claim of "all the masters" that the separate complexions ascribed to the various parts of the body could be differentiated by touch. He pointed out that,

> [if] a living animal that has been cut into and eviscerated while it is still alive is touched, the innate complexion [of each part] will not be apparent to you, since the actual heat of all the organs [together] will be apparent, therefore you won't be able to judge by touch that the nerves and ligaments and bones are of cold complexion, because these are very hot to the touch in a living animal.[38]

(Gentile's remarks should not be taken as evidence for any regular practice of vivisection by fourteenth-century physicians.)

The perception of difficulties did not lead to the abandonment or any general overhaul of complexion theory. The intellectual habits that governed the outcome of critical insights such as Gentile's are well illustrated by his own explanation of the imperceptibility of the differences in the complexion of various internal organs. He accounted for it by making a distinction between two different kinds of complexion—one arose from the mixture of the elements, was very different in different bodily parts, and was imperceptible to sense; the other was brought from potentiality to actuality by the vital heat of blood and *spiritus*, was the same throughout the whole body, and was perceptible to sense. Gentile, in short, used observation and critical acumen, not to repudiate medical theory but to refine it with the aid of ideas derived from Aristotelian philosophy. More far-reaching in its implications than his critique of complexion theory was his clear appreciation—unusual in a fourteenth-century writer on any aspect of natural science—of the difference between repetition of authoritative statements to the effect that something is known by experience and actual experience.

The Humors

The concept of humors—that is, specific bodily fluids essential to the physiological functioning of the organism—originated at a very early stage of Greek medicine. Various Hippocratic treatises mention one or more of these fluids; *On the Nature of Man* presents what was to become the standard set of four: blood, phlegm, bile (also termed choler, or red or yellow bile), and black bile (or melancholy). The theory of the humors probably developed because bodily fluids of all kinds played a large part in ancient, and subsequently medieval and Renaissance, physiology, diagnosis, and therapy. Treatises in the Hippocratic corpus include explanations of physiological change in terms of the behavior of real or imagined internal fluids, assume that the physician's supervision of his patients involves monitoring all forms of excrement, with special attention to consistency, and occasionally advocate therapeutic bloodletting. Also of importance for the subsequent development of humoral theory was the uniquely significant role ascribed to blood in Aristotle's works on animals. Aristotle classified animals into blooded or bloodless types, asserted that blood nourishes the body, and considered that the quality of blood was responsible for psychological characteristics. According to Aristotle, courage and intelligence were a consequence of the possession of hot, thin, clear blood. And as with so many other topics, Avicenna provided a handy systematic review of the doctrine of the four humors, with some elaborations. He divided each of the four into good and bad, or unnatural, varieties (bad blood, phlegm, and biles being "superfluities" that should be eliminated) and added various secondary humors.[39]

The four humors were real bodily fluids to which largely hypothetical origins, sites, and functions were ascribed. Thus, phlegm was a catchall term for more or less any colorless or whitish secretion (except semen and milk); both Galen and his medieval successors stressed that phlegm comes in a number of varieties with different characteristics: sweet, salty, acid, watery, and mucilaginous, to name only a few of those listed by Avicenna. The brain was the special organ most frequently associated with phlegm (presumably the association was originally made because of the color and consistency of brain tissue or cerebrospinal fluid, or both); but "natural" phlegm was also described as merely a stage in the manufacture of the blood.

Red or yellow bile was identified as the fluid found in the gallbladder and said to be manufactured in the liver, along with black bile and blood; black bile, however, was provided with an imagined "receptacle" in the spleen. The ancient distinction between the two biles probably originated in the demands of fourfold symmetry and a desire to match the number of humors with the number of elements and qualities, taken in conjunction with observations of variations in the color of vomitus and feces.

Blood occupied a special place among the humors. The actual fluid found in the veins was considered to be a sanguineous mass consisting of a mixture of the pure humor blood with a lesser proportion of the other three humors; changes in color and partial separation in drawn blood left standing in a container were advanced as evidence of the presence of the biles and phlegm. The other humors were generated as part of the process of the manufacture of blood; and an important function of yellow and black bile—in their "good" form—was, respectively, to purify and fortify the blood. Through the veins, which were considered to be specialized for the reception of blood, it was diffused throughout the entire body.

The humors filled two important functions in the body's economy. In the first place, they were essential to nutrition. Indeed, in Galenic physiology the blood, incorporating with it the other humors, *is* the body's nutrition. Avicenna's account is brief and clear: ingested food, having been transformed into chyle in the stomach, is subsequently transported to the liver and there concocted (literally, "cooked") into blood, the two biles, and phlegm. Various stages of concoction purify the blood of superfluities, which are excreted, and ultimately, part of the blood is refined into semen. Most of the blood, however, is used up in nourishing every part of the body. Hence, the parts of the body were said to be generated from the humors.

Secondly, the humors were in a special way the vehicle of complexion. Like all bodily parts, they were themselves complexionate. But in addition, the four humors collectively were the means whereby an individual's overall complexional balance was maintained or altered. Hence, the balance of humors was held to be responsible for psychological as well as physical disposition, a belief enshrined in the survival of the English adjectives sanguine, phlegmatic, choleric, and melancholy to describe traits of character. Humoral theory is probably the single most striking example of the habitual preference in ancient, medieval, and Renaissance medicine for materialist explanations of mental and emotional states. In late antiquity and the Middle Ages, Christian, Muslim, and Jewish critics all took Galen to task for psychological materialism; they believed that the theory of temperament or complexion implied that material causes (the elements) determined the nature of the human soul and moral qualities, and they objected on philosophical or religious grounds.[40] But complexion was often thought of as a balance of qualities rather than of substances and as only notionally perceptible to sense. From a purely psychological standpoint rather than from religious or philosophical points of view, the ascription of a role in shaping personality to specific bodily fluids is an even stronger assertion of materialism. Whatever the limitations of actual knowledge, medical theory consistently appealed to sensible models of explanation.

Principal Members and Associated Systems

One of the main controversies between Aristotelians and Galenists involved the concept of principal members. Aristotle generally taught that the heart, the source of heat and life, ruled the entire body; the Galenists taught that three principal members—heart, brain, and liver—each governed or provided the originating or ruling principle (*principium*) of, a separate group of organs and functions. The testicles (a term also used for the ovaries, understood as analogous organs in the female) were sometimes added to the list of principal members. The rival concepts were in essence connected with the differing Platonic and Aristotelian views of the soul and were the subject of much learned scholastic disputation. But whether the ultimate principal or principle within the body was considered to be one or several, particular internal organs and humoral fluids were grouped into three distinct systems. To these systems were also ascribed virtues, operations, and faculties. Virtues were general powers of action or sensation belonging to each system. Operations were functions of particular organs; for example, that of the stomach was digestion. Faculties were specific abilities peculiar to various parts of the body; for example, both the nine-month gravid uterus and the intestines had an eliminative or propulsive faculty.

These schemes were simultaneously anatomical and physiological, although anatomy was usually the handmaiden of physiological theory. The influential accounts in Galen's *On the Natural Faculties* and the chapters on the virtues in the *Canon*[41] focused more on physiological function than on bodily parts. Thus, when Avicenna wrote of vital, animal, and natural virtues, he associated each of these powers—or, more properly, clusters of powers—with a particular physiological system or systems and with a particular group of organs. Each set of virtues, system, or group of organs was governed by or took its origin from its own principal member. Avicenna's account was complicated by the fact that he tried to reconcile the essentially incompatible views of Aristotle and Galen by allowing the heart a sort of overriding influence over the entire body while simultaneously subscribing to the Galenic doctrine of several principal members.

The power termed vital virtue, so called because it ensured that life (*vita*) itself was maintained, was associated with *spiritus* (the Greek *pneuma*). Hence the organs involved were sometimes described as spiritual members. The manifestations of this virtue were the rhythms of heartbeat, pulse, and respiration. The organs with which vital virtue was associated were those of the thoracic cavity and the arteries, which disseminated a mixture of blood and *spiritus*, the vehicle of vital virtue, throughout the body. The heart was, of course, the principal member of this system.

Psychic powers were termed animal virtues because they were associated with functions of soul (*anima*, in the philosophical sense). They were responsible for mental activity, motion, and sensation and were localized in the brain, spinal cord, and nervous system, the brain being the principal member. *Spiritus* was conveyed from the heart by the arteries to the *rete mirabile*, where it underwent further refinement into special animal spirits to which were ascribed a role in brain function and the process of vision. These spirits carried the power of seeing (*virtus visiva*) from the brain through the supposedly hollow optic nerve to the eye. Medical writers devoted considerable attention to the eye and vision; a work that was especially influential in the medieval West was *Ten Treatises on the Eye* by Ḥunain b. Isḥāq (d. 873), or Johannitius, which was translated into Latin before the end of the eleventh century. Following Galen, Ḥunain discussed the anatomy, physiology, and diseases of the eye and the nature of sight, stressing the role of spirits within the eye and adopting Galen's (and Plato's) view that vision occurred by means of extramission of rays from the eye. Medical discussions of the eye and sight contributed to a subject that evoked lively interest in the thirteenth-century West. In treatises on what was termed *perspectiva*, a variety of topics relating to vision and optics were discussed. The composition of these treatises was stimulated by ancient and still more by Islamic contributions to the subjects of psychological and cognitive aspects of vision and of mathematical optics, notably by the work of the mathematician Ibn al-Haitam (d. 1041), whom the Latins knew as as Alhazen. An important issue in the medieval literature on optics was whether vision occurred by extramission of rays from the eye, as Plato and subsequently Galen had believed, or by intromission, as Aristotle and subsequently Avicenna, Averroes, and in a more complex version Alhazen had held. The opinion adopted on this issue did not, however, necessarily affect the physiological role ascribed to spirits within the eye.

The natural virtues were more or less the same as the powers attributed by Aristotle to the nutritive, or vegetative, aspect of soul: nutrition, growth, and reproduction. The powers of nutrition and growth were, of course, associated with the digestive organs and the veins that disseminated the body's nourishment in the form of blood. Of these organs, the liver was the principal member. The demands of symmetry led to the idea that specialized natural *spiritus* served as the vehicle of the natural virtues.

An essentially similar picture from a somewhat more anatomical point of view is presented in Mondino de' Liuzzi's *Anatomy*. Mondino described the triple division in terms of three containers in the body: a superior ventricle containing the "animal members" (that is, the skull enclosing the brain and associated parts), a middle ventricle containing the "spiritual members" (that is, the thorax enclosing the heart and lungs), and an inferior ventricle containing the "natural members" (that is, the abdomen, containing the liver and other viscera).

This scheme of separate systems provided a means of distinguishing and classifying different aspects of physiological activity. The resulting arrangement was hierarchical; thus, Mondino de' Liuzzi, who was emphatic in his assertion of the nobility of the human body as a whole, also made it clear that some parts were intrinsically superior to others. He supplied two reasons for beginning dissection with the abdominal viscera—because of the rapidity with which they putrefied and because, in every branch of knowledge, one should begin with the most confused and least noble and proceed toward the higher and better organized.[42]

Classification of activity in turn determined the way structure was understood; the case of the blood vessels provides a well-known example. For *medici* in the Galenic tradition, as we have seen, the venous and arterial systems were entirely distinct.[43] Except for the small amount of blood that allegedly crossed through the supposed pores in the central septum from one side of the heart to the other to mix with the *spiritus*, the content of the two types of vessels was believed to be different; the veins contained blood, the arteries a mixture of *spiritus* and blood. They were associated with different principal organs, namely, the liver and the heart, and their purposes—nutrition in one case, the dissemination of *spiritus* conveying vital virtue in the other—were also quite separate. Differences in the actual structure and contents of veins and arteries would accordingly, and rationally, be interpreted as visual confirmation of received physiological theory. However, one would not expect to find any signs of recognition that the theory might have been devised in the first place in order to explain the appearance of body parts and fluids.

The History of Human Life

Medieval physiological ideas not only provided a rational and ordered account of the complexity of human bodily function at any one moment but also yielded a narrative of the progress of the human organism through time, from conception and embryological development through various defined stages of life to natural death. Note has already been taken of the presence of the power of growth among the natural virtues and of the concept of progressive complexional change throughout life, leading ultimately to natural death when innate heat and radical moisture have both been used up. The idea expressed in Plato's *Timaeus* of man as microcosm encouraged linking the stages of human life with stages or constituents of the universe as a whole. Several Hippocratic treatises pointed out links or analogies between stages of human life and various sets of four: the seasons, the elements, the primary qualities, and the humors. In the Middle Ages, the concept of a four-stage human life cycle interacting with other fourfold aspects of the universe was frequently expressed in the form of a diagram. The most influential general medical textbooks—the *Pantegni*, the *Canon*, and the *Isagoge*—all divided life into four ages. However, astrological tradition stemming from Ptolemy's *Tetrabiblos* held that the sun, the moon, and the five known planets each influenced a different stage of human life and therefore postulated a life cycle of seven ages.[44] Astrologically minded physicians such as Pietro d'Abano made use of this scheme as well as of the fourfold cycle; Pietro, who evidently preferred the seven-age scheme, noted that it coincided with assumptions about the capacity of different ages made by legal writers.[45] The various other six-age, five-age, and three-age schemes developed by patristic authors and subsequent Biblical exegetes, theologians, preachers, and moralists seem not to have affected medical ideas on this issue.

Human reproduction received much attention in the medical literature. The issues raised were far from trivial, even though the only way they could be treated was by inconclusive and repetitive verbal debate. Among the questions discussed, for example, were the respective roles of male and female parents in conception and the origin of semen and its vivifying power. On the former topic, Aristotle had held that the male alone contributed sperm containing an active principle to conception, the female providing only the matter of the fetus; by contrast, the Galenist view was that both male and female contributed sperm, so that the offspring could have characteristics from both parents (this is a much simplified account).

Discussions of embryology took up the issue of how and in what sequence the fetal organs took shape and how the fetus was nourished in the womb. Since the development of the human embryo involved its emergence as a separate living organism, endowed not only with complexion, virtues, and so on but also, at some point, with a soul, metaphysical and astrological considerations also played a part in embryology. The theological aspects of the subject were usually avoided by *medici*, who were also less preoccupied than philosophers and theologians with defining the precise way in which the Creator of each individual rational soul cooperated with the "informative virtue" of the paternal semen in forming and enlivening a new human being. But the astrological ideas that by the early fourteenth century were beginning to be widely diffused in some sections of the medical community often included the belief that heat, light, and occult influences emanating from the heavenly bodies assisted in the generation of life on earth. Also known was Aristotle's view of the importance of the sun for the generation of all living beings, including humans. Pietro d'Abano, a physician famous for his astrological learning, asserted that informative virtue was the virtue that gave life; a substance in semen with the power of receiving this virtue, "is the first spirit, bringing celestial heat." He added that informative virtue had two instruments, celestial heat and elemental heat. The first was "worthier" and played a role in the generation of "nobler" beings, bringing them to life in some kind of conformity with the heavens.[46]

In addition to the general influence of the heavenly bodies (figure 21), the horoscope at conception or birth was also considered to signal or predispose the physical and mental constitution of each individual down to the most minute detail; Pietro d'Abano held the stars responsible for his own dislike of, or possibly allergy to, milk. Horoscopic astrology thus had a place in reproductive theory as well as in medical practice, in which its main uses were in selecting regimen and treatment (see chapter 5). It could also provide a form of reproductive planning: the Emperor Frederick II (d. 1250) delayed sexual intercourse with his bride until his astrologers told him the propitious moment for the generation of a male had arrived; immediately after the marriage had been consummated according to the astrologers' recommendations, the emperor confidently informed the empress that she was now pregnant with a son. According to the chronicler Matthew Paris, who reported the story, the astrologers had given the right advice, and nine months later the empress duly gave birth to a boy.[47]

Medical texts as a rule presented sexual physiology in morally neutral terms and, following Galen, endorsed sexual activity as essential for the continuation of the species and, in moderation, as healthful for the individual. For the most part, Latin translators and commentators transmitted with little modification views that had originated in societies not influenced by the religious attitudes of medieval western Europe. For example, the monk Constantinus Africanus opened a medical treatise on male sexuality (probably translated from the Arabic) as follows:

> The Creator, wishing the race of animals to remain firmly established and not perish, disposed that it would be renewed by coitus and by generation. . . . Therefore he shaped for the animals the natural members which are apt and proper for this work, and provided them with such wonderful virtue and lovable pleasure that there is no animal

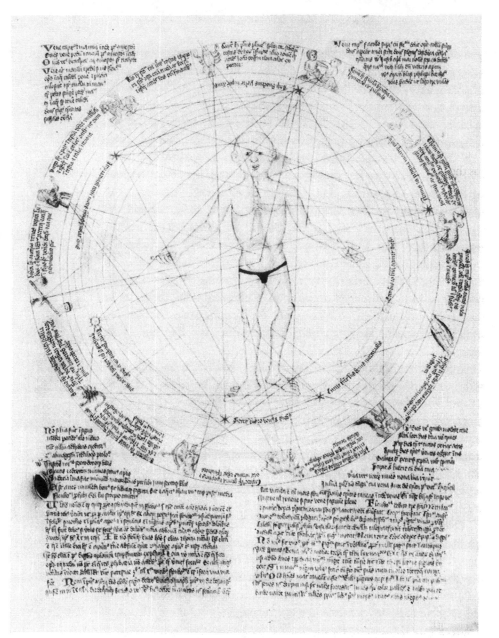

Figure 21   The stars and the human body. This diagram is intended to illustrate the relationship between the heavens and appropriate times and sites for bloodletting, but it also presents a fine general image of the all-embracing influence of the heavenly bodies and zodiacal signs on both human physiology and the diseases to which the human body is subject. Specific information about the particular influences affecting an individual patient at a given time had to be obtained by drawing up an astrological chart based on the use of astronomical tables. Here, man is shown surrounded by and as the focus of celestial influences. Each zodiacal sign has special power over a different part of the body and the diseases peculiar to it; for example, Pisces is linked to the feet and hence to diseases of the feet such as gout. (Courtesy the Wellcome Institute Library, London, MS 49 [Wellcome Apocalypse], ca. 1420, fol. 41ʳ.)

that does not excessively delight in coitus. Because if animals hated coitus, the race of animals would certainly perish.[48]

The fundamental idea that the power to reproduce is a gift of the Creator can of course also be found in the work of medieval Christian theological writers, although always placed by them within the bounds of Christian morality and often accompanied by praise of celibacy. One twelfth-century example of a positive approach on the part of an author who wrote mainly on theological subjects is Alan of Lille's *Plaint of Nature* (ca. 1160–65). In this literary work's alternating passages of poetry and prose, Alan used ingenious grammatical metaphors to present marital procreative sexuality as the work of Nature carrying out God's plan and to contrast it with a fiercely condemned homosexuality. The stress on the reproductive usefulness of pleasure in the passage just quoted is more specifically medical and is not an isolated example; a recent study has underlined the extent to which similar ideas about human sexuality and sexual pleasure (female as well as male) characterized the medical literature in the Galenic tradition that was disseminated or composed in Latin during the twelfth, thirteenth, and fourteenth centuries.[49]

In the realm of sexuality, medical ideas thus constituted only one ingredient, and by no means necessarily the most important, in the attitudes embodied in medieval and Renaissance literate culture. The same may be said of medical ideas about physiology and anatomy in general. While it seems highly likely, for example, that medical teaching about the complexionate differences between men and women reinforced stereotypes about women, it is as a rule difficult to disentangle a specifically medical component in general cultural attitudes.[50] Nor is it easy to isolate the influence of fourteenth- or fifteenth-century cultural norms or assumptions about the human body in the language authors or translators of that period chose to transmit physiological information.[51] Of course, interaction among popular beliefs, religious teachings and influences, medical, and, from the thirteenth century, Aristotelian philosophical ideas permeated the way the human body was described and understood at many levels and for many purposes, both within and outside the medical community.

In the foregoing summary, the limiting conditions of physiological and anatomical knowledge among western European *medici* and literate surgeons between the twelfth and the fifteenth centuries are apparent. Mastery of the subject meant in large part mastery of texts; and a methodology that would permit much addition to knowledge or change in theory was not yet available. But the reliance upon Islamic syntheses of ancient medical teaching and the introduction of aspects of scholastic Aristotelianism into medical discourse—both often denigrated by Renaissance humanists and modern historians of medicine alike—were initially useful resources, in that they facilitated the assimilation of information from a variety of texts and the connection of medicine to areas of broader inquiry in contemporary natural philosophy. And the *medici* who used these means to study physiology accomplished results that were, in their time, significant: the assimilation of part of ancient science; the recognition, following the lead of Avicenna and Averroes, of differences between the physiological doctrines of ancient authorities; the introduction of dissection of the human cadaver into medical education; and, above all, the endorsement of the study of the human body as an intellectually respectable, useful, and dignified pursuit.

FIVE

DISEASE AND TREATMENT

here were many and varied discussions about my case among the medical practitioners in attendance. And although what they were saying didn't seem very reasonable to me, I gave in to them. I have used the diet and medicines they recommended for almost three months already, but up to now I feel very little, indeed scarcely at all, better." Detailed reports from highly articulate patients are a rarity in the early history of medicine, so one is grateful for the dissatisfaction with the treatment he was getting that led Peter the Venerable, Abbot of Cluny (d. 1156), to describe his experience in a letter to a *medicus* called Bartholomeus in the hope of getting better advice. Peter's letter provides a glimpse of the ways in which an intelligent and well-informed patient and medical experts interpreted and managed his ill health in the light of the concepts and procedures of Galenic medicine.[1]

As a learned monk, Peter was no doubt much more familiar with medical ideas and terminology than the average patient and correspondingly readier to second guess his medical advisers. His letter to Master Bartholomeus explains that owing to pressure of monastery business he had postponed his regular bimonthly bloodletting. Meanwhile, he suffered an attack of "the disease called catarrh," to which he was subject, and so he postponed venesection yet again because he had been told that bloodletting during an attack of catarrh would cause the patient to lose his voice and perhaps even be life threatening. But Peter's catarrh did not improve, and he began to fear that overabundance of blood and phlegm was bringing on a fever. Finally, after four months he did not dare to postpone bloodletting any longer and twice had large amounts of blood drawn off within three weeks. Thereafter, just as prognosticated, the catarrh still did not go away, and Peter's voice suffered. At the time he wrote this letter just quoted, his voice had been adversely affected for three months; in addition, his chest felt heavy and he continued to cough up a lot of phlegm. Peter was particularly concerned about the loss of his voice, which prevented him from celebrating the liturgy and especially from preaching.

Peter further reported that the *medici* he consulted locally (were they other monks of Cluny, or practitioners from outside the monastery?) attributed his continued ill health to the loss of the heat of the blood in bloodletting, which left cold and "sluggish phlegm diffused through the veins and vital channels." It was this unpleasant-sounding substance that was oppressing both his chest and his voice. Their prescription was to use heating and moistening foods and medicines. Peter objected to this recommendation on rational grounds; following the Galenic theory of cure by contraries, he thought that a cold, moist disease ought to be countered by hot and dry, not hot and moist, remedies. The *medici* replied that the throat, arteries (*arterias*—most likely the *arteria aspera*, that is, the trachea) and "some other parts whose names I don't know well" ought to be soothed with moist things, not irritated with dry things. He was also worried about the consequences of continuing to omit his regular bloodletting. The medicines Peter took without obtaining any relief included hyssop, cumin, licorice, or figs steeped in wine and syrups of tragacanth, butter, or ginger.

Historians disagree as to whether Bartholomeus is to be identified with a famous Salernitan physician by that name,[2] but wherever he came from, Bartholomeus was an expert, thoroughly informed about medical theory and cognizant of up-to-date medical literature emanating from the Salernitan milieu. In his reply Bartholomeus for the most part endorsed the judgment of the local *medici*, although he tactfully avoided directly contradicting his distinguished patient. He advised against bloodletting until after the catarrh was better, but for Peter's headache, he suggested repeated cautery of the head ("don't worry about it damaging your sight"). He drew on a sophisticated version of Galenic complexion theory for his explanation that a medicine that was actually moist might be "potentially" dry and so suitable for use against a moist disease, supporting his assertion with an example from a learned medical text based on the writings of Constantinus Africanus. The allusion to actuality and potentiality may also suggest that Bartholomeus had some knowledge of Aristotelian philosophical ideas, then beginning to penetrate Salernitan circles from indirect sources. And he recommended hot baths, inhaling medicated steam, poultices for the chest, lozenges to dissolve in the mouth, gargles, and, for good measure, a laxative.

The story of Peter the Venerable's upper respiratory infection reveals much about the way medicine based on Greco-Islamic tradition worked in practice as a therapeutic system. This particular case belongs to the winter of 1150–51, a time when medical knowledge still had a significant place in general monastic learning. Concepts of formal medical qualification and the development of specialized centers of medical education were still at an early stage of their development. Consequently, Peter the Venerable probably had more self-confidence in challenging his medical attendants on the basis of his own medical knowledge than would an equally learned and authoritative person after, say, the end of the thirteenth century. For example, Petrarch was a highly articulate and opinionated patient; but his verbose objections to the advice of his friend and medical attendant, the university professor of medicine Giovanni Dondi, to avoid fresh fruit and to drink wine in preference to water, were based on personal preference (fruit) and religion and morality (wine), not on a claim to specialized medical knowledge.[3] Nonetheless, the opinions, explanations, advice, and treatment proferred by the various people involved in Peter the Venerable's case illustrate aspects of medical and patient thinking and behavior that are illuminating for the entire period covered by this book.

In the first place, Peter, his local medical attendants, and the learned consultant all conceived of his ill health as essentially a kind of imbalance in the body. This imbalance was located primarily in the humors; so the task of therapy was to restore them to their proper equipoise. Bloodletting, cautery, and the hotness or coldness of foods and medicines were all ways of regulating the quantity and temperamental quality of the humors. The balance required constant monitoring and regulation in health as well as in sickness. Peter's frustration and anxiety mounted when the special conditions of his illness obliged him to miss the regular bloodletting that was part of his normal health routine.

The notion of generalized disturbances of the balance of temperament coexisted with the concept of individually named diseases. Peter was quite sure that he suffered from "the disease (morbus) called catarrh," but this means only that he and his medical advisers were confident of their ability to attach a name to a set of symptoms. They certainly did not think in terms of an underlying invasive entity with specific, determinate, and persisting identity; on the contrary, neglected catarrh might turn into a fever, which would be another "disease."

We may note, too, that the practicing medical experts were flexible and pragmatic in their application of medical theory. It was the patient who wanted the theory of cure by contraries to be rigidly followed, even if it meant irritating his sore throat; and it was the patient, not the physicians, who was convinced of the virtues of bloodletting in heroic quantities in sickness and in health. What both the local medici and the distant consultant actually recommended were simple, soothing remedies that would bring some comfort and do no harm to a sufferer from bronchitis or a similar complaint. And Master Bartholomeus used his superior academic philosophical and medical learning and knowledge of the new Arabo-Latin sources to lend weight to the recommendation of grandmotherly forms of treatment that still seem to help relieve sore throats and unblock stuffed nasal passages.

In short, except for the recommendation of cautery, Peter the Venerable was probably better off in the hands of his medical advisers, near and far, than left to his own devices. His experiences illustrates several ways in which medicine in the Greco-Islamic tradition could help patients. Its practitioners decoded and named collections of symptoms and placed them in the context of a logically satisfying, general explanation of ill health. Taught to esteem prognosis, some of them evidently developed genuine prognostic skill (Peter did lose his voice as the *medici* predicted he would, although presumably not for the reasons they adduced), and their practical experience enabled them to select medications and procedures that were simultaneously justifiable in terms of medical theory and usually innocuous or in some instances actually helpful in reducing discomfort. But although a severe bronchial infection in a man of nearly 60 years is not trivial, and although loss of voice is a serious matter for someone whose occupation calls for public speaking, Peter's recovery after a few months shows that his complaint was self-limiting and not life threatening.[4] No means existed whereby medicine could alter the course of acute, life-threatening, or serious chronic disease.

Since the maintenance of health and the treatment of disease were the central tasks of medicine, a very large and diversified body of written and some pictorial material came into being to guide the practitioner. By the late thirteenth or early fourteenth century, material in use included Latin versions of lengthy treatises by Galen on diseases, symptoms, and treatment; synoptic works used as academic textbooks, each of which acquired its own body of commentary (for example, the section on fevers in Avicenna's *Canon*); general treatises on practical medicine; collections of opinions on specific cases by famous physicians (*consilia*); guides to medical terminology; manuals on techniques of phlebotomy; directories of ingredients for medicines; collections of medicinal recipes; color charts to aid in diagnosis by inspecting urine; calendars and tables for use in astrological medicine; and handbooks on particular subjects such as poisons or theriac.

The last-named substance was a compound of vipers' flesh and other ingredients and was supposedly a universal antidote to poison as well as a remedy for diseases caused by an excess of melancholy and phlegm (figure 22). Descriptions of theriac (which had been invented in antiquity) by Avi-

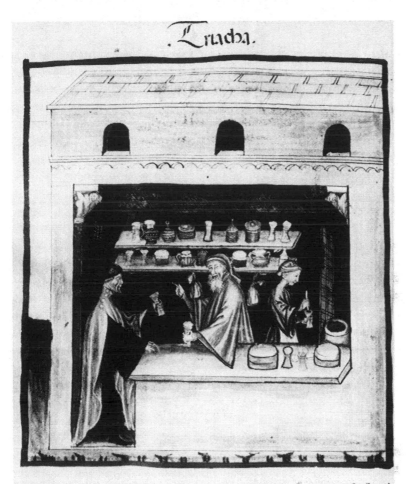

Figure 22   Preparation and sale of theriac. The pharmacist who sells this marvelous
substance appears scarcely less dignified and finely dressed than his customer, who
is perhaps a learned physician buying a supply for his patients. Compare the appearance of the customer, evidently a patient himself, in figure 33, which comes from
the same manuscript. (Courtesy Bild-Archiv der Österreichischen Nationalbi-
biothek, Vienna, MS ser. nova. 2644, end of the fourteenth century, fol. 53ᵛ.)

cenna and Averroes stimulated especially keen interest among medical masters at Montpellier in the late thirteenth century; they discussed principles
of medicinal action through which theriac was supposed to work and the
basis for determining dosage, and they gave practical directions for its use.[5]

Although essentially similar medical ideas are found throughout, some parts of this body of writing about disease and treatment are obviously much nearer to the world of actual practice than the rest. Only a few of the most learned or pretentious physicians would be likely to consult Galen's *On the Technique of Healing*[6] or an academic commentary on Avicenna in the course of treating patients, whereas many practitioners might find constant use for a short handbook, a pictorial diagram, or a collection of recipes for medicinal remedies.

Yet the medical booklets and pictures that appear most directly related to actual practice are still prescriptive texts rather than a record of what was actually done. Even the collections of *consilia*, or advice given by leading physicians in individual cases, show signs of being edited for didactic or other purposes. Only on rare occasions can one determine with certainty what was done to a patient and with what results. There can be no doubt that the teaching conveyed in medical books guided actual practice, at any rate up to a point, but the scanty available evidence suggests that, just as in the case of Peter the Venerable, the application of theory was often modi-fied or simplified according to the needs of the empirical situation, the availability of ingredients for remedies, or the practitioner's preferences. Hence, the following brief account of the principles according to which health and disease were understood and managed necessarily conveys only part of the realities of practice.

Medical theory asserted that the human body exists in either health, sickness, or a neutral state between the two. Deviations from health were classified into congenital malformations (in medieval Latin, *mala compositio* of the body), complexional imbalance (*mala complexio*), and trauma (*solutio contin-uitatis*, or break in the body's continuity).[7] This classification placed almost all internal illness in the domain of complexional imbalance. Relatively little attention was paid to the first of these three categories, and when surgery emerged from medicine as a separate occupation and discipline in the West during the twelfth and thirteenth centuries, the management of trauma became the characteristic task of the surgeon. Hence, the care offered by medical practitioners other than surgeons consisted primarily in the man-agement of the body in health (that is, the maintenance of a good temper-ament) and the treatment of internal and some external illnesses attributed to complexional imbalance.

As a result medical care, at least ideally, consisted as much in a preventive health regime as in the treatment of disease. The physician was supposed to maintain health by regulating the non-naturals, that is, by tailoring the pa-tient's diet, exercise, rest, environmental conditions, and psychological well-being so as to maintain him or her with the optimum complexion (figure

23). In one form, this concept was applied to groups; thus, regular prophylactic venesection was prescribed for entire monastic communities, and regimens were suggested for categories of people such as children or the elderly, or the residents of a particular place. Michele Savonarola's pediatric handbook, already mentioned, takes the form of a regimen of health for pregnant women and children under seven in the city of Ferrara.[8]

But since complexion differed in each individual, a really satisfactory health regime would have to be tailored to individual needs. Obviously, in existing social conditions such fine tuning was possible only for the wealthy. One example of an individual regimen is the diet book Savonarola wrote in Italian around 1450 especially for his patron and patient Borso d'Este, ruler of Ferrara. The individuality is somewhat illusory, since much of the advice comes from Avicenna (indeed, some of the dietary recommendations can be traced back to Hippocrates); but the learned medical author was careful to introduce distinctions between foods suitable for nobles such as Borso and their courtiers and those appropriate for lesser mortals.[9] Increased variety and refinement of foods and methods of food preparation available to the wealthy in later medieval and Renaissance Europe may have fostered interest outside the medical profession in ancient medical theories about the relation between food and physical health; perhaps not coincidentally the period was also one in which some women ascetics laid great emphasis upon abstinence from food in their search for spiritual health.[10]

Indeed, food and medicine shaded into each other. Avicenna declared, in a passage frequently cited and discussed by Latin medical writers, that the formal distinction between them was that food was assimilated by the body, whereas medicine assimilated the body to itself. But both food and medicine were complexionate and affected the complexion of the person who ingested them; in practice, not only spices but also various vegetables counted now as one and now as the other. Lettuce, for example, frequently crops up as an ingredient of cold complexion in medicinal recipes; Petrus Hispanus recommended a concoction of lettuce leaves for toothache and lettuce seed to cool excessive libido.[11] The emphasis on dietary regulation as the key to health was one of the most ancient components in medicine, since it was a central feature of the Hippocratic tradition. The more-or-less systematic classification of foods according to complexion theory was a later contribution. Although careful attention to diet is a characteristic of premodern medicine that may seem enlightened to readers in the diet-obsessed late twentieth century, the types of foods actually recommended were largely determined by textual tradition and were not always those now thought of as especially conducive to health. In particular, patients

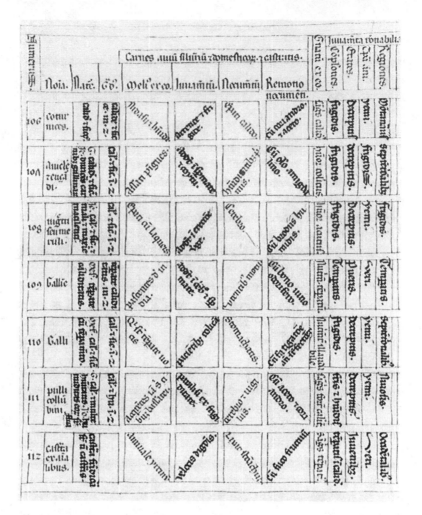

Figure 23   A chart from the *Tacuinum Sanitatis*, or *Tables of Health*, a handbook of regimen based on an eleventh-century Arabic original. The *Tacuinum* summarized in tabular form the benefits and contraindications for different types of patients in different circumstances of items of diet, environmental factors, and various forms of activity. This particular example forms part of a large collection of Latin medical works copied in Italy, probably as a commission for a practitioner from Bohemia, before 1326. The page shown deals with poultry. Item no. 110, reading across from left to right, informs us that roosters are dry and hot, that they have these qualities in the second degree, that the best kind to eat are those that crow temperately, that their meat is especially good for patients suffering from colic, that it may cause irritation of the stomach that can be avoided if the birds are tired out before they are slaughtered, that it provides nourishment engendering the humor bile and is recommended for people of frigid complexion, in old age, in winter, and in northern regions. (Courtesy the Yale Medical Library, MS 28 (Codex Fritz Paneth), p. 718.)

were frequently urged to avoid fresh fruit and some vegetables. Michele Savonarola warned Borso d'Este that apples and pears were "hard on the stomach." Onions clouded the intelligence and were therefore not a suitable food for people who needed to use their minds or be alert—such as Borso's falconers.[12]

If the boundaries between food and medicine were not strongly and clearly drawn, those between good and bad complexional balance were equally vague. As noted previously, good complexion—that is, good health—lay somewhere within a range, or latitude, that differed in each individual and could never be precisely measured; and there was thought to be a neutral state between health and sickness. But when the management of health obviously failed, it became the physician's task—with the cooperation of nature and the patient—to manage illness. The immediate causes of most forms of disease were attributed to shifts in the patient's complexional balance. These changes might in turn be set off by harmful changes in the non-naturals, especially food, drink, air, and water. The idea that the environmental air itself could become infected, or putrefy, served as a useful explanation of epidemic illness that affected many people at the same time and place. In this way the ancient concepts of the influence on health of region, climate, and weather, which were as central to Hippocratic medicine as diet,[13] were brought into the theories about the balance of the four qualities in the humors of the human body systematized by Galen. In the version of the whole complex of ideas that was elaborated in Islam and, subsequently, in the West, celestial influences were often considered responsible for variations in the health or sickness of the body, either directly or via changes they brought about in the air. As Rhazes put it: "Wise men among the *medici* agree that everything relating to times, the air, and waters, and complexions, and diseases is changed by the motion of the planets."[14] The planets supposedly exercised this power through light, heat, and their individual special characteristics.

Diagnosis

Diagnosis of disease was achieved by using the concept of complexional imbalance as a fundamental explanatory mechanism to interpret clinical manifestations. Ancient medicine had laid substantial emphasis upon the careful, detailed observation and recording of clusters of symptoms and the way they changed and developed over the course of an illness. As a result, some remarkable clinical observations were achieved, as can be seen in the

Hippocratic *Epidemics*, a collection that contains numerous individual case histories as well as reports of epidemics. This observational tradition survived to an extent into the Middle Ages, especially in the Muslim world; a famous medieval example is Rhazes' description of smallpox, which distinguished its symptoms from those of other epidemic diseases causing skin eruptions such as measles (this description was first translated into Latin by fifteenth-century humanists).[15] In the Latin West, some *consilia* of thirteenth- to fifteenth-century physicians contain descriptions of clusters of symptoms in individual cases witnessed by the author. However, many other *consilia* either omit descriptions of symptoms and explanations of the diagnostic process entirely in favor of merely naming the disease and prescribing remedies, or they are based on second-hand reports about the patient's condition.

When it took place, observation consisted primarily of taking visual note of the patient's external appearance, listening to the patient's own narrative of the illness, and inspecting and smelling his or her excreta. Not all these forms of observation necessarily took place together or completely in any one case. As just noted, physicians prescribed for patients they had not seen in response to written inquiries from colleagues or from the patients themselves or their friends. While physicians considered the patient's narrative valuable, they also felt obliged to mistrust it because of the medical ignorance they imputed to those not trained in their own learning and craft.[16]

Even the examination of excreta—to which much importance was attached because they were considered to contain "superfluities" or "bad humors" thrown off by the sick body—was often only partial. Major textbooks urged the physician to consider variations in the color, odor, and consistency of all the excreta. The survival of a few independent short Latin and vernacular tracts giving rules for diagnosis or prognosis by inspection of fecal matter,[17] not to mention jokes about the medical preoccupation with feces, suggest that some *medici* practiced this form of diagnosis. Blood drawn in venesection was also included among the substances to be examined for diagnostic purposes. A work on phlebotomy, attributed to the twelfth-century Salernitan author Maurus, gives careful instructions for observation before, during, and after coagulation; characteristics to be noted, (in addition to those named above), included viscosity, hotness or coldness, "greasiness" (*unctuositas*), taste, foaminess, rapidity of coagulation, and the characteristics of the layers into which drawn blood separated. As a final step, the practitioner was supposed to wash the coagulated blood and once more feel its texture. Blood that was greasy or showed certain characteristics after washing was a particularly ominous sign that suggested a diagnosis of *lepra*. Essentially similar instructions are included in a number of thirteenth- and fourteenth-century medical writings, influential general Latin works on practical medicine and surgery as well as vernacular manuals of practice.[18]

However, the proliferation of brief handbooks and color charts giving rules for diagnosis by inspection of urine leaves little doubt that, in actuality, many practitioners relied primarily and perhaps exclusively on such observations of urine (figure 24; see also figure 5 in chapter 2). A common condition in contracts drawn up for practitioners hired by towns was that they inspect the urine of all citizens who wished it. The ubiquitous presence of the urine flask as a convenient symbol of the medical practitioner in medieval art is a convention, but it is one that reflects reality. Observation of the urine was not always accompanied by observation of the patient; Arnald of Villanova took it for granted that the practitioner might be asked to diagnose urine that had not been excreted by the person who delivered it, and also that the person who came for a consultation might be deliberately testing the practitioner by giving a false account, or no account, of the urine's source. Arnald suggested that the best way for a practitioner to deal with the latter situation was to develop the art of putting leading questions.[19]

Standard works also taught various forms of diagnosis by touch, although it is of course impossible to say how often these were put into practice. For example, Rhazes, following Hippocrates, noted that one of the signs of dropsy was the characteristic sound made when the abdomen was percussed; he also stated that one of the signs of a "hard aposteme" (abscess, swelling, tumor) of the liver was a hard mass under the ribs that could be felt by touch.[20] Of course, the manual art of surgery always involved diagnosis by touch (see chapter 6). Unquestionably, however, the most common use of touch in medical diagnosis was taking the pulse (see figure 7 in chapter 2). Since the arteries were held to distribute life-bearing vital spirits along with blood throughout the body, and since the movement of the arterial pulse was manifestly affected by some forms of disease as well as by exertion and emotion, the act of taking the pulse put the physician in a profound and literal sense in touch with the ebb and flow of vitality in his patient.

Learned physicians expounded a complex theory of pulse that was first developed by Herophilus and enunciated by Galen. Variations of the pulse were analyzed into several different components: the dimensions of the arteries, of which there were nine simple and twenty-seven composite varieties—an example of composite dimensions being "long, narrow, and deep"; strength; rhythm; and according to whether the beats or the pauses

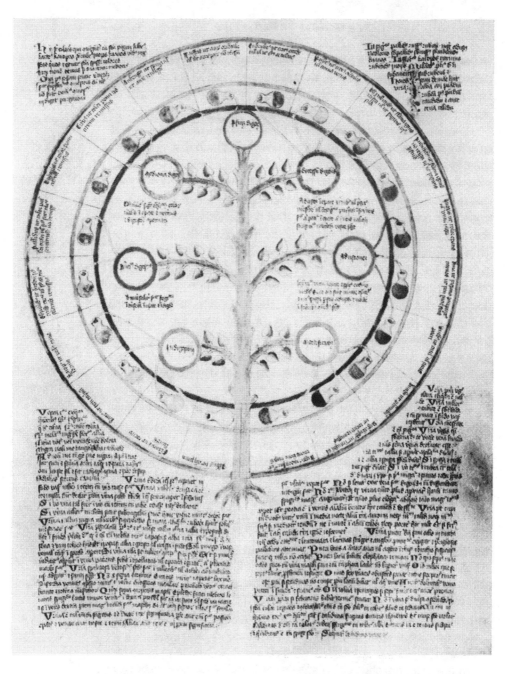

Figure 24 An aid to diagnosis by inspection of urine. This exceptionally elaborate and elegant wheel of urines was drawn in the early fifteenth century. The flasks contain urine of different colors, as the color variations were considered a source of diagnostic and prognostic information. The legend just inside the outermost circle describes the color of each flask. The seven small circles hanging from the tree describe different stages of "digestion" of urine, a perfect state being represented by the circle at the top. (Courtesy the Wellcome Institute Library, London, MS 49 [Wellcome Apocalypse], fol. 42ʳ.)

126

between them were under consideration. Pulses were also described as equal or unequal, ordinate or inordinate, rhythmic or arrhythmic, and as soft, hot, or full. A set of standard adjectives was used to describe individual instances of pulse that supposedly combined specific variations in all ten categories; these terms included a number of comparisons with the motion of animals—for example, pulses were said to be antlike, goatlike, or wormlike.

As will have become evident, most of this pulse theory essentially involved codifying the description of qualitative impressions. However, in describing the rhythms of pulse, the terminology of musical proportion and metrical verse was also applied. The meter of pulse was supposed to vary with age; according to Pietro d'Abano, the pulse beat in dactyls in infants and in iambs in the old. Various influential authors, among them Avicenna, asserted that specific musical proportions existed in pulse and that the practitioner could identify them by touch. In the West, the idea of musical proportion in pulse was sometimes linked to the ideas about "human music" (*musica humana*, an otherwise undefined category excluding audible vocal or instrumental music) and "world music" (*musica mundana*, including the music of the spheres) transmitted via Boethius' (d. 524 or 525) *On Music*, a standard musical treatise.

Few practitioners can have known the details of this arcane pulse lore or attempted to put them to use. Learned exponents of the theory of pulse themselves expressed doubts as to whether analysis of the pauses between pulsebeats or identification of specific musical rhythms in pulse was possible in practice. Yet the existence of a complicated body of theory must have strengthened the general perception among *medici* that pulse was a highly significant, albeit difficult to interpret, bodily sign. As Pietro d'Abano remarked, the ten varieties of pulse and the more-or-less infinite number of individual pulses could all, loosely speaking, be reduced to one—whatever kind of knowledge the *medicus* gets out of it. No doubt, in reality experience gave some practitioners considerable sensitivity to minute variations in pulse and the ability to relate them to the patient's general condition. Pietro also pointed out a prosaic practical advantage of relying on the pulse in the wrist as a means of diagnosis: it avoided the necessity of asking the patient (especially the female patient) to undress.[21]

In principle, the observation of symptoms led to the identification of disease. Moreover, a rich vocabulary of names for disease conditions was available. But both the relation of symptom to disease and the distinction of symptom from disease remained problematic even for the few careful observers in the world of medieval Islamic and Western medicine, as it had been in antiquity. To be sure, Galen had stressed the importance of carefully distinguishing between disease and symptom, but it is hard to see how he imagined this could be achieved in practice. One of Galen's medieval interpreters, Arnald of Villanova, reworked the exhortation to suggest that it is only important to distinguish disease from symptom in situations in which it can be shown that such a distinction is relevant to treatment. Criticism of the adequacy of Galen's definitions of disease, symptom, sign, and related terms and concepts began in the sixteenth century, but even then there was still no real possibility of replacing them.[22]

Furthermore, until well into the early modern period, European medical descriptions of disease were strongly influenced by ancient and, until the sixteenth century, Islamic textual tradition. Disease descriptions frequently echo earlier texts; in many instances one cannot be sure whether physician–authors actually encountered either the diseases they listed and described in more or less detail in their handbooks on the practical aspects of medicine or even the symptoms they attributed to individuals. Of course, conditions described in earlier texts might recur in a practitioner's own experience; but even when personal observations were made, textual tradition was likely to govern the understanding and interpretation of what was seen.

And, as is always the case, observations of new phenomena were likely to be interpreted in the light of existing theory. In the medieval context, the most striking example is provided by plague. In fourteenth-century Europe, plague was effectively a "new" disease characterized by highly distinctive symptoms (at any rate in its bubonic form) and overwhelming, catastrophic impact. The experience of plague was sufficiently novel and terrifying to generate a new variety of medical literature, the plague tractate; 281 of these treatises giving explanations for the causes of plague and recommending treatment or precautions are known to have been composed between the mid-fourteenth century and 1500.[23] But the writers usually found it more acceptable to stretch existing categories of disease to encompass plague (often assimilating it to various types of fever) than to allow for the existence of a disease not described in authoritative medical textbooks and not susceptible of rational explanation.

The spread of plague was accordingly explained as a result of corruption or infection of the air that altered for the worse the complexion of those who breathed it; the precipitating cause of the bad air was often, but not always, said to be astrological. In astrological theory, the precipitating cause of outbreaks of epidemic disease was usually held to be adverse conjunctions of the planets; various medical and other writers produced tracts attributing the outbreak of the Black Death, which arrived in Sicily and southern Italy in 1347 and swept across different parts of Europe until 1351, to the conjunction of the three superior planets said to have occurred in 1345.[24] Variations in individual complexion or horoscope were called on to explain why, when a whole community breathed the same air, some people got sick and others did not. This type of explanation was not as much at variance as is sometimes supposed with the belief in contagion from person to person, and from infected goods, held by those outside the medical profession and implicit in the quarantine regulations that began to be imposed by some public authorities before the end of the fourteenth century. Physicians recognized clearly that proximity to plague victims made one liable to get plague—hence the precautions they took when visiting the sick—and some of them termed it a *contagium*, meaning that it passed rapidly from one person to another.[25] The theory of corruption of the air provided an underlying mechanism. Medical explanations of the causes of plague, whether or not they invoked astrology, were, of course, consonant with the idea that the primary cause was God's will. Nor would medical explanations necessarily have been perceived as at variance with explanations, much favored by preachers and moralists, that attributed the plague to God's displeasure with general human sinfulness. But the learned medical explanations seldom gave support to the popular prejudice that laid the blame for plague epidemics on deliberate poisoning and used this hostile fantasy as a pretext for intensified persecution of Jews during times of plague.

The treatments and precautions recommended for plague were wholly rational in terms of the explanations provided; physicians recommended flight, if possible, from regions where plague had broken out; dietary regimen and medication to regain complexional balance; and measures to counter the bad air—fumigants, carrying strong- or sweet-smelling spices in one's clothes, and the like. Physicians followed their own advice in regard to prophylactic measures; although some fled, others recognized a responsibility to visit the sick and remained to do so.[26]

Partly as a result of the spread of syphilis from the 1490s, the issue of the possible existence of diseases inexplicable in terms of complexion emerged more clearly and was the subject of intensive discussion during the sixteenth century. By that time there was somewhat greater readiness to admit the possibility of idiosyncratic, specific diseases—but the innovative explanations that were devised still took as their starting point ideas formulated by ancient authors. The theory that some diseases might affect the "total substance" of the body rather than its temperament was a different application of an explanation originally provided by Galen for the idiosyncratic action of a few medicinal substances; the famous theory of contagion via "seeds of disease" developed by Girolamo Fracastoro (1478–1553) owed much to ancient atomism as expounded by the Roman poet Lucretius (first century B.C.).[27]

From the standpoint of the actual history of disease in human populations, descriptions of morbidity in ancient Greek and medieval Islamic or Western medical or other narratives are thus of limited value. It is frequently difficult or impossible to identify in modern medical terms conditions described solely by selected external symptoms and conceptualized within the framework of complexion theory. Various instances of continuity in terminology often compound the problem by masking the radical discontinuity between the ancient and nineteenth- or twentieth-century understanding of disease. For example, *lepra* was described by numerous medieval authors, both Arabic and western. The list of its symptoms was long and grew longer as time went on, doubtless as a result of the elaboration of a textual tradition, but possibly also in some instances because *medici* were charged by public authorities with the heavy responsibility of determining whether individuals were leprous or not—a positive verdict would result in the unhappy patient's total social isolation. Some of the symptoms listed appear to refer to the disease now known as leprosy, but others do not; so it is clear that the term *"lepra"* encompassed a variety of conditions producing lesions of the skin. Secure knowledge that leprosy was present in medieval Europe, at any rate at some times and places, rests on paleopathological and other evidence, not on the descriptions in medical texts.[28]

But if the range of diseases described, or prescribed for, in the medical literature is not a useful guide to historical epidemiology, it is a rich source of information about the way in which ill health was understood and recognized, and about the kinds of problems practitioners were prepared to treat. Theoretical writers analyzed diseases according to their complexional characteristics. Considering only conditions that affected the entire body, rather than those peculiar to various bodily parts, Pietro d'Abano classified fevers as hot; paralysis, epilepsy, and apoplexy as cold; wasting and cancer as dry; and dropsy as wet. Again, these terms are not necessarily to be equated precisely with the conditions now known by the same names.[29]

Among conditions regarded as diseases of the whole body, fever, the paradigmatic example of a hot "disease," occupied a special place. The subject of fever came to constitute almost a separate branch of pathology; among much-used textbooks and works of reference, a major section of Avicenna's *Canon* (Book 4, Fen 1) and the whole of Book 10 of Rhazes' general treatise on medicine, known in the West as *Almansor*, were devoted to fevers. As might be expected, the main source of ideas about fever was once again Galen, whose principal treatise on the subject, *On Different Kinds of Fevers*, was also studied directly.[30] In these works fevers were elaborately subdivided into different varieties (quartan, tertian, hectic, ephemeral, and others), and much attention was paid to the concept of periodic rhythms in fevers.

Another kind of classification of diseases that was followed in many practically oriented manuals, presumably because it was useful, emphasized the concept that different diseases were peculiar to different parts of the body by adopting a head-to-toe arrangement. Although they were accepted as part of rational, learned medicine, such manuals were essentially empirical in their approach, since they simply listed symptoms and remedies in standard diagnostic categories. These books varied significantly in sophistication and complexity. The ninth book of *Almansor* was frequently used as a university textbook of practical medicine until the sixteenth century. Indeed, Vesalius, the most famous of Renaissance anatomists, found the work of sufficient interest to edit or paraphrase the twelfth-century translation. Each of the book's 115 chapters is devoted to a different condition, ranging from headache to pains in the feet. The materialist psychology associated with the concept of complexion and humoral qualities ensured that, in the *Almansor* and similarly arranged treatises, mental complaints (frenzy, melancholy) were interspersed among other afflictions of the head. Thus, too, physicians included passionate love (*amor hereos*) among the physical diseases and enumerated the languishing lover's physical symptoms.[31]

In the *Almansor*, most chapters begin with a description of the symptoms; in many cases this account is fairly complex and detailed and employs a technical vocabulary allowing for subtle, if not always clear, distinctions; recommendations for treatment follow. For example, Rhazes distinguished between the symptoms of kidney and bladder stones thus:

> Stone in the bladder manifests itself by continual itching of the patient's private parts, so that he or she is always touching them and experiences frequent sexual arousal followed by sudden relaxation, and excretion of urine with difficulty and pain; in this condition, too, the rectum, being compressed by the stone in the bladder in the meanwhile, usually falls forward. But the symptoms of stone in the kidneys are great difficulty in urinating, violent pain in the kidneys and the vessels which carry the urine from the kidneys to the bladder and the surrounding parts, pain in the groin, and a constricted stomach, and nausea from food.[32]

By contrast, Petrus Hispanus composed his *Treasury of Poor Men* in simple Latin around the mid-thirteenth century for working practitioners who did not have access to the resources of higher learning that he himself enjoyed. Petrus Hispanus' little book survives in 70 manuscripts, and versions of it were printed over 50 times in Latin and various vernacular languages between the late fifteenth and the early seventeenth century. This wide dissemination no doubt, is in part a tribute to the distinction of the author, but it also suggests that the book may legitimately be regarded as representing the level to which the understanding of disease was reduced in much medical practice. The original work consisted of 50 chapters, each listing the remedies recommended by medical authorities for a different health problem (a short treatment of fevers and various appendices were subsequently added). Neither description nor complexional analysis of the various conditions is provided; the reader is expected either to be able to recognize them or to acquire the ability to do so on his own. However, the preface urges the reader to consider "the species of infirmity and the nature of the patient, and study diligently to know the natures of things and complexions and substance, and, to the extent possible, the hidden virtue of each thing," before administering any medication.[33]

More than a quarter of the 50 chapters in the original *Treasury* are devoted to easily recognizable complaints, among them falling hair, headache, earache (figure 25), toothache, nosebleed, fainting, nausea, diarrhea, stomachache, hemorrhoids, arthritis, and worms. Obviously, while some of these problems could be symptoms of severe illness or be acutely painful, in many instances they would be manifestations of minor and self-limiting conditions. Fourteen chapters are given over to gynecological problems and sexual dysfunction. In one of them, the future pope compiled 34 recommendations of remedies to protect against impotence or excite sexual desire, a number of them magical or at any rate intended to ward off magic. The use of magical remedies against impotence was widely recommended, presumably because of the general acceptance of the idea that impotence not caused by a permanent physical or mental defect was likely to be the result of sorcery or spells.[34] In Petrus Hispanus' treatment of the problem, Christian morality was preserved by the clear indication that the prescriptions in this chapter were intended for the married. The remaining chapters are more problematical, since they are given over to internal conditions only vaguely defined by terms such as "oppression of the liver," "oppression of the spleen," "diseases of the chest," or "lesion of the lung," or to evidently serious problems such as bladder and kidney stones and inability to urinate.

A practitioner who confined his activities to diagnosing and treating the conditions listed in the *Treasury of the Poor* could expect to have fair success in a good many minor cases and with some of the sexual problems in which a psychological component was involved; such success might well be sufficient to build a medical reputation. Users of Rhazes' more sophisticated manual, however, would have been able to name a wider range of disease conditions and to provide much fuller and more complex descriptions of the symptoms and course of illness associated with each.

Prognosis

The prediction of the course and outcome of disease was an important aspect of the physician's skill. In a medical system in which diagnosis was often problematic and the ability to cure was very limited, prognosis must frequently have emerged as the most valued and actually most useful aspect of medical attendance for both practitioner and patient. Skill in prognosis was a prerequisite for following standard advice urged on practitioners by various writers. This advice included avoidance of hopeless cases; in those

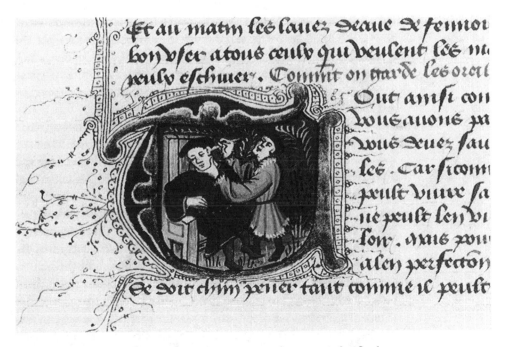

Figure 25   Treatment of the ear. The practitioner grasps the patient's chin firmly while inserting a probe into his ear. This illustration is included in a mid-fifteenth-century copy of a health handbook compiled in French during the thirteenth century. (Courtesy the Pierpont Morgan Library, New York. MS M. 165, Aldobrandino da Siena, *Régime du corps*, fol. 53ᵛ, detail.)

taken on, careful manipulation of the hopes and fears of patients and their relatives so as to ensure confidence in the physician—viewed as a psychological asset to recovery—and the prompt payment of fees. For some patients, a hopeful prognosis may indeed have aided recovery; unfavorable prognosis would be a signal to turn to religious means of physical healing, to set one's affairs in order, or simply to seek religious consolation. Examples noted elsewhere in this book (pp. 41, 166) indicate that practitioners did indeed on occasion inform patients that their cases were hopeless.

There is no reason to doubt that experienced practitioners gained very considerable expertise in recognizing signs of recovery or signs of impending death, forecasting the likely progress of illnesses characterized by particular symptoms, and differentiating between dangerous and harmless pains, swellings, and so on. Nonetheless, prognostication was obviously a fallible art. Like the astrologer, the physician used his arcane knowledge to predict, and, like the astrologer, the physician became expert in identifying by the light of hindsight the conditions that had invalidated his predictions. When Taddeo Alderotti attended the count of Arezzo, he found the patient improving; accordingly, he prescribed medicines but left junior colleagues or medical students to administer them and watch the patient during the night. On returning next morning and finding the patient at the point of death, Taddeo neatly shifted the blame away from his medicines and onto his junior colleagues by pointing out that they had omitted to close an open window and thus had caused an unfavorable environment.[35]

The importance attached to prognosis meant that endeavors were made to identify criteria that would enable the practitioner to know when disease was to be expected and what its course would be. Pulse-taking and inspection of urines were used as means of prognosis as well as initial diagnosis. The Hippocratic *Prognostics*, one of the standard texts studied in advanced medical education, taught its readers to consider signs presaging recovery or death and provided numerous examples. Other Hippocratic works provided precedents for associating the onset of certain types of diseases with particular types of climate, weather, or seasons of the year. In addition, horoscopes could be cast to determine when disease was likely to occur or what diseases were likely to be prevalent over a particular period of time. The "judgments of the year," which the professor of astronomy and astrology at the University of Bologna was required by university statute (1405) to provide without charge for students, must have contained such predictions. Of course, horoscopes could also be cast retroactively to identify the planetary aspects that had brought about disease that had already broken out; this second use may in fact have been more common.[36]

In prognosticating the course of disease, learned physicians invoked quasi-mathematical theories about periodicity and favorable or unfavorable days. The original basis for such theories was the frequent inclusion in case descriptions in the Hippocratic *Epidemics* of information about the number of days from the onset of illness to the day on which particular phenomena occurred, as well as the behavior of recurrent fevers such as malaria. Data of this kind, initially derived from observation, were subsequently interpreted in the light of beliefs held in antiquity about the properties of numbers and auspicious or inauspicious calendar dates. Galen's treatises *On Crisis* and *On Critical Days* provided a very full treatment of the whole subject, which was subsequently taken up by various Muslim medical authors and further developed in Latin scholastic medicine.[37] Acute diseases were held to have a crisis, or turning point, which usually took the form of a sudden excretion of "bad humors"—a characteristic example would be a heavy sweat during a fever, but crisis might also be marked by a bout of vomiting, or diarrhea, or even the onset of menstruation. A crisis should be good or bad, that is, it could mark a turn toward recovery or a turn toward death, and it could be strong or weak. Two things determined the nature and the outcome of the crisis: the state of the patient's own body and whether or not the crisis fell on a favorable day. But opinions differed as to the intervals at which favorable days recurred and from what point one should start counting.[38] Thus, the identification of such days and the proper means for determining them became subjects of medical debate.

Because it involved calendar dates and thus the motions of the moon, the theory of critical days was a branch of medical astrology. Although the term "medical astrology" normally implies nothing more than the use of astrological techniques for medical purposes, the doctrine of critical days included an astrological concept peculiar to medicine, namely, that of the "medicinal month." Galen had postulated that critical days were to be calculated on the basis of a "medicinal month" of 26 days and 22 hours, which he arrived at by averaging the 27-1/3 days of the period of the moon's return in longitude with the 26-1/2 days of its period of visibility. And this "medicinal month" was accordingly taken as a basis of calculation by various subsequent medical writers.[39]

The different levels of astronomical competence among practitioners of medical astrology in general, and medical prognostication by astrological means in particular, are revealed by Pietro d'Abano's views on the subject of critical days. Pietro, who taught and wrote on astrology and astronomy as well as on medicine, thought that the treatment of the theory of critical days by medical writers, including Galen himself, was marked by sloppiness and superficiality. In Pietro's words, "Assignment of the cause of critical days is almost always in error, because the subject leads the *medicus* away from his own art, since it has more to do with astrology than natural philosophy." Pietro's objections were to the qualitative approach and astronomical ignorance of medical writers on critical days, exemplified by their ascription of special importance to the visibility of the moon and their failure to grasp the complexity of its motions. He explained to his own readers that all of the planets affected crisis in human illness through each of four different types of variation: position in the zodiac, relation to the cardinal points (ascendant, descendant, and upper and lower midheaven), position on the epicycle, and conjunctions and aspects (position in regard to other planets). Since the moon was the heavenly body primarily affecting critical days, a correct theory would have to be based on a full understanding of the several motions of the moon as described by Ptolemy and on an accurate knowledge of the different periods required to complete return in each. Pietro expressed his doubts whether precise prediction of critical days could in fact ever be achieved. In any case, Galen had lacked the necessary astronomical understanding or information; therefore his "medicinal month" was "a fantasy." Thus, medical astrology provided the occasion for one of the few instances before the sixteenth century in which a learned physician was prepared to disagree, openly and sharply, with Galen.[40]

The art of prognosis thus ranged from the type of intuitive response to symptoms made possible only by experience to the application of highly artificial and abstract astrological theories. Neither approach can be said to have belonged exclusively to any one category of practitioner. Although it is evident that only the learned would have engaged in the kind of discussion of critical days embarked on by Pietro d'Abano, abundant evidence exists in the form of miniature calendars, astronomical tables, and the like designed for medical use to indicate that ordinary practitioners based their conclusions on simplified astrological calculations.[41] And in the course of treating their numerous patients, some learned physicians doubtless acquired an intuitive recognition of the progress of disease that influenced their application of prognostic theory in particular instances.

Treatment

The ultimate goal of the treatment of disease was, of course, cure. But cure was not necessarily conceived of as a rapid, immediately recognizable return to total health. A more vague and diffuse concept of recovery was the concomitant of the complexional interpretation of health and disease and the similarity between the medical regimen for sickness and the dietary regimen for health, as well as of actual health conditions that must have involved much chronic illness, weakness, malnutrition, and lasting aftereffects of injuries. The Galenic idea of a neutral state between health and sickness surely accorded with the experience of medical practitioners.

Learned practitioners knew and discussed the fact that the relation between medical theory and medical practice was uneasy and ambiguous, although very few showed any signs of readiness to modify theory in the light of experience.[42] And, as noted in chapter 2, medical practitioners of all kinds had no monopoly on the administration of medical treatment. With or without medical guidance, patients practiced self-help in the form of self-medication, visits to medicinal baths, pilgrimages, or prayer; and religious shrines offering alternative forms of healing were omnipresent. In many instances, any of these endeavors was as likely to be successful—or unsuccessful—as the most skilled medical attention.

Operating within these constraints, practitioners treated mental and physical illness with three main types of therapy, traditionally classified as the three "instruments of medicine": diet, medication, and surgery.[43] Diet was an important component in the treatment of illness as well as in the maintenance of health; but because dietary principles were essentially the same in sickness and in health, no further discussion seems called for. Surgery, in the sense of treatment by incision, cautery, or physical manipulation, was from the thirteenth century normally relegated to surgeons, barber-surgeons, and barbers, although the division of labor was far from complete (see chapter 6). Two minor surgical procedures, cautery and phlebotomy, were, however, frequently prescribed by physicians as part of the treatment for complexional illness and will therefore be discussed in this chapter.

The use of cautery for complexional disorders (that is, internal complaints such as headache), as distinct from its surgical use for wounds, was predicated on the notion that actual cautery with a heated metal instrument or "potential" cautery by the application of heated cups or caustic substances to the skin could be used to direct good or bad humors to different parts of the body (figure 26; see also figure 37 in chapter 6). Cautery was an ancient technique that probably became more widespread in the medieval West after the influential surgical manual of Albucasis, which devoted much attention to the subject, became available in Latin during the course of the twelfth century (see chapter 6).

Knowledge of phlebotomy was part of medical skill, not only because some medical practitioners performed bloodletting themselves but also because an important part of any physician's task was to judge when and how

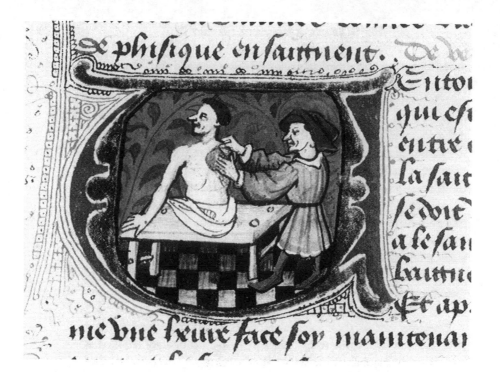

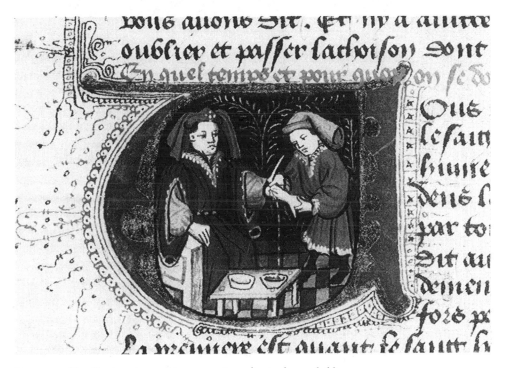

Figure 28   Bloodletting. A practitioner wearing a short robe, probably a surgeon or barber-surgeon, performs phlebotomy on a seated patient. A basin has been placed to catch the blood, which may subsequently be examined for purposes of diagnosis and prognosis. (Courtesy the Pierpont Morgan Library, New York, MS M. 165, mid-fifteenth century, fol. 19ᵛ.)

Figure 26 (Opposite, top)   Cupping. A practitioner places heated metal cups on a patient's skin in order to draw the humors to the body part being treated. (Courtesy the Pierpont Morgan Library, New York, MS M. 165, mid-fifteenth century, fol. 24ʳ.)

Figure 27 (Opposite, bottom)   A guide to bloodletting. The captions list the sites and, in some instances, the names of appropriate veins to incise for different complaints; lines link each caption with the body site in question. Thus, the sixth caption from the top on the left informs the reader that the basilic vein in the arm should be incised for complaints of the liver and spleen, and a guide line leads to a site on the inner arm just above the elbow. This chart comes from the small practitioner's handbook shown in figure 3. (Courtesy the Wellcome Institute Library, London, MS 40, a. 1463.)

phlebotomy should be performed (figure 27). Phlebotomy was unquestionably one of the most frequently used forms of general therapy; presumably its less painful character made it more tolerable to patients than cautery. The principle behind this ancient and long-lived therapeutic procedure was that bloodletting drew off corrupt matter from the body (figure 28). Each of the four humors, all of which were contained in blood, was capable of being transformed by disordered complexion into a harmful secondary humor that had to be removed if the patient was to recover (or maintain) health. Galen was influential in systematizing and elaborating these concepts as well as so many others.

Simple phlebotomy tracts circulated in western Europe during the early Middle Ages; but when the works of Haly Abbas, Avicenna, and Albucasis and some of Galen's own writings on the subject became available in Latin, they provided much fuller accounts of Galenic theories about phlebotomy and considerably more detailed practical instructions. The Arabo-Latin encyclopedic accounts formed the basis of subsequent Latin and vernacular treatises on phlebotomy. At least in the opinion of Pietro d'Abano, who reviewed the technical literature on phlebotomy available in Latin about 1300, the Arabic medical writers who transmitted Greek phlebotomy doctrine were somewhat more conservative in their recommendation of venesection than their Greek sources had been. Pietro thought that the difference in emphasis might have been because the Arabs wrote in a hot climate, where the local diseases would be of a kind for which phlebotomy would not be useful. By contrast, the Greeks, although they wrote "for the whole world and not just for Italy," provided directions suitable for the robust constitutions found in temperate climates such as that of Italy.[44]

Practitioners could inform themselves from the technical literature as to conditions for which bleeding was appropriate, together with the correct vein to incise for each. Most commonly, blood was drawn from one of three major veins of the arm (named the cephalic, median, and basilic); but other veins were opened for particular conditions—for example, melancholy might call for bleeding from a vein in the forehead. Bloodletting was normally performed by surgical venesection, although leeches were also used on occasion. Textbooks and manuals also gave fairly detailed directions for ligating the arm, making an incision, recognizing and avoiding nearby nerves and arteries, and stemming bleeding. Also provided were rules and recommendations regarding the patient's diet before and after the procedure and appropriate seasons of the year, phases of the moon, and times of day for performing the operation in different types of patients and cases.

Phlebotomy called for the practitioner to exercise both theoretical and practical judgment. Fundamental theoretical issues were whether it was preferable to draw a large quantity of blood at once (removing much noxious humor, but possibly causing the patient to faint) or a series of small amounts and whether it was preferable to bleed on the side of the body nearest or the side of the body furthest away from the part afflicted—that is, whether the bad humors should be drawn off directly from the site of the disease or encouraged first to migrate away from that site. The second of these issues, important in the ancient literature and well known in the Middle Ages, took a fresh lease on life in the early sixteenth century under the stimulus of a fuller knowledge of both Greek medical texts and human anatomy and inspired a controversy in which Vesalius was an active participant.

At a more immediately practical level, practitioners had to consider the possible hazards of phlebotomy, hazards of which they were well aware. Routine advice was that small children, pregnant women, the old, and very weak patients should not be phlebotomized. The author of one phlebotomy manual, who wrote probably at Montpellier at some time between about 1150 and 1225, firmly repudiated the notion that it was ever desirable to remove such a large quantity of blood that the patient fainted; he frankly gave as his reason fear of the opinion of ordinary people outside medicine. The translator of a Middle English version of the same text made about 1400 added a series of dire warnings about the damage unskilled phlebotomy could do, especially by inadvertently cutting an artery or by causing the arm to become so swollen that death ensued (presumably as a result of the introduction of infection by the knife or lancet).[45]

Of the three instruments of medicine, medication was the principal form of active intervention by which physicians sought to combat disease. The choice of appropriate medicinal substances and their compounding in the proper proportions were central areas of medical knowledge (figure 29). The foundation of medieval European pharmacy—as of traditional herbal medicine in other societies—was the attribution of medicinal powers to commonly available substances, usually plants and often those that might also be used in cooking. Sharp taste, pungent aroma, and unusual texture as well as readily perceptible action of some kind (for example, as a laxative or opiate) were all properties that might lead to the classification of a plant as medicinal. Unquestionably, consistent use of certain common European plants as medicines began in antiquity and had a continuous history thereafter. But in western Europe, even in the early Middle Ages, this simple "kitchen-garden" medicine was never purely empirical, local, folkloric, and handed down by oral tradition—although these characteristics must surely have been present to some extent—but seems always also to have contained elements derived from Greek medicine by way of written sources.[46] From the early Middle Ages to the high Renaissance, medicinal recipes were the commonest form of medical writing.

The new medical literature that began to become available from the late eleventh century included much technical pharmacology. Principal items included an alphabetized and enlarged version of an older Latin translation of the collection of materia medica by Dioscorides, a lengthy treatise by Galen on medicinal simples (that is, individual medicinal substances), and long sections on simple and compound medicines in the Arabic encyclopedic works.[47] One compilation of lasting influence, produced in Salerno, was the *Antidotarium Nicolai,* a work that listed remedies for particular complaints with little attention to pharmaceutical theory.

Practitioners studied these materials, and other works based on them in lengthy or abbreviated, complex or simplified, Latin or vernacular versions, depending upon the reader's educational level and whether his or her immediate purposes were academic or practical. The knowledge thus gained was in some sense applied in practice, but the relation between the data and theories contained in the books and the practitioner's actual experience of the effect of various substances on the body can seldom have been direct or unambiguous. In addition to inevitable variations in individual patient response, nomenclature and identification of medicinal substances, pharmacological theory, and actual sources of ingredients all presented problems.

Botanical pharmacology was a major area of Arabic medical science and one involving notable original contributions beyond those made by the Greeks. At both the eastern and the western ends of the Islamic world, in

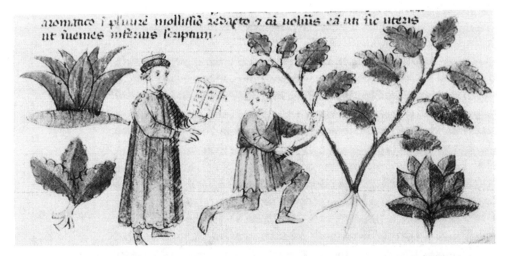

Figure 29   Medicinal botany is represented as part of a learned tradition in this imaginary author portrait of "Apuleius," garbed as a long-robed physician and giving instructions from his herbal to someone cutting medicinal plants. (Courtesy the Yale Medical Library, MS 18, *Herbarium Apulei,* ca. 1400, fol. 6r.)

Persia and in Spain, botanical investigation contributed the names of more plants than had been known to Dioscorides or Galen; from eastern Islam, too, came knowledge of the names of plants from India and China.[48] Hence the improved knowledge of Greek and introduction of Islamic pharmacology represented, in principle, a very significant addition to the botanical information available in western Europe.

Any potential practical usefulness in medicine was, however, offset by the increased possibilities of confusion in substance identification and nomenclature provided by the multiplication of translated or transliterated plant names.[49] Plant naming was of course unsystematic in all of the languages involved. European practitioners were faced with a multitude of plant names of Latin, Greek, Arabic, and vernacular origin. The rendering of names from Greek and Arabic into Latin was accomplished in some instances by translation, in others by transliteration; different authors might choose different ways of rendering the same name. As a result, the same plant might be known by several different names, or a completely different plant might be identified with one mentioned by an ancient or Islamic author. Nor did visual images provide any consistent means of controlling nomenclature. Manuscripts of herbals and similar works were by no means always illustrated; and although a few notable examples of naturalistic plant depiction are to be found before the fifteenth century, there was no securely established tradition of naturalistic illustration to aid in plant identification (figures 30 and 31).

Medical practitioners were acutely aware of these difficulties, as is shown by the compilation of medical glossaries and by Gentile da Foligno's complaints about the incomprehensibility of some of the transliterated Arabic terms in a collection of medicinal recipes that forms Book 5 of the *Canon* of Avicenna.[50] Furthermore, recognition that some ingredients described in books of Greek or Islamic origin were unavailable led to the compilation, under the general title *quid pro quo*, of lists of permissible substitutions, although it is by no means clear on what basis it was decided, for example, that oregano was an acceptable replacement for *abrotano*.[51] But it also seems likely that practitioners improvised substitutions or made them unknowingly. By the late fifteenth and early sixteenth centuries, this complex of problems gave rise to vigorous controversies over the proper identification of substances mentioned in the texts (from the pedestrian rhubarb to the exotic mummy), and, ultimately, to demands for a revised and purified pharmacopoeia characteristic of various forms of sixteenth-century medical neotericism.

Although information about medicinal substances came chiefly, albeit

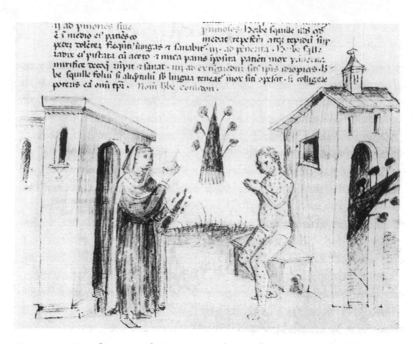

Figure 30   A medication and its uses. According to the caption, among the uses of
the herb squill was treatment of complaints causing itching, one of which is vividly
illustrated here. A highly stylized depiction of the herb itself appears three times in
the picture, presumably to emphasize its shape: it is shown once in relatively natural dimensions in the practitioner's hand and twice greatly enlarged. (Courtesy the
Yale Medical Library, MS 18, *Herbarium Apulei*, ca. 1400, fol. 23ʳ.)

Figure 31 (Right and opposite)
Naturalistic plant illustrations in a
manuscript copied near Venice in
the mid-fourteenth century. The
book contains pictures without text
except for substance names, and it
has been variously identified as intended to accompany the Salernitan
work on remedies known as *Circa in-
stans*, or the Latin alphabetized version of Dioscorides, or as a model
book for illustrators of herbals.
Plants shown on these pages include
shepherd's purse, crocus, and sting-
ing nettle. Glass-blowing, already a
Venetian specialty in the fourteenth
century, is presumably shown in a
manuscript devoted mainly to medicinal plants because of the association of medical practitioners with
glass urine flasks. (Courtesy the Pierpont Morgan Library, New York,
MS M. 873, fols. 20ᵛ, 27ʳ, 90ʳ.)

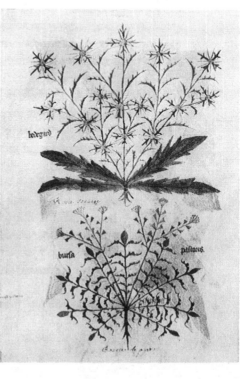

often indirectly, from Dioscorides and from the Arabic authors, Galen was the principal source of the pharmaceutical theories of the later Middle Ages. The large body of data available from the twelfth century could not be assimilated without the aid of unifying theoretical principles. These were provided by Galen's incorporation of simples into the theory of primary qualities and complexionate balance; simple medicines were hot or wet or cold or dry, and their action depended on these qualities. In Galenic medicine, therefore, rational treatment consisted of finding a medicine with qualities that counterbalanced the patient's complexional disorder—hence the idea of cure by contraries. In the simplest possible example, a cold medicine would cure a hot disease.

This formulation left two areas open for further discussion, adumbrated by Galen and greatly elaborated by Islamic and, after the mid-thirteenth century, by Latin medical writers. One was how to explain the action of various substances that, for whatever reason, were not considered to act by virtue of the primary qualities. Avicenna, in the *Canon*, was influential in enlarging the idea suggested by Galen that some medicines, simple or compound, had particular, individual effects due not to the primary qualities but to a purely idiosyncratic "specific form." The paradigmatic example of action by specific form—which was regarded as an occult property in the

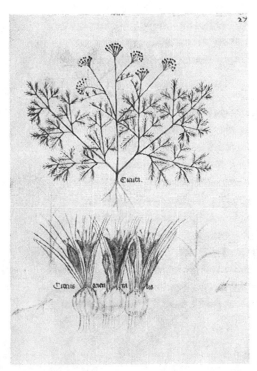

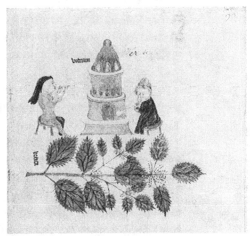

sense of natural but not susceptible of rational explanation—was the action of a magnet. (This was considered an example of action at a distance of a kind not allowed for by Aristotelian laws of motion.) The powers attributed to theriac were explained as being due to its specific form. The idea of "specific form" was useful in that it gave practitioners an alternative to explanations couched in terms of the primary qualities and complexion, and later it suggested the analogy of diseases with specific, idiosyncratic action; however, it also facilitated arbitrary assertions about the occult powers of supposedly medicinal substances.

The second area of inquiry was the problem of defining, measuring, or describing varying intensities of qualities in individual medicinal substances and how one might determine the overall effect of combining ingredients of different qualities in different intensities into a compound medicine. In a broader sense, the issues involved were current in contemporary natural philosophy as well as in medicine. As far as pharmacy was concerned, Galen had taught the existence of four "degrees" of strength of the primary qualities in medicines. Subsequently, two Arabic authors, Alkindi (Al-Kindī, d. ca. 873) and Averroes, discussed ways of devising mathematical rules to determine the complexion of a compound medicine based on the quantity and degree of each of its ingredients. This notion was taken up and elaborated by Arnald of Villanova at Montpellier during the 1290s. Arnald's rules for determining the complexion of a compound are of interest for their role in the development of ideas about quantification in the period; but Arnald himself seems to have thought them too complicated for use in practice, as his own simple prescriptions show. In this instance, the increasing sophistication of theory removed it almost entirely from influence upon practice.[52]

Finally, the very urban and commercial developments that in so many ways fostered the growth of the medical community distanced some medical practitioners from personal familiarity with medical ingredients. Although practitioners in the early Middle Ages presumably obtained and put together their own materia medica and doubtless continued to do so in rural areas, by the second half of the thirteenth century, tradesmen who made a specialty of compounding and selling medicinal substances were to be found in Italian cities (see figure 22); for example, the grandfather of the anatomist Mondino de' Liuzzi owned a pharmacy in Bologna about 1270. Recent studies have shown that in fourteenth- and fifteenth-century Florence and sixteenth-century Venice, individual physicians associated themselves with particular pharmacies (see figure 2 in chapter 2); in Florence, in some instances, physician and pharmacist had a contractual arrangement

whereby the practitioner made himself available for consultation with patients on the pharmacist's premises (and prescribed the pharmacist's medications).[53] Furthermore, there was a flourishing Mediterranean trade in materia medica; Venice, in particular, was a major entrepôt for the import of
medicinal substances from the Middle East. The actual content of some of
these exotica could have been known neither to the pharmacists who sold
them nor to the practitioners who prescribed them. For example, the medical reformer Giambatista Da Monte (d. 1551) pointed out that the mummy
(*mumia*) sold in Venetian pharmacies in the early 1540s was certainly not the
authentic substance, which he defined as an aromatic exudate from corpses
of the spices that had been used in embalming them, gathered from ancient
tombs in Arabia.[54] Late fifteenth- and early sixteenth-century critics of academic physicians and Arabo-Latin medicine attacked the practice of relying
on pharmacists to compound medicines precisely because it took direct
knowledge and control of medicinal ingredients out of the hands of the
practitioner.

In reality, medical prescription was probably often a simpler matter than
some of the technical literature, and certainly than pharmaceutical theory,
would lead one to suppose. The prescription of local herbs for local diseases,
much advocated by sixteenth-century Paracelsian reformers of pharmacy,
was probably always the norm for empirics and their patients, if only on
economic grounds. On occasion, physicians tailored their prescriptions to
the patient's ability to pay—cheap, easily obtainable ingredients for the
ordinary patient; exotic drugs, gold, or precious stones for the rich. The
medical faculty of the University of Paris recommended that the king and
queen preserve their health against the plague with a smelling "apple" of
pure ambergris of the finest quality; on grounds of cost, the faculty prescribed other aromatics for the king's subjects. Gentile da Foligno thought
the poor should use any strong-smelling herbs for the same purpose.[55] It
would be unnecessarily cynical to suppose that either the Paris faculty or
Gentile believed that medications for the rich were significantly more effective than those for the poor, or vice versa. Possibly exotica inspired greater
confidence or hope in the patients, since some of them had a fairly realistic
idea of the results to be expected from simple forms of medication with
local products. Several people who had sought out the ministrations of St.
Francesca Romana assured the commission of inquiry into her sanctity that
their recovery must have been due to a miracle since the saint's home remedies—"ordinary oil," wine, rue, marjoram, and an ointment made from
lard and zinc oxide (*tucia*)—could not possibly have cured complaints ranging from a seriously burned hand to plague.[56]

Recipe collections, *consilia*, and elementary manuals such as the *Treasury of the Poor*, although still removed from actual practice, may be a better guide than more sophisticated medical literature to the kinds of medicines most frequently prescribed. Medicines were normally compounds, but the number of ingredients was not necessarily very large; some, such as oil or wine for liquid medicines and wax or grease for ointments, served only as a base. Moreover, in various manuals and textbooks, medicaments were classified on the basis of function—for example, cleansing, strengthening, pain-relieving (*sedantes dolorem*), stupefacient—as well as in terms of the primary qualities. These examples come from a handbook of medicines compiled in the late thirteenth century, which opened with a triple classification of simples: by function, by the part of the body or condition for which they were useful, and alphabetically.[57]

Frequently used remedies included wine, employed since antiquity for cleansing wounds, and various laxatives and emetics (figure 32), prized because they removed superfluities or bad humors. Most ingredients came from plants (figure 33), a fair number from animals (figure 34), and a few from minerals (figure 35). Emphasis on the medicinal use of excreta make some of the recipes using animal ingredients unappealing to a modern reader—another of the remedies collected by Petrus Hispanus suggested that the application of pig dung would stop a nosebleed—but in general it seems likely that the great majority of remedies were entirely harmless. A medication new to Europe in the thirteenth century was alcohol, in the form of aqua vitae. To Taddeo Alderotti, aqua vitae seemed an exceptionally powerful and effective remedy; he wrote with enthusiasm about its usefulness for external application to cleanse wounds, as a pain reliever on an aching tooth, and as a medium for cordials, and he noted approvingly its cheering psychological effect.[58]

Although the range of substances actually likely to have been in common use included a few that could be relied upon to produce fairly consistent, perceptible results, the ability of practitioners to produce predictable effects by medication was limited. The only means available of controlling the amount or concentrations in which medicines were administered were rough and largely intuitive or empirical. Physicians discussed dosage to some extent, at any rate in the abstract, but although some medicinal recipes specify quantities, a great many do not. Means of preparation, when they are described or alluded to, more often suggest the kitchen than the laboratory. Moreover, although in some instances commonsense, empirical, and naturalistic folk medicine doubtless lay behind the repeated prescription of some common plants for many conditions of very different kinds, in other cases the original basis for favoring particular plants was not naturalistic but magical (figure 36). Thus, a modern scholar has noted that vervain, or verbena (*Verbena officinalis*), a common plant with a magical reputation but no noteworthy therapeutic properties, was variously recommended for the bite of a rabid dog, as a painkiller, as a diuretic, to bring on menstruation, to reduce fever, restore a nursing mother's milk, stop bleeding, and keep away the plague.[59]

The notion that certain herbs had a magical effectiveness was one of several ways in which magical beliefs and practices played a part in therapy. It should be emphasized, however, that the vast majority of remedies and therapeutic practices was entirely naturalistic. Furthermore, although belief in the existence of demons and malign magic was general, these were seldom blamed for ill health except, as already noted, in the case of impotence. The conviction that witchcraft and demonic possession posed substantial and ever-present dangers to health was a feature of the witch panic that afflicted parts of Europe in the sixteenth and seventeenth centuries, not before.

A few traces of beneficent therapeutic magic can be found in some written collections of remedies; magic doubtless played a wider role in the practice of empirics. For example, certain substances noted for their magical properties—peony was one of them—were frequently called for in medical recipes. The normal mode of using supposedly therapeutic substances was to ingest them or apply them to the skin in the form of ointments, poultices, and so on; sometimes, however, they were placed in amulets or administered to the accompaniment of recited charms. This simple magic can best be regarded as a form of folk healing, even though the remedies to which magical powers were ascribed often derived from ancient medicine (which itself had a folkloric component) and the charms were Christian.

At a more learned level, magic and astrology were both essential, and at bottom inseparable, components of the view of the natural world transmitted from late antiquity and Islam. Since celestial forces were believed to govern all things on earth, they were naturally held to affect plants, animals, and stones—that is, medicinal ingredients—and, of course, the human body itself. Both astrology and learned magic might be used in therapy but in very different ways. From the fourteenth century, medical practitioners routinely sought to assist therapy by finding out when a favorable alignment of the heavens would occur and timing their activities accordingly; thus, they consulted astronomical tables to find out when the position or phase of the moon was best for gathering medicinal plants, administering medicines, or performing phlebotomy. Such practices, like the other forms of

Figure 32 (Below) A female attendant holds the forehead of a vomiting female patient. Although this picture may simply represent someone with a bilious attack, the administration of emetics was included, along with bloodletting and purging, among the standard procedures for evacuating harmful humors. (Courtesy the Pierpont Morgan Library, New York, MS M. 165, mid-fifteenth century, fol. 33ʳ.)

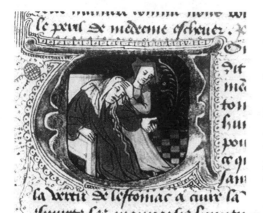

Figure 33 (Above) A patient who is pointing expressively to his chest buys oil of almonds for his cough. This image comes from an illustrated *Tacuinum sanitatis*. Some copies, made for wealthy clients, present the same information found in the tabular version in the form of pictures and accompanying captions or brief text. The caption describes the uses, characteristics, advantages, and disadvantages of oil of almonds according to just the same categories as those in figure 23. (Courtesy the Bild-Archiv der Österreichischen Nationalbibliothek, Vienna, MS ser. nova. 2644, end of the fourteenth century, fol. 91ʳ.)

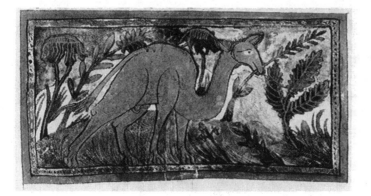

Figure 34 Although the remedies derived from exotic animals such as this camel, depicted in a copy of the work of Sextus Placitus in the same codex as figure 36, can seldom have been used in western Europe, medicines were made from locally available animal substances of various kinds. (Courtesy the Wellcome Institute Library, London, MS 573, mid-thirteenth century, fol. 80ʳ.)

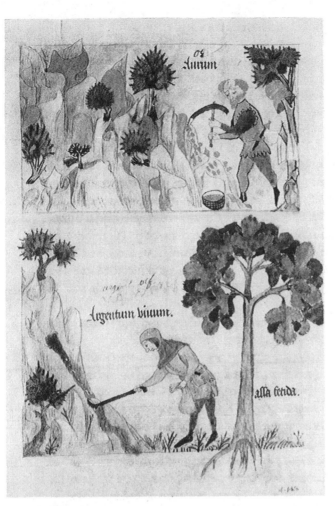

Figure 35   Most medieval medications were herbal, but mineral substances were also used. Another page from the manuscript containing the illustrations reproduced in figure 31 shows somewhat fanciful depictions of mining for gold and quicksilver (mercury). (Courtesy the Pierpont Morgan Library, New York, MS M. 873, mid-fourteenth century, fol. 1ᵛ.)

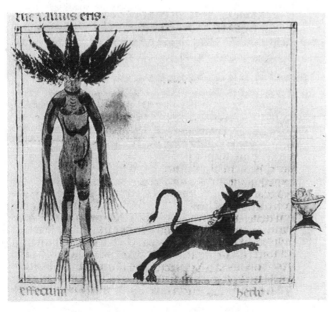

Figure 36   A magical plant remedy and procedure. The legend of the mandrake plant, illustrated here from the herbal of Apuleius in a collection of works on remedies copied in Italy in the mid-thirteenth century, asserted that the mandrake screamed in a human voice when uprooted and that whoever pulled it up would die. Consequently, the approved procedure was to tie a dog to the mandrake root and tempt the dog to pull up the plant with an offer of meat held at a judicious distance. (Courtesy the Wellcome Institute Library, London, MS 573, Antonius Musa and others. De herba vettonica, fol. 35ᵛ.)

astrological medicine that have been mentioned so far, were wholly rational and considered entirely reputable from both a religious and a scientific standpoint. By contrast, therapeutic magic involved direct attempts to control or manipulate celestial or occult forces and was regarded with suspicion by both Jewish and Christian religious authorities. One form of learned therapeutic magic was to engrave astral images on precious stones that the patient would then wear as a talisman, a practice tried by Jewish and Christian physicians at Montpellier in the early fourteenth century.[60] Interest in the beneficent manipulation of astral and occult forces for therapeutic purposes intensified in the fifteenth century. It was widespread at the University of Padua, then a major center for the teaching of practical medicine, and one of the most famous and influential Renaissance accounts of astral magic occurs in a work largely devoted to astrological medicine, the *Three Books on Life* (1489) by the Platonic philosopher and learned physician Marsilio Ficino.[61]

Obviously, in attempting to evaluate medieval and early Renaissance therapeutic knowledge and techniques, the measure cannot be that of modern standards of physical effectiveness; nor can one expect to find either progressive accumulation of scientific knowledge or sustained and systematic endeavors to test and modify theory by experience. In these respects, neither the greatly enlarged body of knowledge received in the eleventh and twelfth centuries nor the experience of plague brought any improvements, or much change. Nonetheless, during this period the branch of medical knowledge known *as practica* (dealing with particulars of disease and treatment) underwent one important development; it became the focus of serious intellectual attention at major centers of learning. Especially in the late fourteenth and the fifteenth centuries, discussion of specifics pertaining to disease and treatment seems to have absorbed an increasing amount of the time and energy of the most highly educated physicians. The outpouring of plague literature testifies to this, as do developments in the fifteenth-century University of Padua, where many of the best-known professors and medical authors taught the branch of the curriculum known as *practica* or wrote on practical subjects (again, Michele Savonarola is a leading example).[62] The increasing attention to astrological and magical aids to therapy can also be associated with the same trend. The bent toward the particular and the specific manifested in the interest in *practica* of fifteenth-century Italian medical professors and their students was part of the background of later innovations already mentioned: critiques of Arabo-Latin pharmacology, new theories about disease, and the new anatomy.

SIX

SURGEONS AND SURGERY

ccording to Pietro d'Abano, some people alleged that the only part of medicine that offered any certainty was surgery, because surgery alone yielded obvious physical results.[1] The enthusiasts for surgery whose views Pietro came across in professional and intellectual circles at Paris or Padua in the decades around 1300 were probably educated and ambitious surgeons. Demand for surgical knowledge and the production of specialized technical writing on surgery had been a marked characteristic of literate medicine in Italy since the late twelfth century and at Montpellier since the mid–thirteenth century; by the time Pietro wrote, a similar emphasis was emerging among some literate practitioners at Paris.

Almost contemporary with the view of surgery recorded by Pietro d'Abano was the response of Vito and Letizia da Villa Casale, a modestly prosperous married couple of Montefalco. When their thirteen-year-old son developed what was probably an inguinal hernia in 1308, they called in a *medicus* who prescribed surgical intervention ("touching and cutting"); the anxious parents jointly decided not to allow the operation but to take their Giovanillo to the shrine of Chiara da Montefalco instead (Chiara was, posthumously, especially renowned as a healer of hernias). The reasons for Vito and Letizia's choice of treatment and the choices of the other early fourteenth-century parents in the diocese of Spoleto, who arrived at a similar decision, can only be guessed at.[2] But some patients who refused recommendations for surgical treatment in favor of visits to shrines expressed fear of the pain of the knife; further, some forms of surgical treatment of hernia practiced in the fourteenth century might entail castration.[3]

These two very different glimpses of surgery in the decades before and after 1300 reflect extremes of enthusiasm and avoidance in extreme situations: rival claims of expertise by physicians and surgeons in the first instance, and in the second the prospect of submitting a child to one of the more risky operations performed by early surgeons. By contrast, in less extreme situations, the daily reality of much surgical practice appears to have involved—in addition to phlebotomy—the routine and doubtless usually more or less successful treatment of injuries such as broken limbs, sprains, dislocations, burns, scalds, cuts, bites, and bruises as well as the treatment by medication of all kinds of swellings or eruptions on the surface of the body. Practitioners who possessed knowledge of bonesetting, bandaging, suturing, and bloodletting provided valuable services for which there was always a social need. Between the twelfth and the fifteenth centuries, surgical literature in Latin and in European vernaculars underwent a richly complex evolution that is in many respects parallel to and entwined with the history of medical writing in general. In the same period, surgery as an occupation was, to a greater or lesser extent at different times and places, separated from the rest of medical practice, and it developed distinct forms of organization and hierarchies of practitioners. But these intellectual and professional developments, which are the subject of this chapter, were possible only in the context of a successfully transmitted craft tradition of simple surgical techniques and of widespread demand for and appreciation of at least some forms of surgical intervention.

Surgery was at once a branch of knowledge conveyed in technical writing, an occupation, and a form of physical manipulation of the human body. As we shall see, "surgery" was considered to include, and surgeons carried out, much treatment by medication as well as procedures involving manipulation and surgical incision or repair. Early surgery developed in the absence of adequate means to control serious pain, bleeding, and infection. The consequent realistic assessment by surgeons of what was possible limited the scope of actual surgical intervention to more or less the following list, essentially unchanged between antiquity and a period long after that covered by the present book: crisis intervention for injuries inflicted by external causes; treatment, often by externally applied medication, of chronic complications resulting from such injuries, notably ulcers or fistulas arising from infected wounds; treatment by incision, excision, cautery, or medication of swellings and blemishes on the skin; and couching for cataract. In addition, as already noted, venesection, cautery, and cupping were employed as treatments for internal disorders. Outside these categories, surgical intervention was likely to be attempted for only a handful of immediately life-threatening or acutely painful conditions, among them urinary obstruction, vesical calculi, and carious teeth.[4]

Physical realities and technical limitations governed not only the range of conditions that could be surgically treated but also the range of possible procedures. This consideration applies to both tools and techniques. Although surgeons had had specialized tools since antiquity, Western manuscript illustrations from the twelfth to the fifteenth centuries suggest that in this period such tools were in most instances not very highly differentiated or sophisticated (figure 37). According to Guy de Chauliac, the essential equipment of the surgeon consisted of knives, razors, and lancets for making incisions, cautery irons, grasping tools, probes, needles, cannulae, and a tool for trepanation (the last may seldom have been put to use).[5] The very similar collection of a late-fifteenth-century surgeon appears in figure 38. To this list may be added sutures, pads, and bandages.

As far as technique is concerned, the physical manipulations involved in the treatment of fractures and dislocations and the suturing (figure 39)—as distinct from the dressing and medication—of wounds, demand manual dexterity and a measure of anatomical knowledge. Hence, procedures effective in principle (that is, provided infection or uncontrollable bleeding did not occur) could readily be developed by ancient surgical craftsmen and their medieval successors. Such procedures offered relatively little incentive or opportunity for technical or theoretical elaboration. For example, a depressed skull fracture confronted the surgeon with the evident necessity of removing fragments of bone and, to the extent possible, protecting or limiting damage to the dura mater. The tasks themselves were imposed by the situation, and options for varying techniques were few. Consequently, similar simple techniques would presumably be developed independently at different times and places. The procedure of setting a broken limb with splints and stiffened bandages need not have varied very much, regardless of whether the operator learned it by reading a textbook based on ancient sources or by watching a skilled surgeon and then practicing under his supervision, although the latter method might well yield a greater ability actually to perform the procedure. In the case of surgery, even more than for other aspects of therapy, it thus becomes peculiarly difficult to weigh the relation between technical writing and actual techniques.

As with the rest of medicine, the expectations of both surgeons and their patients helped to delimit the scope of surgery and to define success and failure. Surgeons frequently expressed pride and confidence in the value of surgical knowledge; as will become apparent later in this chapter, some of them vaunted their own skills and professional successes in no uncertain terms. But they were also highly conscious of the limited range of surgery and of its risks; there seems to have been much cautious avoidance of intervention in serious cases. In this way, surgeons sought to protect themselves as well as to avoid inflicting pointless additional pain and raising false hopes. Textbooks taught the recognition of some malignant tumors, notably breast cancer, and contained lists of organs to which wounds were likely to be

Figure 37 Surgical instruments from a fifteenth-century manuscript of a translation into Middle English of Guy de Chauliac's work on surgery (fol. 164ᵛ). Illustrated are knives, pincers, and cautery irons of various shapes. Compare this relatively realistic presentation with the highly stylized depiction of the same subject in figure 41. (Courtesy of the New York Academy of Medicine Library.)

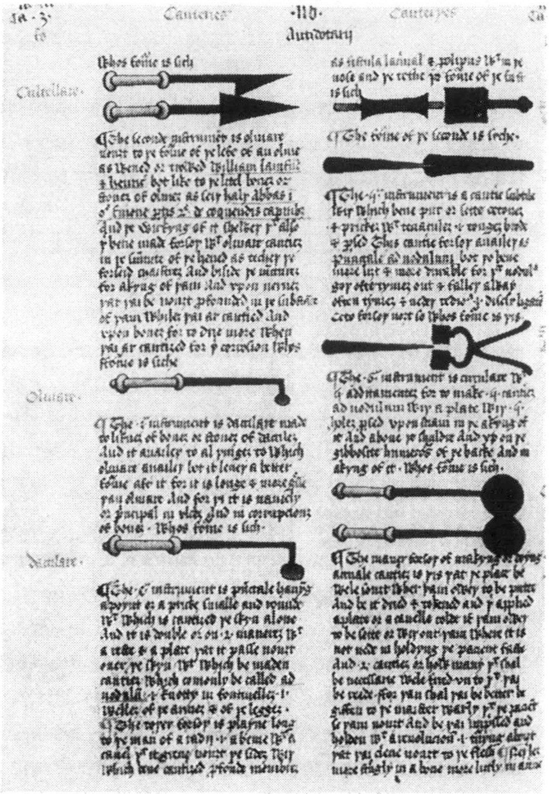

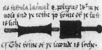

Figure 38 Surgical instruments illustrated in an edition of Hieronymus Brunschwig's German *Buch der Chirurgie*, printed in 1497 (fol. XIXʳ). Among the instruments depicted are tongs, pincers, a saw, and scissors. (Courtesy the New York Academy of Medicine Library.)

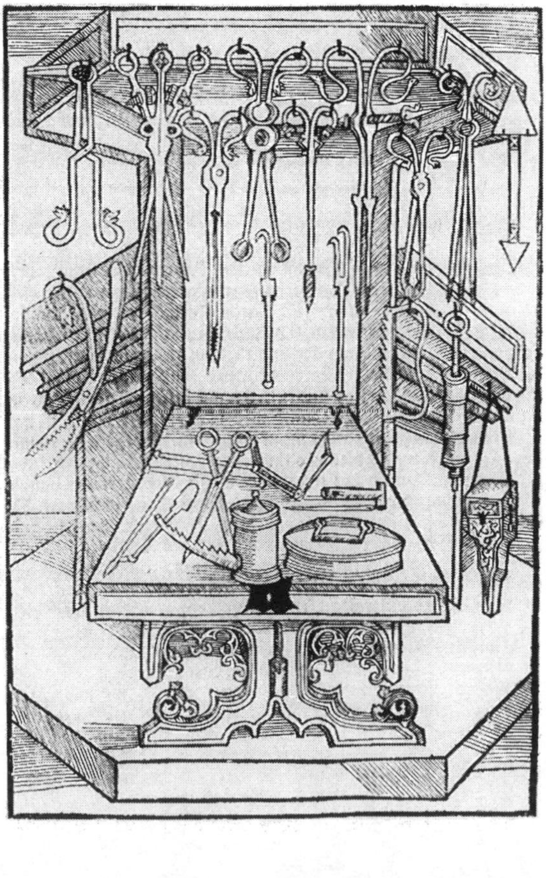

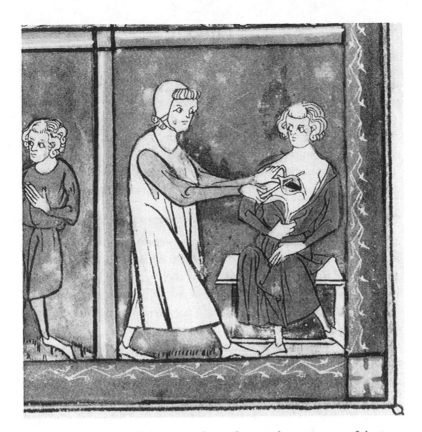

Figure 39   Suturing. In this miniature from a fourteenth-century copy of the *Surgery* of Roger, the size of the wound has been exaggerated to show the procedure clearly. Although not realistic, the picture is technically informative. (Courtesy of the British Library, MS Sloan 1977, fol. 6ᵛ.

mortal; the object was to warn against attempting treatment. Some books emphasized that tooth extraction should be undertaken only as a procedure of last resort.[6] The confident butchery ascribed by a Muslim witness to a "Frankish physician" present in the Holy Land in the mid-twelfth century cannot have been characteristic. According to this report, the European practitioner treated a patient's abscessed leg by summoning a knight to amputate it with an axe, with the result that the patient had a massive hemorrhage and died immediately. In reality, amputation of limbs through living tissue was probably rare before the sixteenth century.[7]

By contrast, the anxieties that could beset a conscientious and thoughtful surgeon are vividly conveyed by an example (possibly hypothetical) in an early thirteenth-century manual for confessors: "A surgeon came and confessed that he often performed lithotomies, and after the operation many of his patients died; but he really didn't know whether he was the cause of their deaths or not."[8] For the author of this manual, lithotomy provided a classic example of a surgical operation involving high levels of risk that had to be weighed against the severe pain and danger of the condition it was designed to relieve. Stone in the bladder was apparently a fairly common condition in the ancient and medieval world (both East and West), as it certainly was in early modern Europe. The frequency with which lithotomy was actually performed before the sixteenth century and the rate of success or failure are unknown. However, lithotomists, who were often itinerant, certainly practiced, and a procedure for the operation was described in surgical textbooks. Albucasis, following ancient authors, called for the surgeon to insert his finger into the patient's rectum in order to work the stone down toward the neck of the bladder and then to make a perineal incision through which the stone could be extracted. Evidently such an operation demanded a high level of dexterity and a good working knowledge of complex regional anatomy.

Clearly, surgery, much more than any other form of therapy practiced, called on occasion for the practitioner to make difficult decisions that had immediate and highly obvious consequences for the patient's survival, or future health or impairment. And despite, or because of, their schooled caution, skilled surgeons evidently believed their knowledge equipped them to make such decisions. The practitioner and university professor of medicine and surgery Dino del Garbo would probably have had little patience with the scruples of the lithotomist referred to in the last paragraph; writing around 1308, Dino explained that in choosing the appropriate treatment in individual cases of skull fracture the surgeon should take into consideration the risks inherent in each of two possible procedures, the patient's general health, and the precise nature of the injury. He evidently assumed that a well-trained surgeon ought to be capable of making such an informed judgment.[9]

Moreover, the facts that surgery flourished as a craft and a branch of knowledge and that patients sought out surgical treatment and paid the surgeons' fees surely indicate that, by and large, the accomplishments of surgery satisfied prevailing social expectations. Although some people such as the couple from Spoleto mentioned at the beginning of this chapter refused surgery, many others willingly underwent surgical procedures that were known to be potentially dangerous as well as painful. Doubtless this was so because most of the patients who endured major surgical intervention (herniotomy, lithotomy, repair of large wounds, treatment or fractures of the skull or compound fractures, for example) were already suffering from painful, disabling, and in some instances—as in the case of wounds involving extensive loss of blood—immediately life-threatening conditions. In such circumstances, surgery would appear either essential or, at the very least, an option well worth considering.

A natural desire to avoid painful treatments if possible may, however, have provided patient as well as expert endorsement for the use of internal and external medications as an alternative to surgery in treating conditions such as tooth decay and anal fistulas.[10] Dino del Garbo noted that it was widely believed that skull fractures could be cured by the use of plasters alone, without the procedure recommended, in one form or another, by most authoritative textbooks, which called for enlarging or, if necessary, making an incision in the scalp; smoothing the edges of the opening in the skull and, if need be, enlarging it; elevating any depressed bone; and removing any bone fragments. Dino attributed the belief in the efficacy of plasters used alone to the extreme willingness of the public to believe in such cures and to the ignorance or deceit of empirics. Dino was evidently well aware of the difficulty of diagnosing head wounds by palpation and observation; he asserted that the empirics either themselves genuinely could not tell skull fractures from other head wounds or else inflated their own powers by claiming that any head wound they had cured was a skull fracture. Dino's own opinion, based on his experience, was that the cure of fractures by plasters alone might indeed take place, but only very occasionally.[11]

In the context of these techniques and the expectations of surgery outlined above, the successful repair of a major abdominal wound (figure 40) was an unusual feat worthy of commemoration. In his surgical textbook, completed in 1276, Guglielmo da Saliceto recounted a claimed success with pardonable pride (and perhaps some exaggeration of the severity of the wound). When Giovanni da Pavia was wounded in the belly, the practitioner first summoned, Guglielmo's friend Master Ottobono da Pavia, saw the intestines hanging out of the wound and said, "He's a dead man." Nonetheless, Ottobono tried and failed to put the gut back in place. Then he and the patient's friends rushed to the Palazzo Comunale to fetch Guglielmo himself. When Guglielmo saw the condition of the patient, he was extremely anxious, especially since (according to him) the intestines themselves were injured and fecal matter was escaping. As an emergency measure, there being no time to send for medications, Guglielmo washed the intestines in heated wine and succeeded in restoring them in place. The wound was sutured, Ottobono undertook postoperative care, and "after he recovered the patient married and had children and lived for a long time."[12]

The sketch of surgery just presented reflects physical realities common to all early surgical practice but assumes the social context of the developed surgical craft, occupation, and learning that existed in western Europe in the late Middle Ages and early Renaissance. Let us now turn to examine the origins and course of the developments that allowed surgery to emerge as a well-organized, distinct occupation and that fostered the expansion in technical writing about surgery in both Latin and vernacular languages in the twelfth to the fifteenth centuries.

Despite intractable physical realities, surgery fully shared in the striking

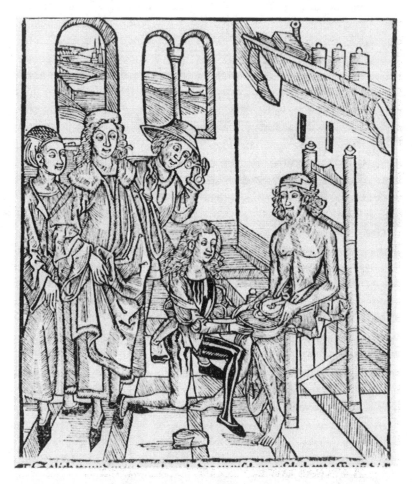

Figure 40   Treatment of an abdominal wound. The patient's calm demeanor is a reminder that, despite the naturalistic effects, the illustration is purely decorative; it is neither realistic nor technically informative. (Courtesy the New York Academy of Medicine, Hieronymus Brunschweig, *Buch der Chirurgie* [1497], fol. LXXVIIIʳ.)

intellectual, social, and professional development of all aspects of medicine that began in the late eleventh century. Before then, of course, simple surgery was included among the forms of healing practiced in the early Middle Ages, as both skeletal and written evidence attests. Yet, with the exception of brief tracts on phlebotomy and sites for cautery (the former being considerably more numerous), most of the medical handbooks available in the Latin West between the sixth and the eleventh centuries had little or nothing to say about surgery. Furthermore, surgery was not distinguished from the rest of medical practice.[13]

As with the rest of medicine, the stimulus for the development of literate surgery came from social and economic growth that fostered new crafts and techniques and from the reception of written material that gave a fuller account of ancient Greek and Islamic achievements. In the case of surgery, books by Arabic authors were the most important vehicles of new information. Greek surgery had given rise to a substantial technical literature, but in western Europe this literature remained largely inaccessible to direct knowledge or use until the fifteenth and sixteenth centuries. Some of the most important items were treatises in the Hippocratic collection on injuries to the head and on fractures and dislocations; these were a principal source for long sections on surgery in the general works on medicine by the Roman encyclopedist Celsus (first century A.D.) and the Alexandrian Greek physician Paul of Aegina (seventh century A.D.). The case of Celsus serves as a striking reminder that the simple nature of early medieval medicine was not solely due to the absence of translations. Celsus' work was written in Latin and copied three times in northern Italian monasteries in the ninth and tenth centuries, but it was too long and complicated to be of practical use to early medieval western *medici*.[14]

However, the Arabic translation of Paul of Aegina made in the ninth century proved of great interest to sophisticated Muslim medical scholars. Book 6, which has been described as "the most detailed account of ancient surgical practice to have come down to us," was extensively utilized by all the major Arabic medical encyclopedists: Rhazes, Haly Abbas, Albucasis, and Avicenna.[15] Their works thus provided the West with a substantial amount of technical writing on surgery, much of it ultimately deriving from the Hippocratic corpus. Albucasis' *Surgery* (actually part of his medical encyclopedia, although it circulated in the West as a separate work) was especially influential after its translation into Latin in twelfth-century Spain. For surgical content, Albucasis drew heavily on Paul of Aegina, but the organization and emphasis were strikingly original. Cautery was made the subject of a lengthy special section; and the entire exposition was accompanied by numerous illustrations of surgical instruments, which were copied with greater or less fidelity in the various Arabic and, subsequently, Latin manuscripts (figure 41).[16] In addition to the Arabic works, Galen's *On the Technique of Healing* provided another source of information about surgery. Sections on wounds, ulcers, and fractures sometimes appeared separately in Latin manuscripts under the title *Galen's Surgery*.[17]

Practitioners and teachers in the West rapidly responded to the new material. The first people to show special interest in the writings on surgery, the learned monk Constantinus Africanus (whose *Pantegni* included a version of the surgical section of Haly Abbas' medical encyclopedia) and, subsequently, practitioners in mid-twelfth-century Salerno, were in no sense surgical specialists.[18] But the existence of a body of specialized knowledge preserved in learned sources soon helped to bring about the emergence of literate surgery as a distinct discipline. Once this material was available, Latin literacy became an important asset for working surgeons. It provided the key to authoritative technical literature, command of which was taken as a mark of competence and intellectual status and hence was closely connected with enhanced social position and economic opportunity.

However, the actual information about ancient and Muslim surgery contained in the translated works was by no means easy to use. There were numerous obstacles to the understanding, let alone the practical application, of much of the surgical doctrine reported by the Arabic authors. Obscurities of terminology, confusions, and repetitions abounded. The long lists of conditions and procedures were more or less faithfully reproduced from the ancient sources and did not necessarily reflect the relative prevalence of particular problems in the actual experience of the Islamic compilers, let alone in the medieval West. Although the reader was only sometimes warned off by direct injunctions, some of the more elaborate procedures repeated from ancient sources were probably never intended by the Arabic writers to be performed.

As a result, a series of surgeons tried their hands at producing new Latin textbooks of surgery. Among the first was Roger Frugard, who practiced and taught surgery at Parma around 1170. As noted in a previous chapter, his activities and those of his colleague Guido Arezzo the Younger show that Parma was an early center of expanded and intensified medical instruction in northern Italy. Roger drew on the Arabic tradition, probably directly or indirectly via Constantinus Africanus, but also on Salernitan practice and his own experience. Roger's *Surgery*, organized into a book by Guido Arezzo the Younger about 1180, provided a repertoire of techniques for treating injuries in a head-to-toe arrangement. This extremely influential book generated a

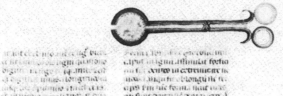

Figure 41 Surgical instruments from an early fourteenth-century Latin manuscript of Albucasis' *Surgery*. The artist has treated the instrument as decorative elements on the page, so little trace of realism or technical information remains. (Courtesy the Yale Medical Library, MS 28 [Codex Fritz Paneth], p. 559.)

large derivative literature. In the late twelfth and the thirteenth centuries, Roger's work was widely used as a basis of Latin instruction in surgery. As a result, practitioners in Salerno, northern Italy, and Montpellier early on began to produce glosses and commentaries, necessary aids for the understanding of Roger's highly compressed and often somewhat cryptic presentation. Some time in the early thirteenth century, Roger's pupil Rolando (or Rolandino) of Parma left his native city for the newly flourishing medical center of Bologna. There his teaching was based on Roger's work; ultimately Rolando produced a new edition of Roger's book that became known as the *Rolandina* and was influential in its own right. At Montpellier, Guillaume de Congenis, who was active in about the middle of the thirteenth century, based his teaching on the *Surgery* of Roger Frugard, although Guillaume's own book shows that he also knew Rhazes' treatment of surgery; Guillaume's book was in turn the subject of a pupil's explanatory notes.[19] Moreover, other independently composed Latin books on surgery showed strong traces of Roger's influence.

By the late thirteenth century, in circles in which texts on surgery were read in Latin, Roger's work had been largely supplanted by newer books composed in Latin or by the direct study of translations of Galen or the Arabic authors, especially Albucasis, whose work had not yet reached Italy when Roger taught. But the *Surgery* of Roger Frugard nonetheless continued to have widespread influence on surgical practice in the fourteenth and the fifteenth—and even in the sixteenth—centuries. From around the late thirteenth or the early fourteenth century, the emergence of a substantial class of practitioners who were literate but without Latin, or more at ease in the vernacular, created a demand for technical writing on surgery, as well as on other aspects of medicine, in vernacular languages (figure 42, with figures 38, 40, and 43, comes from a fifteenth-century surgery printed in German; see also figure 37). The compendia on various aspects of practical medicine, manuals on surgery, collections of recipes for the use of surgeons, and so on that supplied this demand continued, with few exceptions, to incorporate material from the *Surgery* of Roger and works derived from or based upon it.[20]

Following Roger and Rolando until the end of the thirteenth century, surgeons associated with northern Italian cities produced a notable series of Latin books on surgery. These surgeons included Bruno Longoburgo of Calabria, whose major work was written at Padua in 1252; Teodorico Borgognoni of Lucca, who received his training at Bologna and wrote before 1266; Guglielmo da Saliceto, who divided his career between the community of teaching and practicing surgeons in Bologna and practice in Pavia, Verona,

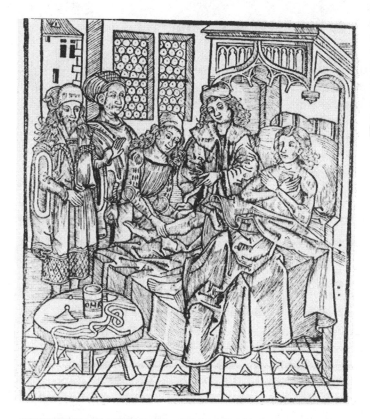

Figure 42 A late fifteenth-century artist's representation of treatment of a compound fracture by surgeons. (Courtesy the New York Academy of Medicine, Hieronymus Brunschweig, *Buch der Chirurgie* [1497], fol. XCIIIIʳ.)

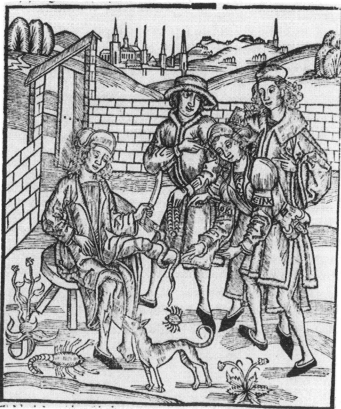

Figure 43 The domain of surgery including the treatment of bites and stings. In this schematic representation, a venomous snake, a scorpion, a spider, and a possibly mad dog are all to be found. (Courtesy the New York Academy of Medicine, Hieronymus Brunschweig, *Buch der Chirurgie* [1497], fol. XXXVᵛ.)

Cremona, and Piacenza and who completed the final version of his book on surgery in 1276; and Lanfranco of Milan, who, exiled from his native city, finished his major work at Paris in 1296 and thus helped to transmit the new forms of surgical literature and training to northern France.[21] Leading surgeons continued to write major Latin treatises on their art in the fourteenth century; two of the most important were Henri de Mondeville and Guy de Chauliac, both of whom had associations with Montpellier and with Paris.[22]

Thereafter, until the sixteenth century, most of the Latin and vernacular writing on surgery produced in Europe drew on traditions of form and content that had been established in the series of surgical books extending from the work of Roger Frugard to that of Guy de Chauliac. In particular, the work of Guy de Chauliac joined the complex of texts generated by the work of Roger as a standard source of information about surgery. Whereas Roger's influence often appears in short sections or specific recommendations for the treatment of particular conditions (for example, dental problems)[23] in later practical compendia compiled from a variety of sources, Guy's massive tome, completed in 1363, provided a single systematic and comprehensive overview of the whole discipline of surgery, reviewing and evaluating the teaching of the principal learned authorities. The author's Galenic learning, historical consciousness, and extended treatment of anatomy were doubtless among the features that kept Guy's *Great Surgery*, as it was termed by some of its early editors, in demand into the second half of the sixteenth century. It was translated into various European vernaculars soon after its composition; among the editions issued after 1500 were printings in Dutch, French, Italian, Spanish, and an English adaptation as well as the original Latin.[24]

Records other than the writings of surgeons sometimes provide descriptions of actual surgical treatment. When Sofia of Spoleto had abscesses (*apostemata*) in both her arms and legs "so that the bone showed," the *medicus* extracted a number of fragments of bone. When a "horrible aposteme" appeared on the head of eight-day-old Andreuccio, son of Francesca and Mattiolo of Spoleto, they had the *medicus* incise it; he made a large wound in the baby's head and inserted a pad (*tasta*) as long as a finger, while at the same time letting the parents know that he had given the infant up for dead. The baby did not die, but his subsequent recovery was attributed to a miracle of Chiara of Montefalco. Practitioners in Rome successfully treated Petrarch for a wound in the leg caused by the kick of a horse. The wound was severe enough to bare the bone, but the poet continued on his journey for three days before getting medical attention. By the time he was treated, Petrarch wrote to Boccaccio, "So troublesome was the odor from the neglected wound that often I would turn away violently, with an incredible inability to tolerate it." Less fortunate was Rosso della Tosa, a leader of the Black Guelf party in Florence whose long and tumultuous career of civil strife ended when, at the age of 75, he tripped over a dog, fell, and broke his knee. The wound became infected and he died "martyred by the doctors," an event recorded with some satisfaction by the chronicler Dino Compagni (d. 1324), who disapproved of Rosso della Tosa's politics.[25] Other collections of miracles from saints' shrines, personal letters or memoirs, and chronicles yield other examples of such incidental narratives about surgery and confirm its widespread practice. Yet most of what we know about the content and teaching of surgery—as distinct from the professional organization, employment, and fees of surgeons—depends not on such occasional anecdotes but on the books surgeons themselves wrote. It is therefore worth considering some characteristics of these books.

In the first place, these works are simultaneously highly derivative and in significant ways individual and innovative. In the case of the Italian authors, most of the content unquestionably comes from the various Arabo-Latin sources indicated above. Moreover, the later authors incorporated material from the earlier ones—the prefaces of Teodorico Borgognoni and Bruno Longoburgo parallel one another almost word for word: Henri de Mondeville explained that on wounds he was following Teodorico and, for ulcers, Lanfranco.[26] Guy de Chauliac was exceptional in that he made considerably more direct use of Galen than most other writers on surgery. In particular, Guy knew and used Galen's comprehensive treatise on anatomical physiology, *On the Usefulness of the Parts of the Body*, translated in full from Greek into Latin for the first time in the early fourteenth century.[27] The full version of the lengthy, complex, and theoretically oriented *On the Usefulness of the Parts* is a superior source of Galen's teaching, but its sophistication precluded much attention to it even in the university milieu before the sixteenth century.

Yet in the twelfth and thirteenth centuries the idea of treating surgery in a separate, specialized textbook was in itself an innovation in western medicine; each author plainly gave serious and independent consideration to the objectives of his book, the arrangement of its contents, and the emphasis to be given to different topics. Bruno Longoburgo thought that what was needed was a compilation that would bring together in a single work the opinions of the main authorities. Lanfranco included among his priorities the need to explain differences in nomenclature among the various sources. Teodorico focused on the idea of the mutual authentication of current surgical practice and ancient authority; he treated as specially and equally authoritative his own master (and probably father), Ugo of Lucca, and Galen, "who we know differs with the aforementioned man [that is, Ugo] in no respect." Ugo of Lucca, engaged by the municipal government of Bologna as town surgeon in 1214, was a renowned practitioner but not a medical author. Teodorico's equation of Ugo and Galen was thus a conscious endeavor to integrate craft and learned aspects of surgery as well as a startling expression of family pride and professional confidence.[28]

Organization and emphasis were as diversified as goals. By combining, selecting from, adapting, and adding to organizational schemes found in their sources, the various authors produced their own solutions to a range of questions. Should the book be arranged according to parts of the body or according to type of injury? How much anatomy ought a surgeon to know? Should the anatomy taught be regional or systemic? And where and how in the book or course should it be presented? Should there be separate sections on medications used in surgery? On instruments? On techniques of cautery and venesection? Some authors or their copyists also gave attention to a further question: Should there be illustrations; if so, of what?[29]

Thus, as noted in chapter 4, some surgical authors chose to emphasize anatomy by treating it in a separate section at or near the beginning of their books. By contrast, although Guglielmo da Saliceto was a pioneer in introducing a separate section on anatomy into a textbook of surgery, he relegated the subject to a few chapters near the end and treated it from a strictly surgical standpoint. Remarking that not all the minute divisions of anatomy were perceptible to sense and that, even if they were, it would be both tedious and useless to enumerate them, he proclaimed his intention to limit discussion to pointing out structures particularly likely to be injured in the course of surgical intervention. Exiguous as Guglielmo's separate anatomical section was, his *Surgery* as a whole is remarkable for the care with which he incorporated regional anatomy into his actual surgical instruction, warning the student of the need to pay attention to the possibility of damage to adjacent structures when treating wounds or performing surgery at particular body sites. Thus, in discussing wounds of the back of the neck, Guglielmo taught his readers to be alert to the danger of spinal cord injury, which could result in paralysis. Similarly, the subject of wounds of the throat led him to point out the hazard of damage to the trachea.[30]

Although normally relying heavily on descriptions and instructions found in their learned sources, the authors of surgical textbooks felt free to add or eliminate detail and to comment unfavorably on the procedures recommended. Thus, each included in his book a section on wounds of the head and skull fractures that closely resembles the treatment of the subject in one or more of the Arabo-Latin encyclopedias. The recommendations in the works of Arabic origin, as we have seen, in turn resemble one another because of their common ancient sources—in this instance ultimately derived from the Hippocratic treatise *On Wounds of the Head*. All works described techniques of trepanation for the purpose of relieving swelling, cleansing, or medicating the dura mater and removing jagged bone or bone fragments. But Lanfranco of Milan, after describing the procedure (manuscripts of his work also illustrate instruments for it) emphatically warned his readers of its dangers and stated that he himself whenever possible avoided using instruments to remove bone.[31] The authors also freely altered the emphasis accorded to particular conditions and procedures. Thus, although cautery continued to be valued to stop bleeding and wound infection and for its supposed effect on internal conditions, the general textbooks of surgery produced in the West did not devote nearly as much attention to it as had Albucasis.

One of the best-known episodes in the history of medieval surgery—the development of controversy over the treatment of wounds—provides yet another example of the way surgeons reworked material from the learned tradition to suit their own needs and analyzed their own procedures in the light of authoritative texts.[32] A major topic in all surgical texts was the cleansing and dressing of wounds and ulcers, procedures that had been assumed since antiquity to include medication with plasters, powders, ointments, or, in the case of ulcers, corrosive substances. Different substances were assigned different functions such as cleansing, rebuilding flesh, reducing scar tissue, and so on. A measure of suppuration was taken for granted as a normal stage in the healing of wounds; surgeons appear to have learned to distinguish between thick white pus, often indicative of an infection that would either heal or form a local abscess, and watery, fetid pus, indicative of a type of infection likely to be followed by gangrene and death. The formation of pus of the first type was therefore considered a desirable development—hence the later expression "laudable pus." Consequently, various ancient and, following them, Islamic sources recommended using unguents to bring on this stage and keeping the wound open until healing by secondary intention—from the depth of the wound to the surface—took place. A similar practice was followed at Salerno and recommended in textbooks emanating from or influenced by the Salernitan milieu.

Ugo and Teodorico Borgognoni and, following them, Henri de Mondeville preferred an alternative course, that of simply cleansing wounds with wine (in itself an ancient practice). After cleansing, they advocated immediate closure in cases where the wound was fresh and there was no significant loss of flesh or skin. They claimed that in this way they could achieve healing by primary intention—from the surface to the depth of the wound— without formation of pus. According to Teodorico, Ugo dressed such wounds with dry bandages only and used no salves. Henri de Mondeville provided a vivid description of the resistance he encountered from his colleagues when he tried to introduce this method of treatment in France, excoriating their conservatism and unwillingness to learn from experience.[33]

No doubt the advocacy of dry healing by Ugo, Teodorico, and their followers was based on their own experience of the outcome, perhaps in cases of sword wounds without much accompanying crushing or bruising. It seems likely that the success or failure of one method or the other would in reality have depended on the type and condition of the wound. But the argument was at least as much about the proper understanding of the substances of pus and blood in wounds as it was about variations in practical treatment; and the views of Ugo and Teodorico, just as much as those of their opponents, belonged within the established conceptual framework and textual tradition. Teodorico explained Ugo's results in Galenic terms, claiming Galen's support for the view that dryness was conducive to healing. Advocates of both positions argued in terms of complexion theory, defending the superior claims of dry or moist. And Teodorico accompanied his recommendation of wine as an external detergent with equally energetic insistence that the wounded should take wine internally (for nourishment and to build good flesh, not as an anesthetic).[34]

One noteworthy feature of the surgeons' books is their willingness to tell stories about themselves, their patients, and their teachers, colleagues, and pupils. Of course, the great bulk of surgical writing is not anecdotal; and anecdotes can also occasionally be found in other kinds of medical writing. Nonetheless, personal anecdote is markedly more prevalent in surgical than in other books, and therefore it is worth considering some of the ways in which surgeons used the stories they told.

In the first place, one would have to be very ingenuous to take such anecdotes at face value as simple reportage. No doubt some stories are to a considerable extent actually grounded in the author's personal experience, but it is usually experience selected or shaped with specific ends in view. In an attack on Rolando da Parma, Teodorico Borgognoni provided a glimpse of the way stories could be constructed or improved. Rolando recounted, with much circumstantial clinical and biographical detail, that he had attended a patient whose lung protruded from a wound between his ribs and whom all the most skilled surgeons in Bologna had given up for dead. According to his own story, Rolando enlarged the wound to release the constriction of the lung and applied medication, with the result that the patient recovered and subsequently went crusading. But according to Teodorico, Rolando had simply appropriated one of Master Ugo's cures at which Rolando had been present only as a witness. Ugo's success, according to Teodorico, had in fact been even more remarkable than that claimed by Rolando, since Ugo's patient's lung had actually been torn by the original wound. Of course, Teodorico's version of the story, with Ugo as hero, is just as likely to have been constructed or improved as Rolando's account.[35]

Surgeons' stories could serve a variety of purposes. One of the most obvious was simply to provide examples of the narrator's success. In this respect, the stories seem almost like secular parallels to one kind of narrative told about miraculous cures. With the authority of an example in the gospel itself, such narratives since antiquity had often included the topos of the patient's prior, and useless, consultation of secular medical practitioners. And the more fully the physical ailment, the expertise of the medical attendant, and the details of physical treatment could be described, the more striking became the contrast between the failure of secular medicine and the triumph of spiritual healing. Hence, the more secular medical activity expanded, the greater the extent to which miracle stories were likely to elaborate medical detail and emphasize access to professional practitioners; such at any rate seems to be the case in the early fourteenth-century miracles of Chiara of Montefalco, from which several examples have been drawn above. These stories show considerable ambivalence about medical or surgical practitioners, ambivalence that no doubt reflected the real feelings of the tellers but that may have been enhanced by the requirements of the dramatic structure of the narrative. Secular specialists appear as wholly authoritative in matters of diagnosis and, except for the intervention of miracle, prognosis; but their treatments are represented as either ineffectual or unacceptably painful and dangerous.

By contrast, as one might expect, surgeons' stories usually present the specialist as successful in both diagnosis and treatment. Great danger is skillfully overcome, but the subject of pain is seldom mentioned. The pupil of Guillaume de Congenis was highly unusual in mentioning a poor scholar who said the removal of his sutures hurt more than the incision, and a poor youth on pilgrimage who refused to allow Guillaume to continue applying corrosives to his chest because of the pain. That surgeons of the period were in reality concerned about the pain their procedures caused, even if they did not always choose to advertise its extent to their readers, is indicated by a number of recipes, the earliest from the ninth century, for soporific mixtures with which to impregnate sponges to be placed in the mouth or nostrils. Despite the narcotic properties of some ingredients, such sponges could not have provided anaesthesia in the modern sense. The extent to which they were used in surgical practice is unknown, but miniatures in surgical manuscripts show that patients were physically restrained.[36]

Like the successes of the saints, surgeons' successes frequently follow or are contrasted with others' failures—not, to be sure, failures of spiritual healers, but failures of rival specialists, or of less highly trained empirics, or of the patient's family and friends. Thus, Lanfranco recounted how he had treated a fifteen-year-old youth who had cut his arm, with injury to a sinew and much loss of blood. Lanfranco wanted to strip the blood vessel and ligate it, but the boy's mother mistrusted this treatment and summoned a "lay surgeon" under whose care the patient worsened until he was at the point of death. In this crisis, a physician friend of the family took the distraught mother to task for exchanging Lanfranco's expert ministrations for those of an untrained practitioner. The physician then instructed the latter to do what Lanfranco had recommended, with the result that the boy recovered.[37] The anecdote manages to combine an *exemplum* of Lanfranco's success with a technical description of one of his preferred methods of treatment, while simultaneously placing him squarely in professional and intellectual solidarity with the *medicus* against the irrationality of the mother and the ignorance of the empiric.

Other anecdotes hit hard at named professional rivals. Again according to Lanfranco, Anselmo of Genoa made a lot of money by his methods of practice but caused the deaths of many people. The element of competition is also plainly evident in Teodorico's remarks about Rolando, mentioned above. Lanfranco also, even less attractively, made a point of including anecdotes showing that he himself succeeded in treating patients whom his own pupils had failed to cure; one such case was that of a fifty-year-old woman of Milan with an abscess in her throat and neck. Lanfranco incised the abscess, drew off much purulent matter, and inserted a silver cannula into the esophagus to allow for the passage of nourishment while the wound healed.[38]

Anecdotes could also serve to indicate the large number and, wherever possible, the social distinction of the patients successfully treated by a surgeon. One suspects such was the purpose of the well-known list of patients whom the English surgeon John of Arderne (1307–after 1377) claimed to have cured of anal fistulas: of nineteen patients named, two were identified as knightly or noble and eight as members of the clergy.[39]

In all the foregoing cases, it seems most likely that surgeons were writing their narratives for other surgeons and perhaps other literate medical men. In some instances, however, anecdotal case histories were evidently designed as teaching devices, much as collections of *consilia* seem to have been. Guglielmo da Saliceto explicitly announced that his *Surgery*, written for students, would be illustrated with examples drawn from cases on which he had worked with his own hands, "because the only proper way of improving this art is through use and [manual] operation . . . and on this account it is correct in teaching surgery as a formal discipline to proceed according to those things which were manifest to me through use and operation over a long time."[40] Thus, Guglielmo carefully selected—and, no doubt, adapted—case histories drawn from his own experience to illustrate principles and information derived from a learned, textual tradition; such a use of personal narrative constituted one solution to the problem of integrating formal, text-based instruction and craft training.

Guglielmo occasionally criticized the ancients in the light of his own experience; for example, he expressed his disapproval of an implied recommendation to perform surgical operations on newborn infants.[41] More characteristic of his method, however, was his choice of three cases to illustrate the point that wounds to the head or neck could result in paralysis if the spinal cord or brain was injured but that such paralysis was not necessarily permanent or fatal. In the first case, Lazzarino of Cremona received a sword wound to the head so severe that at first Guglielmo prognosticated death; the patient survived but three days later became paralyzed and incontinent. Thanks to the healing power of nature and Guglielmo's treatment, however, he ultimately recovered completely and lived another 20 years. The second case was that of a patient wounded by an arrow in the neck; he also became paralyzed, incontinent, and, as a result, deeply depressed. Having been given up for dead, he made a partial recovery under Guglielmo's treatment; this patient survived for 10 years but could only walk with the aid of crutches. In the case of Gabriele da Pirolo, however, the attending *medicus* was unable to prevent the patient's arrow wound from being followed in less than a month by rigor, fever, and death.[42] Guglielmo thus claimed only the more or less successful outcomes for himself, referring the total failure of treatment to an unnamed colleague or rival. Nonetheless, his readiness to admit to an initially mistaken prognosis in the first case and only partial success in the second is exceptional; it provides a good measure of the seriousness of his pedagogical intent and also inspires confidence that his narratives, however much edited, bear some relation to his actual experience.

The treatises on surgery by practitioner-authors associated with northern Italian cities in the late twelfth and the thirteenth centuries were part of the broader general development of literate medicine and medical training and education in the same period. Yet the appearance of these treatises signaled and, no doubt, intensified a measure of disciplinary and institutional separation between surgery and medicine. In the fourteenth to sixteenth centuries, surgery developed and flourished chiefly in the milieu of towns and guilds, where a distinct hierarchy of surgical practitioners grew up. In some instances, as will become apparent, sharp institutional and economic rivalry characterized the relations between surgeons and academically educated physicians.

Conceptually and technically, however, the separation of medicine and surgery always remained in important respects partial and incomplete. Since medicine and surgery shared a common tradition of knowledge derived from essentially the same sources, they also shared a common conceptual framework. As already noted, authoritative general works on medicine, for example, those of Haly Abbas and Avicenna, incorporated long sections on surgery.[43] And both the authors of treatises on surgery and other medical writers continued to share the belief and reiterate the commonplace that surgery was one of the three therapeutic resources of medicine (each was supposed to be tried in turn before recourse to the next, so surgery was the measure of last resort after diet and then medication). The classification of illnesses into malformations, complexional disorders, and "breaks in continuity" embraced conditions treated by surgery: conditions such as bladder stone would probably fall into the first category, and wounds, fractures, and all other forms of trauma fell into the third.[44]

The impact of the turn to Aristotelian logic and natural philosophy characteristic of the thirteenth century is naturally much less evident in books on surgery than on medical theory. Yet surgeons who wrote in Latin, like learned physicians, used Aristotelian terminology to define their areas of expertise. Just as scholastic physicians tried to show that at least some aspects of medicine fitted the Aristotelian definition of *scientia*, so some literate surgeons endeavored to claim surgery as *scientia*. According to Guglielmo da Saliceto, who was well acquainted with Aristotelian works and terminology, as the preface to his general work on medical practice shows, "Surgery is a *scientia* teaching how to operate manually on the flesh, nerves, and bones of man." Guy de Chauliac made the same claim, although he was even more explicit in stating that only the teaching of surgery qualified as *scientia*; surgery in the sense of practice was in Guy's view more properly termed an art.[45]

In actuality, the scope of medical and surgical practice overlapped, so that no sharp boundary between the two could easily be drawn. Although surgery was defined as encompassing all forms of manual operation—surgical authors carefully instructed their readers in the Greek etymology of the word—surgery's actual distinguishing features were that as a rule only the surgeon sutured wounds, used the knife, and set fractures and dislocations. No doubt even these procedures were occasionally performed by all categories of *medici* (certainly this was true in the case of bloodletting). But throughout the period under discussion, a wide range of other forms of treatment was practiced by surgeons and physicians alike in very similar ways. Physicians as well as surgeons provided external medications for diseases or injuries manifested on the surface of the body and so might treat ulcers originating as wounds; surgeons included dietary recommendations and potions to be taken internally among their treatments for wounds and fractures. Surgical treatises included long lists of materia medica, similar to those found in other medical works. One of the most common forms of medical treatment—phlebotomy—was in fact a minor surgical procedure. The *consilia* and writings on practice of some famous scholastic learned physicians of the thirteenth and fourteenth centuries—Taddeo Alderotti, Guglielmo da Brescia (d. 1326), and Gentile da Foligno—show that they recommended medications for cases of hernia, fistula, wounds, and bites (figure 43).[46] The actual practice of many surgeons appears to have been equally eclectic with regard to all kinds of internal conditions, particularly in localities where academically trained physicians were few in number or weak in organization.

In terms of occupational status and self-definition, the situation was also complex. As surgery emerged as a distinct discipline with its own body of specialized technical writing, literate surgeons found it necessary to defend, assert, or explain their positions on three different fronts—in relation to the public at large, in relation to illiterate surgeons, and in relation to learned physicians. As far as the public at large was concerned, literate surgeons were at one with literate *medici* in general in presenting themselves as possessors of specialized knowledge to which the general public could have no access. Guglielmo da Saliceto, who himself practiced both medicine and surgery, aided in the separation of the two fields by writing separate works on each. But his advice to practitioners in both categories was the same: they should not become too familiar with laymen,

> because laymen always disparage the wise, and too much familiarity breeds contempt; and indeed it is unbecoming and inappropriate to decide the cause of the disease and the procedures to be undertaken

in the presence of the patient and laymen . . . it seems better and
more decent that every discussion with a colleague or assistant should
take place in secret.

In the form quoted, this opinion occurs among the commonplaces at the
beginning of Guglielmo's work on general medical practice, which is dedicated to his son; there can be no doubt that he was referring to *laici* as
contrasted with experts, not as contrasted with clergy. When giving essentially the same advice at the beginning of his *Surgery*, he noted that when
the surgeon becomes too friendly with the patient it becomes difficult to
ask for a fee.[47]

In fact, in times of crisis the surgeon's task might be preempted by "the
laity." Possibly few women would have had the resourcefulness, surgical
knowledge, and lack of squeamishness of St. Francesca Romana, who, when
a great hound bit her spiritual daughter Rita Covelli, promptly poured boiling oil into the wound on her friend's leg. The action was standard surgical
treatment for poisoned wounds. In the next century, when the hardened
battlefield surgeon Ambroise Paré abandoned the use of boiling oil in treating bullet wounds—a practice that had been inspired by the belief that
gunpowder was poisonous—in favor of methods that brought better results, he noted the extremely painful nature of the boiling oil treatment
(happily, Rita Covelli believed herself to be the beneficiary of a miracle that
took away the pain).[48] Although some surgeons followed armies (see below),
trained surgeons were certainly not available to all participants in every af-
fray. Knights and men-at-arms perforce learned to help themselves and each
other with rudimentary surgery; hence the presence, already noted, of German knights in Guy de Chauliac's list of categories of practitioners of surgery.

Military amateurs could have gained good practical experience but may
have been less cautious than educated surgeons. The student of Guillaume
de Congenis recorded an instance of failure of primary closure when knights
immediately sutured a wound in a comrade's arm without bleeding or cautery, so that gangrene spread up his arm, and he died.[49] A more optimistic
picture of battlefield surgery by a warrior comes from a knightly poet. In
Wolfram von Eschenbach's *Parzival*, composed in the first decade of the thirteenth century, there is an episode in which Gawan finds a knight wounded
in the chest and drowning in his own blood. Gawan, "who was no fool in
the matter of wounds," diagnoses the wound as not fatal and restores the
knight to consciousness by making a cannula from a tube of linden bark and
instructing the wounded knight's accompanying damsel to suck out the
blood. A few pages later, Gawan notices an herb that is good for wounds
and dismounts to pick it; the haughty lady whom he is escorting sneers, "If

my companion can be both doctor and knight, he can earn a good living, provided he learns how to sell ointment jars." Cannulas for various uses, although not the one described, as well as the need to drain blood from a chest wound are discussed in the surgical textbook of Albucasis. Wolfram may have known that work; he may also have been drawing on his own experience of battlefield first aid.[50]

Among practitioners who gained their entire living, or a substantial part of it, by surgery, the range in terms of education, training, and socioeconomic status was almost as wide as among medical practitioners in general. Skilled, literate surgeons stood at the head of the surgical hierarchy. But surgical procedures were also carried out by medical empirics, by craftsmen who were often itinerant and specialized in a particular operation (couching for cataract, treating hernias, or cutting for the stone, for example), and by barbers, who frequently included bloodletting among their skills. Some of the empiric specialists built up regionally celebrated craft traditions in particular operations. The pupil of Guillaume de Congenis was honest enough to admit that wandering specialists in couching cataract were often more successful than "famous surgeons" because the itinerants got more practice.[51] However, specialists in risky procedures who were itinerant also had the opportunity to avoid confrontations with dissatisfied patients or their surviving relatives.

Surgeons frequently tried by guild regulations or other means to distinguish themselves from barbers and other lesser practitioners.[52] Those who enjoyed the advantages of access to the learned tradition were especially anxious to distinguish the superiority of their own knowledge and skill from the activities of their humble co-workers. As Bruno Longoburgo put it:

> I think scarcely anyone who is illiterate can understand this art, but at the present time . . . those who exercise this art are for the most part ignorant and stupid peasants; and on account of their stupidity the worst possible diseases are generated in people, by which indeed the patients are killed since the surgeons operate neither wisely nor according to certain reasoning, but haphazardly.[53]

Bruno's complaints about uneducated surgeons, echoed in one form or another by various of the surgical writers discussed in this chapter, are very similar in tone and content to the complaints of learned physicians about empiric medical practitioners. Yet the most difficult relation of literate surgeons was probably that with learned physicians, no doubt largely because the two groups were competing for the most prestigious and lucrative patients.

In terms of professional qualifications and common activities, the relations of *medici* and literate surgeons differed widely in different parts of Europe during the later thirteenth, the fourteenth, and the fifteenth centuries. In principle, the separation of medicine and surgery seems to have been least marked in Italy. In the second decade of the thirteenth century, the earliest time at which Bologna appears as a center of medical study and activity, the surgical practice and private teaching of Ugo of Lucca was already an important part of the medical scene there. Moreover, when the university faculty of medicine finally took shape at Bologna, probably around the 1260s, it did so in the context of a flourishing northern Italian regional tradition of literate surgery. Furthermore, university students and their teachers in Italy, unlike university communities in northern Europe, always included a substantial proportion of laymen who were unaffected by the provision of the Fourth Lateran Council forbidding priests, deacons, and subdeacons from practicing "that part of surgery involving burning and cutting." (Clerics could secure dispensations from these prohibitions; Teodorico Borgognoni received papal permission to practice his art and keep the fees when he was already a Dominican friar and probably a bishop.)[54] Perhaps as a result, at Bologna and other Italian universities surgery secured a place, albeit a minor one with few degrees granted, in the curriculum.

The curriculum in surgery prescribed in the statutes of the University of Arts and Medicine at Bologna, issued in 1405 and probably unchanged since the thirteenth century, consisted of Bruno Longoburgo's textbook and selections from Galen, Rhazes, and Avicenna.[55] Although university students of surgery also studied other branches of medicine, their reading in their specialty was thus very similar to that of their literate colleagues outside the schools. No doubt the university students were required to add scholastic and philosophical competence to their technical learning. This combination is certainly to be found, for example, in Dino del Garbo's theoretically as well as practically oriented commentary on the sections of Avicenna's *Canon* on tumors, wounds, bruises, ulcers, injuries to the nerves, and skull fractures. As noted in chapter 2, Dino himself combined a family background in surgery with learning in arts and philosophy and with training in theory and practice of medicine that he had acquired in a university setting. These qualifications enabled him to become a professor of medicine at the universities of Bologna, Padua, and Siena. At Siena he taught "both the theory and practice of surgery magisterially" as part of the regular program of the medical faculty, as he himself was careful to point out. In the proem to his commentary on the surgical parts of the *Canon*, Dino asserted that the teaching (again, as distinct from the practice) of surgery could be considered a form of *scientia* involving theory as well as practice.[56]

Outside the university, too, physicians and surgeons in Italy occasionally found themselves in common organizations; in fourteenth-century Florence, practitioners in both categories were members of the same guild. However, in actuality it was rare for any surgeon in Florence to attain status, property, or breadth of learning equal to that of a university-trained physician. In fifteenth-century Padua, where university physicians and town surgeons traditionally belonged to the same guild and where medical information and books circulated freely among them, relations between the two groups were nonetheless marked by a measure of social separation and by claims to superior learning by the university physicians and superior practical experience by the town surgeons.[57]

The professional separation between medicine and surgery became sharp and strongly enforced in northern Europe, where craft surgical traditions and the academic study of medicine appear to have grown up much more independently of one another than was the case in Italy. As a consequence, physicians and surgeons were usually members of separate guilds or other associations, and surgeons were excluded from the university faculties of medicine. At Paris, the chief center of medical education in northern Europe, the establishment of a university faculty of medicine in the course of the thirteenth century took place before the emergence of a class of self-consciously literate and latinate surgeons in the early fourteenth century. Relations between physicians and the upper echelon of surgeons were particularly poor in fourteenth-century Paris. The rivalry was not solely economic. Literate surgeons were evidently able to secure excellent opportunities for access to wealthy, noble, and even royal clients, but they nonetheless strongly resented the exclusiveness and intellectual pretensions of the physicians associated with the medical faculty; perhaps as a consequence, the Paris surgeons in the 1350s decided to organize their guild into the quasi-academic College of St. Cosmas, patron saint of surgeons.[58]

Naturally, the situation was particularly galling to those surgeons who did in fact possess extensive knowledge of the Latin learned tradition of their discipline. In Henri de Mondeville, this group had an exceptionally vociferous member. Mondeville, who served the French royal court and taught in Paris, although not in the faculty of medicine, was as dismissive of learned physicians as of unlearned surgeons. His attitude to the former is summed up in his remark that God himself had acted as a surgeon when he made Eve from Adam's rib and when Jesus made clay to anoint the eyes of a blind man, but that Scripture nowhere recorded that the Lord engaged in the characteristic medical activities of feeling the pulse and inspecting urine.[59]

At Montpellier, the tensions, although present, were not so marked. As at Bologna, the teaching and study of surgery was part of the medical milieu in the city from an early date. In the mid–thirteenth century, Guillaume de Congenis introduced his students to Latin surgical learning and provided them with clinical instruction in a local hospital.[60] Mondeville himself had both studied and given lectures at Montpellier. But his lectures were not necessarily given publicly in the university, although medical students attended them. Guy de Chauliac, whose Galenic learning certainly equaled or surpassed that of any contemporary university professor of medicine, had studied under a professor of medicine at Montpellier and called himself *magister in medicina*. However, his study of anatomy took place at Bologna, perhaps because he also wished to graduate in surgery, as was possible in Italy. He dedicated his own work on surgery to the physicians of Montpellier, Bologna, and Paris—the three chief centers of medical learning—and of the papal court of Avignon, where he made his own career. But the broad education and academic contacts of Henri de Mondeville and Guy de Chauliac belonged to an early phase in the development of surgery in France and in any case represented the atypical achievements of exceptionally distinguished men. It is clear that most of the surgeons in Montpellier during the late Middle Ages and Renaissance did not have university connections but were members of the surgeon's guild, which had originated in the thirteenth century as an association of barber-surgeons and by 1418 had developed a system of formal examination of aspirants to mastership in the guild. In 1496 the chancellor of the university acquired the right to be present at guild examinations of would-be surgeons.[61]

In northern Europe other than France during the fourteenth and fifteenth centuries, rivalries and attempts at accommodation among physicians, surgeons, and barber-surgeons also manifested themselves from time to time. For example, in London in 1423, leading surgeons were already organized in their own fellowship when they briefly united with physicians in a joint organization. The common interest inspiring this short-lived enterprise was an attempt to regulate the practice of empirics of all kinds and especially to control the barber-surgeons, who were members of the barbers' guild. Doubtless, tensions between physicians and surgeons were responsible for the failure of this joint association to survive.[62]

Mature forms of guild organization are only one type of evidence for the developed state of surgery as an occupation in urban milieus in northern

Europe at the end of the Middle Ages. Another is the prolific production of vernacular surgical books, notably in Flanders and German-speaking regions during the fourteenth and fifteenth centuries. Just as Lanfranco had brought northern Italian surgical techniques and teaching to Paris, so his pupil Jan Yperman carried them to Flanders and the German lands: Yperman's work on surgery, written about 1329, joins "the Roger-tradition with the results of the Bolognese, or Parisian, school."[63]

One of the most important developments affecting the surgical profession as a whole in the fourteenth and fifteenth centuries was indeed the proliferation of translations of books on surgery, as on other aspects of practical medicine, into vernacular languages—French, German, English, and others. Guy de Chauliac's *Surgery* exists in four separate Middle English translations (although only two contain the complete text).[64] These translations and the many vernacular compendia, manuals, collections of recipes, and so on constitute striking evidence for the growth of a community of surgeons literate in a vernacular language but not skilled in Latin who sought the specialized knowledge of surgery available in technical books. As already noted, all surgical and general medical literature written in the later fourteenth and the fifteenth centuries, whether in Latin or in the vernacular, continued to draw heavily on material transmitted from the learned tradition, modified to a greater or lesser extent on the basis of the author's own experience. The process was similar to that by which the twelfth- and thirteenth-century Italian surgical authors had incorporated material from the Arabo-Latin texts into their own books, which then joined the canon of works on which later writers could draw. The body of knowledge constituting the written basis of surgery was thus repeatedly reworked, adapted, and technically and linguistically modified to form a living technical literature suited to the needs of late medieval and Renaissance practitioners.

While the progressively increasing availability of and demand for technical books on surgery that included much general medical information (first in Latin and subsequently in vernacular languages), can be traced from the twelfth to the fifteenth centuries with no difficulty, it is less easy to determine the extent to which opportunities for surgeons to gain practical experience also increased over the same period. It is a truism that war is the best school of surgery. In the twelfth and thirteenth centuries, factional strife in the Italian cities, the crusades, and the general conditions of feudal society certainly provided plenty of opportunities for surgeons to gain experience. One has only to look at Guglielmo da Saliceto's long list of recommended treatments for sword and arrow wounds in different parts of the body to realize that the treatment of injuries received in fights was always a significant part, although certainly not the whole, of surgical practice. In the following two centuries, some rulers in northern Europe brought together armies for their major campaigns that were large by the standards of the time, and some pitched battles unquestionably produced substantial numbers of dead and wounded, as the excavated remains of 1,185 soldiers who fell at the battle of Visby in 1361 testify.[65] But active campaigns were seldom of long duration, and large pitched battles were infrequent. Cannon were introduced in the fourteenth century but were at first few in number; like their predecessors, the large catapults and other medieval war machines, early cannon were used chiefly to breach the walls of beseiged cities. As a recent scholarly study has documented in great detail, real change in the extent and intensity of warfare came at the end of the fifteenth and in the sixteenth centuries, when armies increased significantly in size, campaigns were longer and more numerous, and the use of hand-held artillery in addition to more mobile cannon became general.[66] It was then that the proper treatment of gunshot wounds and methods of limb amputation emerged as major problems in surgery and were addressed by Ambroise Paré (1510?–90) and others less well known.

Throughout the twelfth to the fifteenth centuries, some surgeons followed armies. One Frankish surgeon who went with the crusaders to the Holy Land in the twelfth century has already been mentioned. Ugo of Lucca's contract with the city of Bologna (1214) included the stipulation that he follow the Bolognese army when it went to war; on one occasion, he also accompanied a crusading expedition.[67] Henri de Mondeville, writing in the first decade of the fourteenth century, adduced his battlefield experience as a reason for preferring dry healing of wounds.[68] In the fourteenth and fifteenth centuries, kings on campaign and military leaders commonly included surgeons in their entourages. But since wealthy aristocrats also frequently retained surgeons in their private service at home and in times of peace and since they also took physicians with them in time of war, such engagements even during wartime by no means necessarily imply either that the surgeons in question served the army at large or that they had the opportunity to treat numerous wounds received in battle. However, one expedition that was accompanied by a group of surgeons whose duty was clearly to treat the wounds of the troops was Henry V's Agincourt campaign in 1415. The London surgeon Thomas Morestede successfully petitioned the king for permission to raise a group of twelve surgeons to go with the army at the standard rates of military pay. King Henry also engaged an Oxford-educated physician to accompany him to France on this campaign.[69]

War, then, was one school for surgeons, but by no means all surgeons followed armies; and those who did were not necessarily on campaign for very long. In the fourteenth and fifteenth centuries as in the twelfth and thirteenth, most European surgeons probably gained the greater part of their experience in their local communities by treating victims of the vicissitudes of everyday life, including wounds inflicted in local affrays. Evidently, too, the guild movement played an important part in the transmission of surgical techniques. Guilds or associations of surgeons similar to those at Paris, Montpellier, and London appeared in many more cities in various parts of Europe during the fourteenth and fifteenth centuries. Like other guilds, surgeons' guilds performed the function of preserving craft traditions and techniques and handing them on to each new generation of members.

The inherently technological and pragmatic nature of surgery has often led medical historians and others to inquire whether medieval surgeons can be credited with any original contributions to surgical technique. The question is legitimate, although limiting, but it is probably an illusion to suppose that it is possible to arrive at a definite answer. The gap between claims made in texts—even in personal narratives such as the surgeons' stories, of which examples have already been given—and unrecoverable actual events, is as wide for surgery as for any other branch of medicine.

The areas in which successful innovation on the part of surgeons has from time to time been claimed with some plausibility include the invention of surgical procedures and instruments for the treatment of particular conditions, control of pain, and wound management. In the first category, it is clear that sometimes literate surgeons did add variations to techniques described in textbooks, and that they perceived, or at any rate claimed, the result as a procedure of their own invention. While no thorough investigation has been made of all such claims found in surgical texts, some of the most celebrated examples do not incorporate technical innovations likely to have substantially improved the outcome of the procedure.

Thus, the fourteenth-century English surgeon John of Arderne claimed great success for his own special instruments and treatment for anal fistulas and other deep abscesses in the rectal region (figure 44). Likely causes of such abscesses include cancer of the bowel and other bowel diseases, gonorrhea, tuberculosis, diverticulitis, embedding of a fragment of hardened feces, and complications resulting from hemorrhoids or hemorrhoid surgery. Hence, it is not necessary to assume a connection, as is sometimes done, between a propensity to develop anal fistulas and membership in a knightly class that spent a lot of time on horseback in heavy armor.[70] The most probable reason that John of Arderne developed a special interest in the subject was that

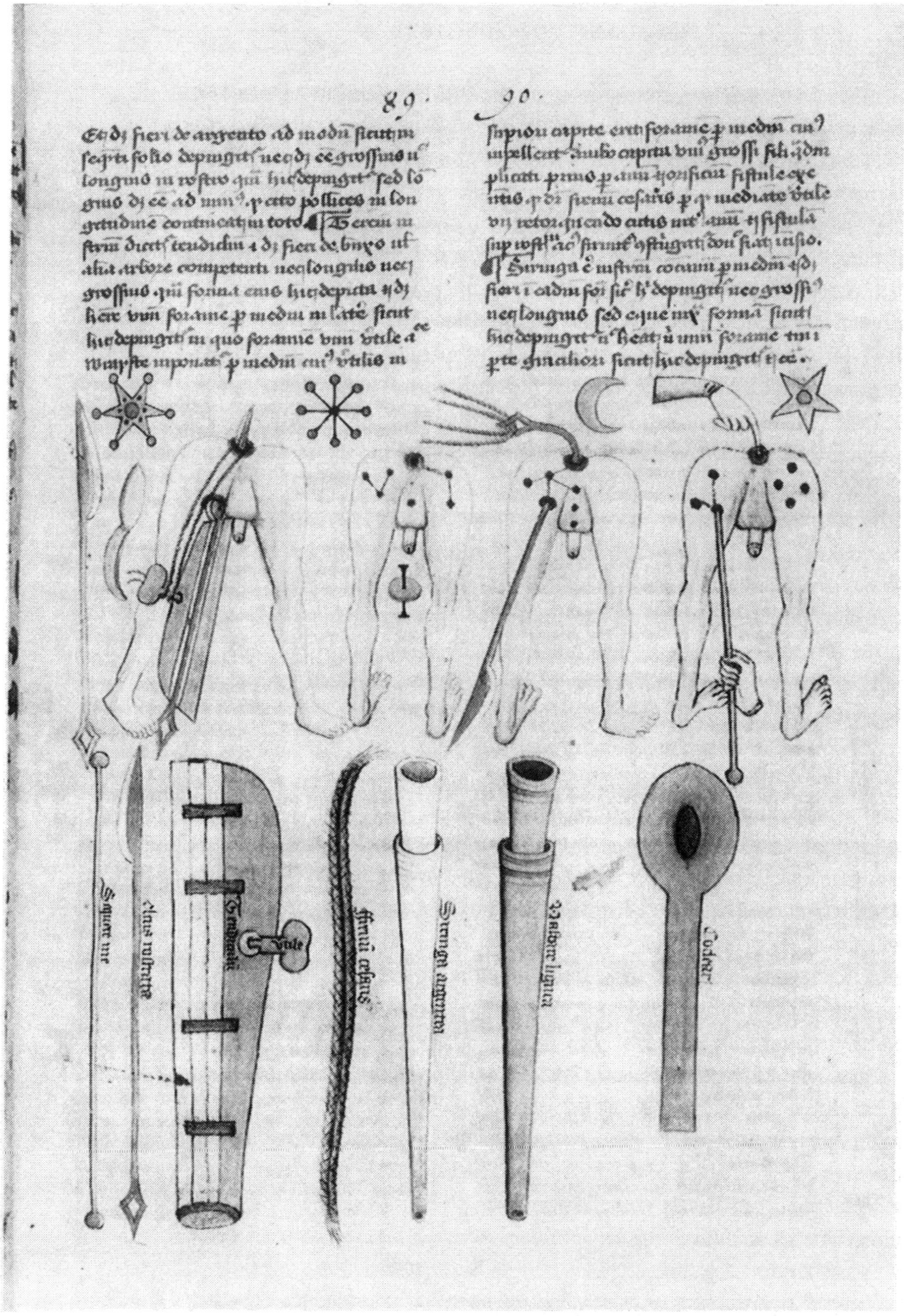

Figure 44 John of Arderne's refinements of the instruments used to operate on anal fistula. The first three instruments on the left in the row at the bottom of the page are John of Arderne's special probe, his "snouted needle," and his bow for tightening the cord passed through the fistula. The row of pictures at the top show how the instruments were meant to be used. (Courtesy the British Library, MS Additional 29301, fifteenth century, John of Arderne, fol. 25ʳ.)

anal fistulas occurred in a number of his patients, whatever their class and occupation, and that the complaint was part of the canon of ailments discussed in all the standard surgical texts. Since antiquity two forms of treatment had been suggested; both, indeed, continued in use until the twentieth century. One involved immediately cutting open the fistula with a knife, and the other involved drawing a thread through from the orifice in the rectum to the orifice on the surface of the body, tying the two ends to form a ligature, and slowly tightening it over a period of several days until the flesh was cut through (the second procedure has been variously credited with being less painful and less likely to produce incontinence). Both procedures are fully described by Albucasis, following Paul of Aegina; and most of the other Arabic and Latin authors mentioned in this chapter described one or both methods. John of Arderne combined the two methods and developed several special instruments, which may have served mainly to complicate the procedure.[71] He may, of course, have achieved the successes he claimed, but it is unlikely that his innovative variations in instrumentation or technique were responsible for them.

Surgeons, like other practitioners, sometimes devised medicinal mixtures of their own. In the case of potions as well as procedures, craft traditions in both medical and surgical practice doubtless encouraged practitioners to develop their own secret or special remedies that they would pass on only to chosen apprentices or successors. Patients could be asked to pay a high fee for such preparations. For example, Ugo of Lucca's special potion for patients with skull fractures originally belonged to the category of remedies that were trade secrets.[72] To write such personal accomplishments down in a Latin book, as Teodorico did with Ugo's recipe, opened them up to a wider public than the practitioner's own apprentices but still confined them within the circle of the learned.

As for wound management and the control of pain, the views of Ugo of Lucca and his followers embodied an insight that may have been useful in some cases of incised wounds. The concept of a soporific device is also impressive, but the absence of evidence to show that either dry healing and primary closure or soporific sponges were generally adopted probably indicates that neither worked sufficiently well in practice to be obviously advantageous. Wider practical usefulness may have resulted from such modest enlargements of the surgeon's repertoire as the availability of aqua vitae as well as wine for cleansing wounds and the use in Italy of locally produced silk thread as an alternative to linen thread for sutures.

In reality, of course, scant justice is done to the rich history of medieval surgery if it is reduced to a few claimed innovations that turn out to be of dubious originality or significance, or both. Equally shallow are endeavors to contrast "practical" surgery with "bookish" medicine. For surgeons as for physicians, books and the heritage of ancient medicine they contained held the keys to privileged forms of knowledge and hence to status and wealth. In addition, authorship was evidently an important road to, or evidence of, career advancement for a surgeon. Moreover, the technical usefulness of the books, although limited, was real: they conveyed some knowledge of anatomy, they provided descriptions of basic procedures, and they frequently directed attention to the dangers involved in ill-considered surgical intervention. But success in actually carrying out the surgical procedures depended chiefly on manual adeptness, good judgment, practice, and luck, none of which books could provide. By the late Middle Ages, European surgeons had both well-developed and long-standing craft traditions and a rich technical literature; both of these, in conjunction with personal experience, were needed to train practitioners who met the standards expected of a skilled surgeon.

EPILOGUE: THE MEDICAL
RENAISSANCE

Medical knowledge, medical practice, the realities of health and disease, and the needs and expectations of patients stood in uneasy relation to one another in the medical world of the thirteenth to fifteenth centuries, as perhaps, in one way or another, they always do. Despite the presence of numerous medical practitioners of one kind and another, despite the value placed on their activities, and despite the efforts of public authorities and religious institutions to regulate medicine, institute quarantine and sanitary regulations, and provide hospitals, medieval and early Renaissance Europe did not have an adequate system of health care. Epidemic disease, malnutrition, and poverty were beyond the control of medical practitioners, public or ecclesiastical authorities, and religious charities alike. Yet the medicine of the period merits serious attention because of the social and cultural influence of medical ideas and medical practitioners, because of the growth of a professional community, and because of the important place of medicine in the history of scholarship, knowledge, and techniques.

This book has attempted to illustrate the reception, diffusion, and transformation of a system of ideas and techniques and simultaneously to trace the formation of a community—or more properly, a series of communities—of practitioners trained in that system. From late antiquity until the sixteenth century, almost all the western European medicine that has left any written record depended for its main concepts and therapies on the medicine of the classical and Hellenistic world. Popular as well as learned medicine drew on the ancient heritage, as an abundance of simplified medical handbooks in vernacular languages testify (of course, local remedies or folk traditions also found a place in popular medicine—and sometimes in the practice of the learned as well).

From one perspective, the history of medieval and Renaissance medicine can be written as a series of receptions of the Greek heritage in various degrees of completeness. Such a formulation tells nothing of social context or of professional development and is grossly inadequate as intellectual history, for it ignores the active and transforming role of the process of reception and takes no account of additions, deletions, rearrangements, and selections for different purposes at different times and places. Nonetheless, the sequence of receptions provides one kind of chronological framework for the development of medicine in medieval and Renaissance western Europe: thus, in the early Middle Ages, scanty knowledge in the West contrasted with the much fuller reception and understanding achieved in the Muslim world. The balance was redressed to some extent by the new translations of Greek and Arabic medical works that began to appear, first from Constantinus Africanus in southern Italy in the late eleventh century and then from the circle of Gerard of Cremona in Spain in the twelfth century. These works formed the basis of a new Latin medical learning that was developed and refined in the milieu of the universities from the thirteenth to the fifteenth centuries. In yet another phase of transmission and reception, Latin medicine provided the conceptual and often the textual basis for a growing vernacular European medical literature produced from the late fourteenth until the sixteenth century. Finally, the endeavors of a handful of medical humanists in the late fifteenth and the sixteenth centuries produced a full knowledge of the surviving texts of Greek medicine in the original language as well as in a fresh round of translations into Latin. The transformation of the ancient authors from living authorities to objects of historical interest began only in the seventeenth century.

The history of concepts of medical qualification and of specialized medical education, both central to the development of medicine as a profession, yields a parallel and related story. The idea of medical licensing first appears in legislation issued in Sicily before the mid-twelfth century; by the fourteenth century, regulations requiring practitioners to obtain some form of authentication or license from guilds, public authorities, or university faculties of medicine had become widespread in Europe. Salerno, a center of medical practice since the late tenth century, developed into a center of medical education in the latter part of the twelfth century. At Salerno, a curriculum of medical textbooks began to be established, and links between medicine and philosophy received a fresh emphasis. By the time faculties of medicine were institutionalized at the universities of Bologna, Montpellier, and Paris in the course of the thirteenth century, the essential components of late medieval and Renaissance advanced medical education leading to a university deree in medicine were all present. An important addition to the curriculum was anatomy taught on the human cadaver, a practice that may have begun around 1300.

Only a minority of all medical practitioners attended universities. In many parts of Europe, university-educated medical practitioners must have been rare before the late fourteenth or the fifteenth century, when their numbers relative to the population presumably increased with the enlargement of the University of Padua and also the addition of German medical faculties, however small. Nonetheless, from about 1300, university training was generally recognized as the highest form of medical education. Texts and theories developed in the world of Latin academic medicine supplied the basis for much of the medical lore and literature used by other practitioners. In addition, the twelfth- and thirteenth-century development of medical education and technical writing in Italy was accompanied by and inseparable from similar developments in surgery at Parma, Bologna, and elsewhere. From Italy, literate surgery passed to Montpellier in the thirteenth century and to Paris by the early fourteenth. Much of the content of this surgical teaching was absorbed by the numerous literate surgeons who flourished in northern Europe during the later fourteenth and the fifteenth centuries but who seldom had social or institutional connections to academic circles.

Many characteristics of the social role and organization of early modern medicine were prefigured in the fourteenth and fifteenth centuries: the appearance of vernacular medical texts; the existence (at least in some cities of southern Europe) of a "medical marketplace," in which a wide range of different types of practitioners competed for patients; the formation of colleges of physicians; the rivalries of physicians and surgeons, and the foundation of hospitals where some medical attention, as well as food and shelter, was available. In these respects, the main differences between the sixteenth and the two preceding centuries probably lie in scale and geographical distribution; to take only one example, the production and dissemination of vernacular medical books greatly increased after the introduction of printing.

Although much of the content of medicine was extremely durable, medical interests changed during the late medieval and Renaissance centuries. Astrology probably played a larger part in medical education and ideas in the fourteenth to the sixteenth centuries than in the thirteenth century. Numerous plague tractates produced in response to the repeated outbreaks of plague that attacked Europe beginning in the mid-fourteenth century attest to medical concern about current health problems. And medical scholarship developed as a sophisticated enterprise, fully responsive to contemporary interests, methodology, and controversies in natural philosophy.

Of course, this same medical scholarship of the thirteenth to the fifteenth centuries has often received a bad press—from humanist critics of scholasticism during the Renaissance, from historians of medical science during the nineteenth and early twentieth centuries, and from modern social historians who are inclined to focus on practitioners without a university education and on patients. Indeed, no one could deny that late medieval university-educated physicians and professors of medicine were involved in scholastic argumentation, that their focus was frequently philosophical as well as medical, and that their arrogance contributed to the denigration and exclusion of other practitioners, notably women and Jews.

However, academic medicine also produced substantial positive accomplishments. These included the establishment of durable institutions for providing formal medical education; an insistence upon the value of human physiology, health, and disease as objects of inquiry; the assimilation of a substantial body of ancient and Islamic scientific writing; the production of a rich, diverse, and complex medical literature; the refinement of a technical vocabulary; the identification of topics of physiological debate (usually discrepancies among ancient authors) that continued to be the focus of attention until the time of Harvey; and the creation of an environment in which the bold innovation of the public dissection of human cadavers could be legitimized.

Latin medical writings of the fourteenth and fifteenth centuries continued to be printed and read during the sixteenth century. In the world of vernacular medicine, treatises, concepts, and remedies translated or compiled from Latin sources before—in some instances, long before—1500 continued to be widely disseminated. By the late fifteenth century, however, medical learning was itself becoming permeated by a humanistic insistence on the superiority of the direct study of ancient Greek authors either in the original language or in modern translation. As a result, learned medical humanists launched a series of scathing attacks on the reliance on medieval translations and medieval Arab authorities in medical teaching. For example, in a work first published in 1521, Giovanni Manardo, a professor at Ferrara, characterized the *Canon* of Avicenna in its twelfth-century Latin translation as filled with "a dense cloud and infinite chaos of obscurities."[1]

Early sixteenth-century critics, however, did not propose to abandon traditional medical ideas, the authority of ancient books, or medical learning focused on arguments about texts. Instead, until about the middle of the sixteenth century, some of the most learned and innovative minds in medicine such as John Caius (1510–73; second founder of Gonville and Caius College, Cambridge, and reformer of the London College of Physicians) concentrated their efforts on improving the knowledge of Greek medicine by searching out and editing Greek medical texts and making or revising Latin translations. In short, they wanted more extensive and more authentic knowledge of essentially the same ancient authorities that their medieval and Islamic predecessors had used. A complete edition of Galen's works in Greek was printed in 1525, and numerous new Latin versions of Galenic and other ancient works on medicine and kindred subjects appeared in the first half of the sixteenth century.

Yet, this intensified enthusiasm for ancient Greek medicine in all its aspects, including related areas such as pharmacology, botany, and comparative anatomy, was also intimately associated with endeavors to expand actual knowledge of the natural world; and fuller knowledge of the writings of the ancients facilitated criticism as well as admiration. But until the late sixteenth century, although many critics claimed to have disproved, added to, or modified particular teachings of ancient authorities or endeavored to replace one ancient authority with another, few or none ignored ancient authority entirely. This was true even of those who made major independent investigations of physical nature. Thus, to take only one very celebrated example, the increased interest in human anatomy and in the practice of dissection, manifested at Paris, Padua, and elsewhere in the late fifteenth and the early sixteenth centuries, was doubtless stimulated by various aspects of Renaissance culture; but among these stimuli was surely Galen's insistence on the importance of the subject. That interest led, in turn, to many other activities, among them the translation into Latin for the first time of Galen's own dissection manual *On Anatomical Procedures* (1531). And the most important original contribution to a new science of anatomy in the sixteenth century, Andreas Vesalius' *On the Fabric of the Human Body* (1543), is intimately involved with Galen's anatomical writings, both as source and as object of attack.

Vesalius's work was perceived by contemporaries as radically innovative, but he was only one of many medical "moderns" or "neoterics"—terms used both in praise and in blame—who in the sixteenth century endeavored to achieve a better understanding of human and comparative anatomy; to reconsider the old disputes over the differences between "the philosophers and the physicians" in the light of the new anatomy; to expand knowledge of medicinal plants by establishing botanical gardens and producing new, more comprehensive, and more accurate herbals; to revise the understanding of disease in order to accommodate such "new" complaints as syphilis; to uncover the "genuine" Hippocrates beneath Galen's widely read commentaries; to introduce clinical instruction in the hospital; and to update the way old textbooks such as the *Canon* were taught or to compose new texts to replace them. In terms of accretion of information, doubtless anatomy and botany were the most successful of these endeavors. In particular, the University of Padua became a noted center of anatomical teaching during the second half of the sixteenth century; as is well known, the milieu of Paduan anatomy provided the early training of William Harvey. With the acceptance of Harvey's account of the circulation of the blood, fundamental tenets of Galenic physiology finally had to be discarded. More generally, the radical revision of physiology that began in the seventeenth century took as its point of departure the anatomical accomplishments of Vesalius and his successors.

Universities provided the milieu for almost all the innovative endeavors described in the preceding paragraph. Thus, institutions in which an essentially medieval curriculum continued to be taught were simultaneously the main centers of Renaissance innovation in anatomy, physiology, and medical education. Old curricula were modified to some extent. At Padua, more time was given to anatomy and to practical medicine and less to medical theory. In some institutions, humanistically inclined reformers succeeded in expelling the *Canon* of Avicenna from the curriculum; this was the case in several German institutions during the 1550s. In some of the Italian universities, the *Canon* was retained as an official textbook until the eighteenth century; but from the 1520s, innovative teachers used their lectures on the *Canon* and other traditional texts to criticize the author or introduce new information. Leading anatomists and botanists freely pointed out the extent to which they had amassed information unknown to or contradicting their predecessors. These themes of renaissance in medicine reflect real change and genuine advances in knowledge, but the changes long involved the modification, not the rejection, of an existing system of knowledge.

Enthusiasts for a revived and purified Greek medicine, which included important works on surgery, believed that it would be of practical use to working surgeons as well as to academically trained physicians. In reality, significant achievements in surgery during the sixteenth century emerged from a social and profssional context largely disconnected from and hostile to academic medicine. The enlarged scale of warfare, together with the widespread use of field artillery and handguns, produced more numerous and more serious battlefield casualties and increased the opportunity for surgeons to gain experience in treating certain types of injury. Ambroise Paré, the most accomplished practitioner of and writer on surgery of the age, was a barber-surgeon who gained much of his expertise in various military campaigns in France. Paré's substitution of ligatures for cautery to check bleeding after amputation increased the chances of survival after amputation of limbs, and this innovation, in his practice and in general, had civilian as well as military applications.

But in the sixteenth century only the German medical practitioner, natural philosopher, and mystic Paracelsus (1493–1541) and his followers made it their objective to repudiate the entire tradition of academic medicine and to replace it with a different system based on folk medicine and craft wisdom, alchemy, and occult practices. Much of this system, if system it may be called, of course involved the reworking of highly traditional concepts, some also derived from learned sources. Paracelsus' ideas about remedies and his emphasis upon the use of mineral ingredients, notably mercury, influenced pharmaceutical practice from the latter part of the sixteenth century. Moreover, vernacular medical writers in Protestant northern Europe were often attracted by Paracelsus' repudiation of academic medicine and his association of reform in medicine with religious ideas and religious reform. Subsequently, Paracelsus' more general religious, philosophical, and physical concepts appear to have influenced some strands of thought in seventeenth-century natural philosophy.

Thus, although the system of medical knowledge and medical practice described in this book flourished throughout the sixteenth century, changes introduced during the sixteenth century surely began the process of bringing down the traditional system of medical knowledge. What has been termed "the medical Renaissance of the sixteenth century" involved both the culmination and the partial rejection of an older medical renaissance that had begun centuries earlier. Many separate developments contributed: the humanist scorn for medicine's recent past; the growth of anatomical and botanical research and the concomitant steady accumulation of information; the apparent proliferation of "new" diseases unknown to the ancients; the critical comparisons facilitated by Renaissance philology, translations, editions, and indexes that for the first time made possible a full knowledge of almost all the surviving sources of Greek medicine; the critiques by Paracelsians; and Renaissance philosophical eclecticism that fostered a search—at first among other ancient sources—for alternatives to Aristotle and Galen. With respect to anatomy and physiology, the links with ancient medicine were finally broken in the age of Harvey, although therapies and materia medica retained traditional elements until a very much later period. But no sharp break separates the medicine described in this book from that of the early modern world.

NOTES

The notes are confined to bibliographical references and make no expository additions to the text. References to ancient sources are identified by subdivisions of the text (e.g., by book and chapter numbers) in order to facilitate the location of material in editions or translations other than those cited. References to Latin texts are accompanied by reference to an English translation whenever possible. (An exception is made in the case of a few well-known works on nonmedical subjects—for example, the *Rule of St. Benedict*—translations of which can easily be located.) If no other translator is indicated, passages quoted in English from Latin texts were translated by me. Some works by Galen are identified, under their conventional Latin titles, by their location in the standard edition of the Greek text, with Latin translation, namely *Claudii Galeni Opera omnia*, ed. C. G. Kühn (Leipzig, 1821–33), abbreviated Kühn. Readers should be aware that the Latin translations printed in Kühn's edition are not necessarily those used in the period covered by this book.

The following abbreviations also are used in the notes.

AMHP	*Acta Medicae Historiae Patavina*
BHM	*Bulletin of the History of Medicine*
CSEL	*Corpus scriptorum ecclesiasticorum latinorum*
CTC	*Catalogus translationum et commentariorum: Medieval and Renaissance Latin Translations and Commentaries*, edited by Paul Oskar Kristeller, et al. (Washington, D.C. 1960–)
EETS	Early English Text Society
JHM	*Journal of the History of Medicine and Allied Sciences*
LCL	Loeb Classical Library (Cambridge, Mass., and London)
MJ	*Medizinhistorisches Journal*
SA	*Sudhoffs Archiv*
WMF	*Würzburger medizinhistorische Forschungen*

CHAPTER ONE

1. For some of the sources of the brief sketch of ancient Greek and Roman medicine in this chapter, and for further information, see the works listed for chapter 1 in the Guide to Further Reading.

2. G. E. R. Lloyd, *Science, Folklore and Ideology: Studies in the Life Sciences in Ancient Greece* (Cambridge, England, 1983), 82–83, 86–111, 129–33.

3. Hippocrates, *Dreams* (also known as *Regimen* 4), chap. 89, in *Hippocrates*, ed. and trans. W. H. S. Jones, vol. 4, LCL (1972; originally issued 1923).

4. *Sense and Sensibilia* 1.436a17–21, translated in *The Complete Works of Aristotle*, ed. Jonathan Barnes (Princeton, 1984), 1:693.

5. *Parts of Animals* 1.1.641a19–20, translated in *Complete Works*, ed. Barnes, 1:997.

6. Galen, *On the Natural Faculties* 2.1, ed. and trans. A. W. Brock. LCL (1979; originally issued 1916).

7. A. Beccaria, "Sulle tracce di un antico canone latino di Ippocrate e di Galeno," *Italia Medioevale e Umanistica* 2 (1959): 1–56; 4 (1961): 1–75; 14 (1971): 1–23. *Iohannis Alexandrini commentaria in librum De sectis Galeni*, ed. C. D. Pritchet (Leiden, 1982), is an early Latin commentary on a work of Galen. John M. Riddle, "Dioscorides," CTC 4 (1980): 20–22.

8. William D. Sharpe, *Isidore of Seville: The Medical Writings, Transactions of the American Philosophical Society* 54, pt. 2 (Philadelphia, 1964).

9. Ambrose, *Exameron* 6.71–72, CSEL 32, pt. 1, pp. 258–59. Cf. Cicero, *De natura deorum* 2.54–55, ed. and trans. H. Rackham, LCL (1933).

10. The subject has recently been surveyed and discussed in Darrel W. Amundsen, "Medicine and Faith in Early Christianity," BHM 56 (1982): 326–50; Vivian Nutton, "From Galen to Alexander, Aspects of Medicine and Medical Practice in Late Antiquity," in *Symposium on Byzantine Medicine, Dumbarton Oaks Papers*, no. 38 (1984): 1–14; and idem, "Murders and Miracles: Lay Attitudes to Medicine in Classical Antiquity," in *Patients and Practitioners*, ed. Roy Porter (Cambridge, England, 1985), 45–53. Amundsen stresses Christian ideas favorable to or compatible with medicine, Nutton emphasizes tensions between faith and secular or physical healing.

11. *The City of God Against the Pagans* [*De civitate Dei*] 22.22, ed. and trans. William M. Green, LCL (7 vols., 1957–72), 7:305, 311–13.

12. Gregory of Tours, *Historiarum libri decem* [*History of the Franks*] 10.1, ed. R. Buchner (Darmstadt, 1955–56), reports Pope Gregory's sermon to the Roman populace on the subject, and his arrangements for public penitential religious exercises.

13. *De civitate dei* 22.8. Peter Brown, *The Cult of the Saints: Its Rise and Function in Latin Christianity* (Chicago, 1981), 77–78.

14. Jerome, Letter 77 in his *Select Letters*, ed. and trans. F. A. Wright, LCL (1933).

15. Augustine, Letter 211, no. 49 in his *Select Letters*, ed. and trans. James H. Baxter, LCL (1930). For Cassiodorus, see n. 18 below. *Regula* [Benedictine Rule] 27, 28, 36, *Sources chrétiennes* 182 (Paris, 1972): 548–52, 570–72. Rudolph Arbesmann, "The Concept of 'Christus medicus' in St. Augustine," *Traditio* 10 (1954): 1–28; Gerhard Fichtner, "Christus als Arzt. Ursprünge und Wirkungen eines Motivs," *Frühmittelalterliche Studien: Jahrbuch des Instituts für Frühmittelalterforschung der Universität Münster* 16 (1982): 1–17.

16. Cassiodorus Senator, *Variae* 6.19, *Corpus Christianorum. Series Latina* 96:248–50.

17. Gregory of Tours, *Historia* 10.15 and 5.6; Darrel W. Amundsen, "Visigothic Medical Legislation," BHM 45 (1971): 553–69. Additional examples of legislation relating to secular medical practice (mostly involving treatment of wounds) in other Germanic law codes are to be found in Annette Niederhellman, *Arzt und Heilkunde in der Frühmittelalterlichen leges* (Berlin and New York, 1983).

18. Cassiodorus Senator, *Institutiones* 1.31, ed. R. A. B. Mynors (Oxford, 1937) ("Dioscorides" may refer to a Latin herbal loosely based on Dioscorides); C. H. Talbot, *Medicine in Medieval England* (London, 1967), 17–21; Linda E. Voigts, "Anglo-Saxon Plant Rem-

edies and the Anglo-Saxons," *Isis* 70 (1979): 250–68; Monica H. Green, "The *De genecia* Attributed to Constantinus Africanus," *Speculum* 62 (1987): 299–323, at 310.

19. Bede, *Ecclesiastical History of the English People* 5.2, ed. and trans. B. Colgrave and R. A. B. Mynors (Oxford, 1969). Jole Agrimi and Chiara Crisciani, *Medicina del corpo e medicina dell'anima: Note sul sapere del medico fino all'inizio del secolo XIII, Episteme* (Milan, 1978), contains a perceptive discussion of the intimate connections between spiritual care, charity to the poor, and health care in the early Middle Ages.

20. Gregory of Tours, *Historia* 5.6. On early medieval ecclesiastical endeavors to limit recourse to folk practices, see Darrel W. Amundsen, "The Medieval Catholic Tradition," in *Caring and Curing: Health and Medicine in the Western Religious Traditions*, ed. Ronald L. Numbers and Darrel W. Amundsen (New York, 1986), 65–107 at 68–81.

21. Fuat Sezgin, *Geschichte des arabischen Schrifttums* 3 (Leiden, 1970): 21–171, provides details regarding translations of medical books from Greek into Syriac and Arabic and dissemination in the Muslim world. On the development of Islamic medicine, Manfred Ullmann, *Die Medizin im Islam* (Leiden, 1970).

22. Bio-bibliographical information on ar-Rāzī, ʿAlī b. ʿAl-Abbās, and Abu l-Qāsim is contained in Sezgin, *Geschichte*, 3:274–94, 320–22, 323–25.

23. Paul Oskar Kristeller, *Studi sulla scuola medica salernitana* (Naples, 1986), 19–49.

24. Darrel W. Amundsen, "Medieval Canon Law on Medical and Surgical Practice by the Clergy," *BHM* 52 (1978): 22–44.

25. John of Salisbury, *Metalogicon* 1.4, ed. C. C. I. Webb (Oxford, 1929).

26. Bernard of Clairvaux, Letter 388 in his *Letters*, trans. Bruno Scott James (Chicago, 1953), 458–59.

27. Marie-Thérèse D'Alverny, "Translators and Translations," in *Renaissance and Renewal in the Twelfth Century*, ed. Robert L. Benson and Giles Constable (Cambridge, Mass., 1982), 421–62. Heinrich Schipperges, *Die Assimilation der arabischen Medizin durch das lateinische Mittelalter*. SA, Beiheft 3 (Wiesbaden, 1964).

28. Guillaume de Conches, *Philosophia mundi* 1.22, ed. Gregor Maurach (Pretoria, 1974), draws on the *Pantegni*, a free translation of Haly Abbas by Constantinus Africanus; in Guillaume's *Dragmaticon* (*De substantiis physicis*, Strasburg 1567, facsimile Frankfurt/Main 1967), written in the 1140s, Book 6 contains a lengthy section on human physiology drawing on Galenic ideas. On Hildegard of Bingen's medical and physiological ideas, see Peter Dronke, *Women Writers of the Middle Ages* (Cambridge, 1984), 144–201, and texts edited at 231–64.

29. S. J. Tester, *A History of Western Astrology* (Woodbridge, 1987), 98–201.

CHAPTER TWO

1. Life of Tommaso del Garbo in Filippo Villani, *Liber de civitatis Florentiae famosis civibus*, ed. C. G. Galletti (Florence, 1847), 29. The passage is quoted from an early Italian version of Villani's book in Katharine Park, *Doctors and Medicine in Early Renaissance Florence* (Princeton, 1985), 131–32. Much of the available information about Tommaso del Garbo is summarized, and bibliography cited, in the same work.

2. The relevant statutes are printed in English translation in *The Liber Augustalis or Constitutions of Melfi Promulgated by the Emperor Frederick II for the Kingdom of Sicily in 1231*,

trans. James M. Powell (Syracuse, N.Y., 1971), 130–31, Title XLIV (1) and Title LXV (23) (1). Kristeller, *Studi sulla scuola medica salernitana*, 51, 62–68.

3. Park, *Doctors and Medicine*, 17–18, 23; Richard Palmer, *The Studio of Venice and Its Graduates in the Sixteenth Century* (Padua and Trieste, 1983), 3–4; Gweneth Whitteridge, "Some Italian Precursors of the Royal College of Physicians," *Journal of the Royal College of Physicians* 12 (1977): 67–80.

4. Vivian Nutton, "Continuity or Rediscovery? The City Physician in Classical Antiquity and Medieval Italy," in his *From Democedes to Harvey* (London, 1988), no. VI, pp. 9–46 (also in *The Town and State Physician in Europe from the Middle Ages to the Enlightenment*, ed. Andrew W. Russell [Wolfenbüttel, 1981]). Amada López de Meneses, "Documentos culturales de Pedro el Ceremonioso," *Estudios de Edad Media de la Corona de Aragón* 5 (1952): 682–84, 690–91, 695–96, 700–701, nos. 16, 25, 31, 37. For discussion of some of these documents, see Luis Garcia Ballester, Michael R. McVaugh, and Augustin Rubio Vela, 1989. *Medical Licensing and Learning in Fourteenth-Century Valencia. Transactions of the American Philosophical Society*, vol. 79, pt. 6 (Philadelphia).

5. F. H. Rashdall, *The Universities of Europe in the Middle Ages*, ed. Maurice Powicke and A. B. Emden (Oxford, 1936; reissued 1988), 1:221, 231. Margaret Pelling and Charles Webster, "Medical Practitioners," in *Health, Medicine, and Mortality in the Sixteenth Century*, ed. Charles Webster (Cambridge, England, 1979), 215.

6. Pearl Kibre, "The Faculty of Medicine at Paris, Charlatanism, and Unlicensed Medical Practice in the Later Middle Ages," BHM 27 (1953): 1–29.

7. Pelling and Webster, "Medical Practitioners," 182–183; Kibre, "The Faculty of Medicine."

8. Nancy G. Siraisi, *Taddeo Alderotti and His Pupils* (Princeton, 1981), 30–31; Park, *Doctors and Medicine*, 152–58; Carol Rawcliffe, "The Profits of Practice: The Wealth and Status of Medical Men in Later Medieval England," *Social History of Medicine* 1 (1988): 61–78.

9. Villani, *Liber de famosis civibus*, 29; Lynn Thorndike, A History of Magic and Experimental Science 2 (New York, 1923): 931–33.

10. Rawcliffe, "Profits of Practice," 66.

11. Ronald C. Finucane, *Miracles and Pilgrims: Popular Beliefs in Medieval England* (Totowa, N.J., 1977), 9, 59.

12. López, "Documentos culturales," 695–96.

13. *I processi inediti per Francesca Bussa dei Ponziani (Santa Francesca Romana) 1440–1453*, ed. Placido Tommaso Lugano (Vatican City, 1945), 261, 264, 266.

14. Danielle Jacquart, *Le milieu médical en France du XIIᵉ au XVᵉ siècle. En annexe 2ᵉ supplément au "Dictionnaire" d'Ernest Wickersheimer* (Geneva, 1981), 363; Luis Garcia Ballester, "Medical Science in Thirteenth-Century Castile: Problems and Prospects," BHM 61 (1987): 185; Irma Naso, *Medici e strutture sanitarie nella società tardo-medievale: Il Piemonte dei secoli XIV e XV* (Milan, 1982), 156; Park, *Doctors and Medicine*, 57; Robert S. Gottfried, "English Medical Practitioners, 1340–1530," BHM 58 (1984): 164–82.

15. Jacquart, *Le milieu médical*, 363; Park, *Doctors and Medicine*, 57.

16. Villani, *Cronica* 11.94, p. 210, quoted in Park, *Doctors and Medicine*, 55; ibid., 55–58; Lauro Martines, *Lawyers and Statecraft in Renaissance Florence* (Princeton, 1968), 5, 41; David Herlihy and Christiane Klapisch-Zuber, *Tuscans and Their Families: A Study of the Florentine Catasto of 1427* (New Haven, 1985), 115, 122, 124.

17. Jacquart, *Le milieu médical*, 155–59, and 380, table 15.

18. M. R. James, *The Ancient Libraries of Canterbury and Dover* (Cambridge, 1903), 138, nos. 1706–14. Nearby St. Augustine's Abbey owned more than 100 medical books in the late fifteenth century; most of them were probably acquired during the thirteenth century (ibid., 332–49). K. W. Humphreys, "The Medical Books of the Medieval Friars," *Libri: International Library Review* 3 (1954): 95–103; this article also lists medical books found in the libraries of twelfth-century English monasteries. Paolo Marangon, "Il rapporto culturale tra università e ordini mendicanti nella Padova del Duecento," *Il Santo* 18 (1978): 129–32, includes references to medical learning and activity.

19. Jacquart, *Le milieu médical*, 383, table 18; Michael Macdonald, *Mystical Bedlam* (Cambridge, 1981), 19–20.

20. Amundsen, "Medieval Canon Law," 40. On Teodorico Borgognoni, see chap. 6.

21. Margaret Pelling, "Occupational Diversity: Barbersurgeons and the Trades of Norwich," *BHM* 56 (1982): 484–511.

22. Siraisi, *Taddeo*, 27–31. *Statuti delle Università e dei Collegi dello Studio bolognese*, ed. Carlo Malagola (Bologna, 1888), 426, 430–32, 438, 466 (doctoral college statutes of 1378).

23. Monica H. Green, "Women's Medical Practice and Medical Care in Medieval Europe," *Signs* 14 (1989): 434–73, summarizes the available evidence regarding female medical practice. John Benton, "Trotula, Women's Problems, and the Professionalization of Medicine in the Middle Ages," *BHM* 59 (1985): 30–53. Dronke, *Women Writers*, 171–82, esp. 180–82.

24. Green, "Women's Medical Practice," 440–41, summarizing data from the prosopographical studies of Jacquart and Gottfried cited above.

25. Luis Garcia Ballester, *Los Moriscos y la medicina: Un capítulo de la medicina y la ciencia marginadas en la España del siglo XVI* (Barcelona, 1984), 64–68.

26. Maimonides, *Medical Writings*, trans. Fred Rosner (Haifa, 1984), introduction, 1–4.

27. Jacquart, *Le milieu médical*, 160–67, 354, and 383, table 18; Garcia Ballester, "Medical Science in Castile," 195–98; Benjamin Richler, "Manuscripts of Avicenna's Kanon in Hebrew Translation: A Revised and Up-to-date List," *Koroth* 8 (1982): 145*–68*; Joseph Shatzmiller, "In Search of the 'Book of Figures': Medicine and Astrology in Montpellier at the Turn of the Fourteenth Century," *AJSreview* (Association for Jewish Studies, Cambridge, Mass.) 7–8 (1982–83): 383–407; idem, "Livres médicaux et éducation médicale: à propos d'un contrat de Marseille en 1316," *Mediaeval Studies* 42 (1980): 463–70. Harry Friedenwald, *The Jews and Medicine. Essays* (2 vols., Baltimore, 1944), 1:146–80, 217–20; 2:551–74, 613–700; Cecil Roth, "The Qualification of Jewish Physicians in the Middle Ages," *Speculum* 28 (1953): 834–43.

28. Jacquart, *Le milieu médical*, 363–64; Park, *Doctors and Medicine*, 75; Naso, *Medici*, 156.

29. Dino's career: Siraisi, *Taddeo*, 55–64. On Bono: A. Corsini, "Nuovo contributo di notizie intorno alla vita di maestro Tommaso del Garbo," *Rivista di storia delle scienze mediche e naturali* 16 (1925): 268.

30. William Eamon and Gundolf Keil, "'Plebs amat empirica': Nicholas of Poland and His Critique of the Medieval Medical Establishment," *SA* 71 (1987): 180–96.

31. Linda E. Voigts and Michael R. McVaugh, *A Latin Technical Phlebotomy and Its English Translation*, *Transactions of the American Philosophical Society* 74, pt. 2 (Philadelphia, 1984), 15. Josep Perarnau i Espelt, "Activitats i fórmules supersticioses de guarició a

Catalunya en la primera meitat del segle XIV," *Arxiu de Textos Catalans Antics* 1 (1982): 47–78, documents 3, 4, and 6. (I am grateful to Michael McVaugh for drawing my attention to this article.)

32. *The Cyrurgie of Guy de Chauliac*, ed. Margaret S. Ogden, EETS, no. 265 (Oxford, 1971), 9–10. The edition is of a Middle English translation of Guy's Latin text; for the Latin, Guy de Chauliac, *Cyrurgia* (Venice, 1498), fol. 3ʳ.

33. Michael R. McVaugh, "Royal Patronage of Medicine: The Kingdom of Aragon in the Early Fourteenth Century," unpublished paper. The author is engaged in a comprehensive study of material pertaining to medicine in the archives of the Kingdom of Aragon.

34. Symon de Phares, *Recueil des plus célèbres astrologues et quelques hommes doctes*, ed. Ernest Wickersheimer (Paris, 1929), v–xii, 14–15, 245–69. Lynn Thorndike, *A History of Magic and Experimental Science*, 4 (New York, 1934): 544–58; Maxime Préaud, *Les astrologues à la fin du Moyen Age* (Paris, 1984), 21–50.

35. Siraisi, *Taddeo*, 48.

36. Park, *Doctors and Medicine*, 85–117, provides numerous examples for Florence.

37. Nutton, "Continuity or Rediscovery," 24–34. Richard Palmer, "Physicians and the State in Post-Medieval Italy," in *Town and State Physician*, ed. Russell, 47; Naso, *Medici*, 156.

38. Park, *Doctors and Medicine*, 104–6; idem, "The Medieval Hospital," FMR 8:127–38. Park is engaged in an ongoing study of the provisions for medical care at Santa Maria Nuova.

39. *Il processo di canonizzazione di Chiara da Montefalco*, ed. Enrico Menestò (Perugia, 1984).

40. Ibid., 270, 435.

41. Ibid., 292–93. The information that Simone da Spello was *medico condotto* of Montefalco is found in an editorial appendix on p. 624.

42. Several witnesses among the nuns gave accounts of this episode; that quoted is ibid., 339–42. All agreed that Suor Francesca actually performed the autopsy, with other nuns acting as her assistants. My account was written before I had seen Piero Camporesi, *La carne impassibile* (Milan, 1983), 11–17, where it is also described.

43. *Processo*, ed. Menestò, 422–23, 445, 455.

44. *Processi*, ed. Lugano, 170–71.

45. *Processo*, ed. Menestò, witness 113, pp. 388–89; witness 119, pp. 395–96; witness 132, pp. 407–8; witness 141, pp. 416–17; witness 158, pp. 432–33; witness 177, pp. 458–59; witness 193, pp. 475–76.

46. The health situation of medieval Europe is well summarized in Katharine Park, "Medicine and Society in Medieval Europe, 500–1500," in *History of Medicine in Society*, ed. Andrew Wear (Cambridge University Press, forthcoming).

47. Luke Demaitre, "Nature and the Art of Medicine in the Later Middle Ages," *Medievalia* 2 (1976): 23–47.

48. Some English examples (mid-fourteenth to late fifteenth century) in Madeleine Pelner Cosman, "Medieval Malpractice: The Dicta and the Dockets," *Bulletin of the New York Academy of Medicine* 49 (1973): 22–47.

49. Matteo Villani, *Chronica* 1.2, in Giovanni Villani, *Cronica: Con le continuazioni di Matteo e Filippo*, ed. Giovanni Aquilecchia (Turin, 1979), 299.

50. Park, *Doctors and Medicine*, 76–84.

51. Amundsen, "Medieval Canon Law."

52. *Chartularium universitatis portugalensis* (1288–1537), ed. A. Moreira de Sá, vols. 1–8 (Lisbon, 1966–81), provides numerous examples under index entries relating to medicine.

53. Darrel W. Amundsen, "Casuistry and Professional Obligations: The Regulation of Physicians by the Court of Conscience in the Late Middle Ages," *Transactions & Studies of The College of Physicians of Philadelphia* 3 (1981): 21–39, 93–112.

54. *Processi*, ed. Lugano, 148–203 and 261–83, especially 156–60, 164–66, 242–43, 261, 264, 272.

55. Francesco Petrarca, *Invectiva contra medicum: Testo latino e volgarizzamento di Ser Domenico Silvestri*, ed. Pier Giorgio Ricci and Bortolo Martinelli (new ed., Rome, 1978), 57. Raimundus Capuanus, *Vita Sanctae Caterinae*, *Acta sanctorum*, April, vol. 3 (Paris and Rome 1866): 898–903 (English translation in Raymond of Capua, *The Life of St. Catherine of Siena*, trans. George Lamb [New York, 1960], 130–49).

56. Texts are cited and discussed in detail in Nancy G. Siraisi, "The Physician's Task: Medical Reputations in Humanist Collective Biographies," in *The Rational Arts of Living*, ed. A. C. Crombie and Nancy Siraisi, Smith College Studies in History, vol. 50 (Northampton, Mass., 1987), 105–33.

CHAPTER THREE

1. The bibliography on the medieval university movement and medieval higher education in general is much too extensive to be indicated here. The standard work on universities, and a good guide to major published collections of university documents, is still Rashdall, *Universities* (see chap. 2, n. 5). Recent studies have added some new collections of documents as well as information about the content of university teaching and the social context.

2. Humphreys, "The Medical Books of the Medieval Friars," which also includes a summary of the holdings of twelfth-century English monastic libraries. Rüdiger Krist, *Berthold Blumentrosts "Quaestiones disputatae circa tractatum Avicennae de generatione embryonis et librum meteorum Aristotelis": Ein Beitrag zur Wissenschaftsgeschichte des mittelalterlichen Würzburgs*, WMF, vol. 43 (Hanover, 1987). Siraisi, *Taddeo*, 34.

3. Tiziana Pesenti Marangon, "La miscellanea astrologica del prototipografo padovano Bartolomeo Valdizocco e la diffusione dei testi astrologici e medici fra i lettori padovani del '400," *Quaderni per la Storia dell'Università di Padova* 11 (1978): 87–106; Tiziana Pesenti, "Generi e pubblico della letteratura medica padovana nel Tre- e Quattrocento," in *Università e società nei secoli XII-XVI. Atti del nono Convegno Internazionale di studio tenuto a Pistoia nei giorni 20–25 settembre 1979* (Bologna, 1983), 523–45, esp. 543–45.

4. Tony Hunt, "Recettes médicales en vers français d'apres le manuscrit 0.8.27 de Trinity College Cambridge," *Romania* 106 (1985): 57–83; Guy de Chauliac, *Cyrurgie*, ed. Ogden, is one example of a lengthy and sophisticated work (for further discussion of its dissemination, see chap. 6); Voigts and McVaugh, *A Latin Technical Phlebotomy*; Beryl Rowland, ed. and trans., *Medieval Woman's Guide to Health* (Kent, Ohio, 1981); Linda E. Voigts, "Editing Middle English Medical Texts: Needs and Issues," in *Editing Texts in the History of Science and Medicine*, ed. Trevor H. Levere (New York and London, 1982), 39–66, esp. 42–43; idem, "Report and Reviews: Old and Middle English Medicine," *Society*

for Ancient Medicine and Pharmacy Newsletter, no. 16 (October 1988), 31–36; idem, "Scientific and Medical Books" in *Book Production and Publishing in Britain, 1375–1475*, ed. Jeremy Griffiths and Derek Pearsall (Cambridge, 1989), 345–402.

5. Krist, *Berthold Blumentrosts "Quaestiones,"* 8. Gundolf Keil, "Das Arzneibuch Ortolfs von Baierland: Sein Umfang und sein Einfluss auf die 'Cirurgia magistri Petri de Ulma'," *SA* 43 (1959): 20–60. Attention is drawn to the importance of vernacular technical medical writings in *Medizin im mittelalterlichen Abendland*, ed. Gerhard Baader and Gundolf Keil (Darmstadt, 1982), 23–44.

6. Luis Garcia Ballester and Michael R. McVaugh, "Nota sobre el control de la actividad médica y quirúrgica de los barberos (barbers, barbitonsores) en los *Furs* de Valencia de 1329," *Homenatge al Doctor Sebastià Garcia Martínez* (Valencia, 1988), document at p. 88. Compare Voigts and McVaugh, *A Latin Technical Phlebotomy*, 38.

7. Nancy G. Siraisi, *Arts and Sciences at Padua* (Toronto, 1973), chap. 5, summarizing information about medical teaching before 1350, when only about a dozen professors of medicine can be securely identified; Tiziana Pesenti, *Professori e promotori di medicina nello studio di Padova dal 1405 al 1509: Repertorio bio-bibliografico* (Padua and Trieste, 1984), for the size and productivity of the fifteenth-century medical faculty.

8. Very few items in Vicente Beltran de Heredia, O.P., *Cartulario de la Universidad de Salamanca* (6 vols., Salamanca, 1970–73) pertain to medicine, or medical teaching, masters, or students before 1500. A few medical books and masters in fifteenth-century Salamanca are noted in Guy Beaujouan, *Manuscrits scientifiques médiévaux de l'université de Salamanque et de ses "Colegios Mayores,"* Bibliothèque de l'Ecole des Hautes Etudes Hispaniques, Fasc. 32 (Bordeaux, 1962), 3, 59–60. Werner Kuhn, *Die studenten der Universität Tübingen zwischen 1477 und 1534* (2 vols., Göppingen, 1971); Gerhard Fichtner, "Padova e Tübingen: La formazione medica nei secoli XVI e XVII," *AMHP* 19 (1972–73): 43–62.

9. Robert Favreau, "L'université de Poitiers et la société poitevine à la fin du Moyen Age," *Les universités à la fin du Moyen Age*, ed. Jacques Paquet and Jozef Ijsewijn (Louvain, 1978), 578, no. 71; 580, no. 102; 582, nos. 120 and 121; Pesenti, *Professori*.

10. Faye M. Getz, "Medicine at Medieval Oxford," forthcoming in *History of the University of Oxford*, vol. 2: *Late Medieval Oxford*, ed. J. I. Catto. Voigts and McVaugh, *A Latin Technical Phlebotomy*, 12–14.

11. The preservation of extensive early matriculation records of the German universities has made possible detailed studies of their size and social composition. Rainer Christoph Schwinges, *Deutsche Universitätbesucher im 14. und 15. Jahrhundert: Studien zur Sozialgeschichte des Alten Reiches* (Stuttgart, 1986), 1, 465–86, and table at 470; James H. Overfield, "University Studies and the Clergy in Pre-Reformation Germany," in *Rebirth, Reform and Resilience: Universities in Transition 1300–1700*, ed. James M. Kittelson and Pamela J. Transue (Columbus, Ohio, 1984), 254. Other examples of small medical faculties: Werner Kuhn, *Die Studenten der Universität Tübingen*, 1:35; Hans Goerke, "Die medizinische Fakultät von 1472 bis zur Gegenwart," in *Die Ludwig-Maximilians-Universität in ihren Fakultäten*, ed. Laetitia Boehm and Johannes Spörl (Berlin, 1972), 1:185–87 (on Ingoldstadt); Erich Kleineidam, *Universitas Studii Erffordensis* (2 vols., Leipzig, 1964, 1969), 1:18–19, 97, 124–25; 2:337.

12. For example, Michele Fuiano, *Maestri di medicina e filosofia a Napoli nel Quattrocento* (Naples, 1973); Naso, *Medici*, with discussion of the medical faculty of the University of Turin (founded 1404, permanently established at Turin only in 1436) at 111–22.

13. Helen Brown Wicher, "Nemesius Emesenus," *CTC* 6 (1986): 39–40, 46–50.

14. Kristeller, *Studi sulla scuola medica salernitana*. Mark D. Jordan, "The Construction of a Philosophical Medicine: Exegesis and Argument in Salernitan Teaching On the Soul," *Osiris* 6 (forthcoming 1990). A. Birkenmajer, "Le rôle joué par les médecins et les naturalistes dans la réception d'Aristote au XIIᵉ et XIIIᵉ siècles," reprinted in his *Etudes d'histoire des sciences et de la philosophie du Moyen Age, Studia Copernicana* 1 (Wrocław, Warsaw, Cracow, 1970): 73–87; Danielle Jacquart, "Aristotelian Thought in Salerno," in *A History of Twelfth-Century Western Philosophy*, ed. Peter Dronke (Cambridge, 1988), 407–28; Brian Lawn, ed. *The Prose Salernitan Questions* (London, 1979). Not all the questions edited by Lawn are either definitely of Salernitan origin or found in Salernitan manuscripts.

15. L. Dulieu, *La médecine à Montpellier*. Vol. 1: *Le Moyen Age* (n.p., n.d. [1976?]). Numerous documents pertaining to the early faculty of medicine are found in *Cartulaire de l'Université de Montpellier . . . Tome 1 (1181–1400)* (Montpellier, 1890).

16. Ernest Wickersheimer, *Dictionnaire biographique des médecins en France au moyen âge* (Paris, 1936), 1:196–97, and its *Supplément*, ed. Danielle Jacquart (Geneva, 1979), 90–91.

17. *Cartulaire*, 1:180–83, document 2; 1:210–13, document 20. Michael R. McVaugh, "An Early Discussion of Medicinal Degrees at Montpellier by Henry of Winchester," *Bulletin of the History of Medicine* 49 (1975): 57–71.

18. Charles Homer Haskins, "A List of Text-Books from the Close of the Twelfth Century," in his *Studies in the History of Mediaeval Science* (2d ed., Cambridge, Mass., 1927), 356–76, with medical books listed on 374–75. The dates given for Nequam's (or Neckham's) stay in Paris are suggested in R. W. Hunt, *The Schools and the Cloister: The Life and Writings of Alexander Nequam (1157–1217)*, edited and revised by Margaret Gibson (Oxford, 1984). Jacquart, *Le milieu médical*, 68; *Chartularium universitatis Parisiensis*, ed. H. Denifle and E. Chatelain (Paris, 1889), 1:517, no. 453. The development of medical studies at Montpellier and Paris is compared in Danielle Jacquart, "La réception du *Canon* d'Avicenne: Comparaison entre Montpellier et Paris au XIIIᵉ et XIVᵉ siècles," *Histoire de l'école médicale de Montpellier. Actes du 110ᵉ Congrès National des Sociétés Savantes (Montpellier, 1985)* (Paris, 1985), 2:69–77.

19. Konrad Goehl, *Guido d'Arezzo der Jüngere und sein "Liber mitis.'* WMF. vol. 32 (Hanover, 1984), 12, 15–31. This adds information to the remarks about the introduction of the *Canon* in Siraisi, *Avicenna in Renaissance Italy* (Princeton, 1987), 44, 52. The dating of the treatise may be problematic, but the unique manuscript was written ca. 1230.

20. Siraisi, *Taddeo*, 13–24, contains a summary of the early history of medical teaching at Bologna, with bibliographical references.

21. Paolo Marangon, *Alle origini dell'Aristotelismo padovano (sec. XII–XIII)* (Padua, 1973). Jacquart, *Supplément* to Wickersheimer, *Dictionnaire*, 232–36 (on Petrus Hispanus); Eugenia Paschetto, *Pietro d'Abano, medico e filosofo* (Florence, 1984) (including bibliography of manuscripts and editions of the *Conciliator differentiarum philosophorum et precipue medicorum*).

22. *Cartulaire*, 1:181, document 2, medical statutes (1220).

23. Siraisi, *Taddeo*, 21, and bibliography there cited. Rashdall, *Universities*, 2:255–56, 282.

24. *Statuti*, ed. Malagola, 477. Giuseppe Pardi, *Lo studio di Ferrara nei secoli XV° e XVI°* (Ferrara, 1903), 85 (referring specifically to the 1530s to 1550s). Roger French, "Medical Teaching in Aberdeen: From the Foundation of the University to the Middle of the Seventeenth Century," *History of Universities* 3 (1983): 127–28.

25. Kibre, "The Faculty of Medicine at Paris, Charlatanism and Unlicensed Medical Practice in the Later Middle Ages"; Denifle and Chatelain, *Chartularium*, 1:185–86, doc. 4 (1239), and 1:234–35, doc. 33 (1316). Mauro Sarti and Mauro Fattorini, *De claris archigymnasii bononiensis professoribus*, ed. Carlo Malagola (Bologna, 1888–96), 2:214–15. Ladislao Münster, "La medicina legale in Bologna dai suoi albori fino alla fine del secolo XIV," *Bollettino dell'Accademia Medica Pistoiese Filippo Pacini* 26 (1955): 257–71, and idem, "Alcuni episodi sconosciuti o poco noti sulla vita e sull'attività di Bartolomeo da Varignana," *Castalia: Rivista di storia della medicina* 10 (1954): 207–15. Anna M. Campbell, *The Black Death and Men of Learning* (New York, 1966; facsimile of original, 1931 edition), 14–17.

26. Christine Renardy, *Le monde des maîtres universitaires du diocèse de Liège 1140–1350* (Paris, 1979), 182.

27. Ronald Ohl, "The University of Padua 1405–1509: An International Community of Students and Professors" (Ph.D. diss., University of Pennsylvania 1980), 59–61.

28. Sarti and Fattorini, *De professoribus*, 2:235 (will of Teodorico Borgognoni); Gentile da Foligno, *Questiones et tractatus extravagantes . . .* (Venice, 1520), question 46, fol. 63ʳ; C. H. Talbot and E. A. Hammond, *The Medical Practitioners in Medieval England: A Biographical Register* (London, 1965), 234–37.

29. Kleineidam, *Universitas Studii Erffordensis*, 1:326–34; 2:339–43.

30. Jacquart, *Le milieu médical*, 364, table 3; 365, table 4.

31. Celestino Piana, O.F.M., "Lauree in arti e medicina conferite a Bologna negli anni 1419–1434," in his *Nuove ricerche su le Università di Bologna e di Parma* (Florence, 1966), 110–74. Naso, *Medici*, 114. Kuhn, *Die Studenten der Universität Tübingen*, 1:35.

32. Ohl, *University of Padua*, 46; *Acta graduum academicorum gymnasii patavini ab anno 1406 ad annum 1450*, ed. G. Zonta and G. Brotto (2d ed., Padua, 1970), 1:3–4, 312–28, 2:312–34.

33. Details and citations regarding Bologna are provided in Siraisi, *Taddeo*, 20–23. Ohl, *University of Padua*, 96–98.

34. Jacquart, *Le milieu médical*, 365, table 4; 390, table 28. Commentaries on these Hippocratic works by known authors of the thirteenth to the fifteenth centuries are listed in Pearl Kibre, *Hippocrates latinus: Repertorium of Hippocratic Writings in the Middle Ages* (New York, 1985).

35. Jacquart, *Le milieu médical*, 393, table 32. Getz, "Medicine at Medieval Oxford."

36. For example Pietro d'Abano, *Conciliator* (Venice, 1565; facsimile, Padua, 1985), fols. 3ᵛ–4ʳ (subsequent references are to this edition). The history of the concept is summarized in Charles B. Schmitt, "Aristotle among the Physicians," in *The Medical Renaissance of the Sixteenth Century*, ed. A. Wear, R. K. French, and I. M. Lonie (Cambridge, England, 1985), 1–15.

37. *Cartulaire*, 1:187, document 5; 1:357, document 68, section 51.

38. Pietro d'Abano, *Conciliator*, fol. 4ʳ.

39. Cecco d'Ascoli, proem to *In spheram mundi enarratio*, edited in Lynn Thorndike, *The Sphere of Sacrobosco and Its Commentators* (Chicago, 1949), 344–46.

40. Préaud, *Astrologues*, provides numerous examples of predictions and judgments by medical astrologers. Talbot, *Medicine in Medieval England*, 125–26; idem, "A Medieval Physician's Vade Mecum," JHM 16 (1961): 213–33.

41. *Statuti*, ed. Malagola, 425, 448. Piana, "Lauree in arti e medicina." Jacquart, *Supplément* to Wickersheimer, *Dictionnaire*, 38.

42. Francesco Petrarca, *Rerum senilium libri*, book 12, in his *Opera* (Basel, 1554; repr. Ridgewood, N.J., 1965), 991–1011; Pesenti, *Professori*, 186–96 (bio-bibliography of Michele Savonarola); many other examples of contacts between medical and literary or hu-

manistic writers are revealed by other biographies in the same volume. On the court of Ferrara, see Werner L. Gundersheimer, *Ferrara: The Style of a Renaissance Despotism* (Princeton, 1973).

43. Galen, *De usu partium*, ed. G. Helmreich (2 vols., Leipzig, 1907–9); English trans., Margaret T. May, *Galen on the Usefulness of the Parts of the Body* (2 vols., Ithaca, 1968).

44. *Cartulaire*, 1:220, document 25 (1309); 1:347–48, document 68, sections 20 and 21 (1340). *Statuti*, ed. Malagola, 274–77 (1405). Siraisi, *Taddeo*, 96–106.

45. Siraisi, *Taddeo*, 14–15. *Cartulaire*, 1:181–82, document 2.

46. *Cartulaire*, 1:187, document 5 (1240); 1:220, document 25 (1309). *Statuti*, ed. Malagola, 274–77.

47. Note 1 to chap. 2; Campbell, *Black Death*, 9–13.

48. Siraisi, *Taddeo*, 30. Manlio Bellomo, *Saggio sull'università nell'età del diritto comune* (Catania, 1979), 104–6.

49. *Dyni florentini super quarta fen primi Avicenne preclarissima commentaria que Dilucidatorium totius practice generalis medicinalis scientie nuncupatur* (Venice, 1514).

50. Jacquart, "La réception du Canon." Luis Garcia Ballester, "Arnau de Vilanova (c. 1240–1311) y la reforma de los estudios médicos en Montpellier (1309): El Hipócrates latino y la introducción del nuevo Galeno," *Dynamis* 2 (1982): 97–158. Siraisi, *Taddeo*, 100–105.

51. On Giacomo and Ugo, see Pesenti, *Professori*, 53–58, 103–12, and bibliography there cited. Danielle Jacquart, "Le regard d'un médecin sur son temps: Jacques Despars (1380?–1458)," *Bibliothèque de l'Ecole des Chartes* 138 (1980), 35–86.

CHAPTER FOUR

1. Avicenna, *Liber Canonis* (Venice, 1507; facsimile reprint, Hildesheim, 1964), Book 1, fen 1, doctrina 1, chap. 1, fol. 1^r. Subsequent references are to this edition.

2. *De viribus illustribus liber Bartholomei Facii*, ed. L. Mehus (Florence, 1745), 35.

3. M. Anthony Hewson, *Giles of Rome and the Medieval Theory of Conception* (London, 1975). Other examples of the treatment of physiological topics by a theologian are collected in Mark D. Jordan, "Medicine and Natural Philosophy in Aquinas," in *Thomas von Aquin*, ed. Albert Zimmerman, *Miscellanea Mediaevalia*, vol. 19 (Berlin and New York, 1977).

4. Galen, *De locis affectis* (Opera, ed. Kühn, 8:1–452). Arnald of Villanova, *Doctrina Galieni De interioribus*, ed. Richard J. Durling, in Arnald's *Opera medica omnia*, vol. 15 (Barcelona, 1985), 306.

5. For one of many examples, *Colliget* 2.11, in Aristotle and Averroes, *Opera* (Venice, 1562), vol. 10, fol. 24^r. The *Colliget* was translated into Latin in 1285.

6. *Burgundio of Pisa's Translation of Galen's Peri Kraseon "De complexionibus,"* ed. R. J. Durling, *Galenus latinus* vol. 1 (Berlin and New York, 1976). Garcia Ballester, "Arnau de Vilanova (c. 1240–1311) y la reforma de los estudios médicos en Montpellier (1309)." Roger French, "*De Juvamentis Membrorum* and the Reception of Galenic Physiological Anatomy," *Isis* 70 (1979): 96–109.

7. On the *Isagoge*, Danielle Jacquart, "A l'aube de la Renaissance médicale des XIe–XII siècles: L'Isagoge Johannitii' et son traducteur," *Bibliothèque de l'Ecole des Chartes* 144 (1986): 209–40.

8. On the use of Book 3 of the *Canon*, and commentaries on it, in anatomical

teaching, see Roger French, "Berengario da Carpi and the Use of Commentary in Anatomical Teaching," in *The Medical Renaissance*, ed. Wear, French, Lonie, 42–74.

9. *De complexionibus*, trans. Burgundio of Pisa (ed. Durling), pts. 1 and 2 (p. 64, for the example cited); Avicenna, *Canon*, Book 1, fen 1, doctrina 3, fols. 2^r–4^v.

10. Henri de Mondeville, *Die Chirurgie des Heinrich von Mondeville (Hermondaville)* ed. Julius Leopold Pagel (Berlin, 1892), introduction to tractatus 1, p. 16. Markwart Michler, "Guy de Chauliac als Anatom" in *Frühe Anatomie*, ed. Robert Herrlinger and Fridolf Kudlien (Stuttgart, 1967), 15–32. Loren C. MacKinney, "The Beginnings of Western Scientific Anatomy: New Evidence and A Revision in Interpretation of Mondeville's Role," *Medical History* 6 (1962): 233–39.

11. Gentile da Foligno, commentary on *Canon*, Book 1 (Pavia, 1510), fol. 51^v. On Gentile's ideas about the proper training of physicians, see Roger French, "Gentile da Foligno and the *via medicorum*," in *The Light of Nature: Essays in the History and Philosophy of Science Presented to A. C. Crombie*, ed. J. D. North and J. J. Roche (Dordrecht, Boston, Lancaster, 1985), 21–34.

12. George W. Corner, *Anatomical Texts of the Earlier Middle Ages* (Washington, 1927), text and translations, 48–66, discussion 19–30.

13. *Anatomia magistri Nicolai*, in Corner, *Anatomical Texts*, 67.

14. Kristeller, *Studi sulla scuola medica salernitana*, 66–68. For the ascription of the *Anatomia vivorum* to a Parisian milieu, Gerhard Baader, "Zur anatomie in Paris im 13. und 14. Jahrhundert," *MJ* 3 (1968): 40–53; other origins have also been suggested for this work.

15. Salvatore de Renzi, *Storia della Medicina in Italia* (5 vols., Naples, 1845–48), 2:249–50.

16. These developments are summarized, with documentation, in Giuseppe Ongaro, "La medicina nello Studio di Padova e nel Veneto," *Storia della cultura veneta*, ed. G. Arnaldi and M. Pastore, vol. 3, pt. 3 (Vicenza, 1981), 92–95.

17. Guy de Chauliac, *Cyrurgie*, ed. Ogden, 1.1, pp. 28–29. In this passage the Middle English faithfully reflects the Latin text.

18. Elizabeth A. R. Brown, "Death and the Human Body in the Later Middle Ages: The Legislation of Boniface VIII on the Division of the Corpse," *Viator: Medieval and Renaissance Studies* 12 (1981): 250–51. MacKinney, "Beginnings of Western Scientific Anatomy," 233.

19. On the principles and practice of medieval scientific illustration, see John E. Murdoch, *Album of Science: Antiquity and the Middle Ages* (New York, 1984).

20. Ynez Violé O'Neill, "The Fünfbilderserie Reconsidered," *BHM* 43 (1969): 236–45; Roger French, "An Origin for the Bone Text of the 'Five-Figure Series,'" *SA* 68 (1984): 143–56.

21. MacKinney, "Beginnings of Western Scientific Anatomy."

22. Mondino, *De omnibus humani corporis interioribus membris Anathomia* (Strasburg, 1513), sig. a3^v; English translation by Charles Singer in [Johannes de Ketham] *The Fasciculo di Medicina, Venice, 1495*, ed. Charles Singer, 2:60. Guy de Chauliac, *Cyrurgie*, ed. Ogden, 1.1, p. 28 (*Chirurgia* [Venice, 1498], fol. 5^v). Roger French, "A Note on the Anatomical Accessus of the Middle Ages," *Medical History* 23 (1979): 461–68.

23. Corner, *Anatomical Texts*, 52; Avicenna, *Canon*, Book 3, fen 18, tractatus 1, chap. 1, fol. 336^{r-v}.

24. Guy de Chauliac commented on the frequency with which Mondino dis-

sected (*Cyrurgie*, ed. Ogden, 1.1, p. 28 *Chirurgia* [Venice, 1498], fol. 5ᵛ). Mondino, *Ana-thomia* (Strasburg, 1513), sig. f iiiᵛ, iᵛ–i iiʳ; Singer, *Fasciculo* (Florence, 1925) 2:83, 94 (and notes 85 and 118, on pp. 106 and 109). Mondino's level of knowledge is evaluated in Fridolf Kudlien, "Mondinos Standort innerhalb der Entwicklung der Anatomie," in *Frühe Anatomie*, ed. Herrlinger and Kudlien, 1–14.

25. Robert Reisert, *Der siebenkammerige Uterus: Studien zur mittelalterlichen Wirkungsges-chichte und Enfaltung eines embryologischen Gebärmuttermodells*, WMF, vol. 39 (Hanover, 1986), traces the history of the concept of the seven-celled uterus. Modifications of Reisert's account are suggested in the review by Ynez Violé O'Neill in BHM 63 (1989): 288–89.

26. Pietro d'Abano, *Conciliator*, differentia 23, fol. 36ᵛ.

27. Danielle Jacquart and Claude Thomasset, *Sexuality and Medicine in the Middle Ages* (Princeton, 1988), 40–41.

28. *Lorenzo Ghibertis Denkwürdigkeiten* (I *Commentarii*), ed. Julius von Schlosser (Berlin, 1912), 1:4, 7, 222; Leon Battista Alberti, *On Painting and On Sculpture*, ed. and trans. Cecil Grayson (London, 1972), 74–75.

29. John B. Schultz, *Art and Anatomy in Renaissance Italy* (Ann Arbor, 1985). The stan-dard edition of Leonardo's anatomical drawings is now Kenneth Keele and Carlo Pedretti, *Leonardo da Vinci: Corpus of the Anatomical Studies in the Collection of Her Majesty the Queen at Windsor Castle* (3 vols., London and New York, 1978–80). Most are also repro-duced in Charles D. O'Malley and J. B. de C. M. Saunders, *Leonardo da Vinci on the Human Body* (New York, 1952).

30. Monica H. Green, "The Transmission of Ancient Theories of Female Physiology and Disease through the Early Middle Ages," (Ph.D. diss., Princeton University, 1985).

31. Gerhard Baader, "Die Entwicklung der medizinischen Fachsprache im hohen und späten Mittelalter," in *Fachprosaforschung*, ed. G. Keil and P. Assion (Berlin, 1974), 88–123; Michael R. McVaugh, introduction to Arnald of Villanova, *Translatio libri Galieni De rigore et tremore et iectigatione et spasmo*, in Arnald's *Opera medica*, vol. 16 (Barcelona, 1981), 11–38.

32. Marshall Clagett, *Giovanni Marliani and Late Medieval Physics* (New York, 1941), 34–100. For other examples, see Per-Gunnar Ottosson, *Scholastic Medicine and Philosophy: A Study of Commentaries on Galen's Tegni* (Naples, 1984).

33. Jerome J. Bylebyl, "Galen on the Non-Natural Causes of Variation in the Pulse," BHM 45 (1971): 482–85.

34. Danielle Jacquart, "De crasis à complexio: Note sur le vocabulaire du tempéra-ment en Latin médiéval," in *Textes médicaux latins antiques*, ed. G. Sabbah, Centre Jean Palerne, *Mémoires*, 5 (Saint-Etienne, 1984), 71–76.

35. Ian Maclean, *The Renaissance Notion of Woman: A Study in the Fortunes of Scholasticism and Medical Science in European Intellectual Life* (Cambridge, England, 1980), 35, 57.

36. *De complexionibus* 2.6, ed. Durling, 86. Ptolemy, *Tetrabiblos* 2.2, ed. and trans. F. E. Robbins, LCL (1964), 120–27. *Airs Waters Places*, chaps. 12–22, in *Hippocrates*, LCL, 1:104–30. The account of complexion theory given in this chapter is based chiefly on *De complexionibus*, ed. Durling (= *On complexions*) and Avicenna, *Canon*, Book 1, fen 1, doc-trina 3, fols. 2ʳ–4ᵛ.

37. Aristotle, *On Length and Shortness of Life* 5.466a17–466b31; Galen, *De complexionibus* 1.3, ed. Durling, 13; Thomas S. Hall, "Life, Death, and the Radical Moisture," *Clio Medica* 6 (1971): 3–23; Michael R. McVaugh, "The 'humidum radicale' in Thirteenth-Century Medicine," *Traditio* 30 (1974): 259–83.

38. Gentile da Foligno, *Tractatus de resistentiis* in his *Questiones extravagantes* (Venice, 1520), fol. 89ʳ.

39. *On the Nature of Man*, chap. 4, in *Hippocrates*, LCL, 4:2–40. Examples (many more could be cited) of emphasis on humors, fluids, excreta in the Hippocratic corpus: *On the Sacred Disease* 7–14, in *Hippocrates* (LCL) 2:154–70, explains epilepsy as a result of a bad kind of phlegm; the assumption that the physician monitors excreta is present throughout the *Epidemics*, in *Hippocrates*, LCL, 1; *Regimen in Acute Diseases* 22, in *Hippocrates*, LCL, 2:80, recommends therapeutic bloodletting. Aristotle, *Parts of Animals* 2.2.647b1–648a35. Avicenna, *Canon*, Book 1, fen 1, doctrina 4, fols. 4ᵛ–6ᵛ.

40. Owsei Temkin, *Galenism: Rise and Decline of a Medical Philosophy* (Ithaca, N.Y., 1973), 87–92.

41. Avicenna, *Canon*, Book 1, fen 1, doctrina 6, fols. 23ʳ–25ʳ.

42. Mondino, *Anathomia* (Strasburg, 1513), sig. [aiiiʳ⁻ᵛ]; Singer, *Fasciculo* 2:60–61.

43. A complete account of Galen's own teaching is found in C. R. S. Harris, *The Heart and the Vascular System in Ancient Greek Medicine* (Oxford, 1973), 267–396.

44. Elizabeth Sears, *The Ages of Man* (Princeton, 1986), 12–20, 25–31, 38–53.

45. Pietro d'Abano, *Conciliator*, differentia 26, fols. 38ᵛ–39ʳ.

46. Aristotle, *On Generation and Corruption* 2.11, 336a36–338b21. Pietro d'Abano, *Conciliator*, differentia 48, fol. 71ᵛ–72ʳ.

47. Matthew Paris, *Chronica majora*, ed. Henry Richards Luard, 3:324 (Rolls Series, vol. 57, [repr. London, 1964]), under the year 1235. The story is mentioned in S. J. Tester, *A History of Western Astrology* (Woodbridge, Suffolk, 1987), 190.

48. Enrique Montero Cartelle, ed., *Constantini liber de coitu: El tratado de andrología de Constantino el Africano* (Santiago de Compostela, 1983), 76.

49. Alan of Lille, *The Plaint of Nature*, trans. James J. Sheridan (Toronto, 1980), 154–57. Jan Ziolkowski, *Alan of Lille's Grammar of Sex: The Meaning of Grammar to a Twelfth-Century Intellectual* (Cambridge, Mass., 1985). Jacquart and Thomasset, *Sexuality and Medicine*, 116–22, 130–38.

50. Vern L. Bullough, "Medieval Medical and Scientific Views of Women," *Viator* 4 (1973): 485–501. Maclean, *Renaissance Notion of Woman*, presents a nuanced view of the interaction and mutual reinforcement of religious, legal, philosophical, and medical stereotypes.

51. M. C. Pouchelle, *Corps et chirurgie à l'apogée du Moyen Age* (Paris, 1983), undertakes to provide such an analysis of the language in a French version of the Latin work on surgery by Henri de Mondeville.

CHAPTER FIVE

1. *The Letters of Peter the Venerable*, ed. Giles Constable (Cambridge, Mass., 1967), 1:379–83, letters 158a and 158b, Peter's letter and Bartholomeus' reply. The passage quoted is on pp. 380–81.

2. For the issues and bibliography, see Constable, *Letters of Peter the Venerable*, 2:302–03, appendix M.

3. Petrarca, *Rerum senilium libri*, 12, pp. 991–1011.

4. For discussion of Peter's health, and his concern about it, see Constable, *Letters of Peter the Venerable*, appendix B, 2:247–51.

5. Arnald of Villanova, *Epistola de dosi tyriacalium medicinarum*, ed. Michael R. Mc-

Vaugh, in Arnald's *Opera medica*, vol. 3 (Barcelona, 1985), 55–91, with historical over-view in the editor's introduction, 57–73; Michael R. McVaugh, "Theriac at Montpel-lier, 1285–1325," SA 56 (1972): 113–44; Thomas Holste, *Der Theriakkrämer: Ein Beitrag zur Frühgeschichte der Arzneimittelwerbung*, WMF, vol. 5 (Hanover, 1976), 1–39.

6. Galen, *Methodus medendi* (*Opera*, ed. Kühn, vol. 10), also known in the Middle Ages as *De ingenio sanitatis* or *Megategni*.

7. The neutral state between health and sickness is postulated at the beginning of the Galenic *Tegni*. The triple classification of ill-health, also Galenic in origin, is used in Avicenna, *Canon*, Book 1, fen 2.

8. Michele Savonarola, *Ad mulieres ferrarienses de regimine pregnantium et noviter natorum usque ad septennium*, ed. Luigi Belloni (Milan, 1952).

9. Michele Savonarola, *Libreto de tute le cosse che se manzano: Un libro di dietetica di Michele Savonarola, medico padovano del secolo XV*, ed. Jane Nystedt (Stockholm, 1982).

10. John Scarborough, "Botany, Pharmacy, and the Culinary Arts," in *The Rational Arts of Living*, ed. Crombie and Siraisi, 161–202, especially 196–202; Caroline Walker Bynum, *Holy Feast and Holy Fast: The Religious Significance of Food to Medieval Women* (Berke-ley, 1987).

11. Avicenna, *Canon* Book 1, fen 2, doctrina 2, summa 1, chap. 15, fols. 33^v–34^v. Petrus Hispanus, *Thesaurus pauperum* in his *Obras médicas*, ed. Maria Helena da Rocha Pereira (Coimbra, 1973), XI.35, p. 145; XXXVIII.23 and 24, p. 243.

12. Savonarola, *Libreto*, 53, 61.

13. This aspect of Hippocratic teaching is the subject of the treatise *Airs Waters Places*.

14. Rhazes, *Aphorismorum libri* 2, in his *Opera* (Basel, 1544; facsimile repr., Brussels, 1973), 524.

15. Rhazes' brief treatise was translated into Byzantine Greek, and thence, twice, into Latin. Early editions of the Latin humanist versions bore the title *De pestilentia*. The first direct translation to Latin was made in 1747, and given the title by which the work is usually known in the West, namely *De variolis et morbillis* (Sezgin, *Geschichte* 3:283). Shortly after its production, the eighteenth-century Latin translation was in turn translated into English, and published with Richard Mead, *A Discourse on the Small Pox and Measles* (2d ed., London, 1755). Eighteenth-century Western interest in Rhazes' writings on smallpox was due to the prevalence of the disease in Europe at that time.

16. Taddeo Alderotti's discussion of the problem is analyzed in Siraisi, *Taddeo*, 124.

17. Konrad Goehl and Gundolf Keil, "Eine Salzburger spätmittelhochdeutsche Stuhlschau," SA 71 (1987): 113–15.

18. The tradition is traced and relevant text excerpts printed in Friedrich Len-hardt, *Blutschau: Untersuchungen zur Entwicklung der Hämatskopie*, WMF, vol. 22 (Hanover, 1986).

19. Arnald of Villanova, *On the Precautions that Physicians Must Observe* [*De cautelis medico-rum*], trans. Henry E. Sigerist, with annotations by Michael R. McVaugh in *A Source Book of Medieval Science*, ed. Edward Grant (Cambridge, Mass., 1974).

20. Rhazes, *Almansor*, Book 9, chap. 69, in his *Opera*, 253; and his *Liber divisionum*, chap. 43, *Opera*, 384.

21. This account of pulse is largely based on Pietro d'Abano, *Conciliator*, differentiae 82–83, fols. 122^v–126^r, a very full discussion of the subject. The ancient sources and other Islamic and Western discussions are cited in Nancy G. Siraisi. "The Music of

Pulse in the Writings of Italian Academic Physicians (Fourteenth and Fifteenth Centuries), *Speculum* 50 (1975): 689–710.

22. Galen, *Methodus medendi* 2.1–3 (*Opera*, ed. Kühn, 10:78–93), and elsewhere. Arnald was discussing a similar passage in *De interioribus* (*De locis affectis*) 1.3; Michael R. McVaugh, "The Nature of Limits of Medical Certitude at Early Fourteenth-Century Montpellier"; Nancy G. Siraisi, "Giovanni Argenterio and the Boundaries of Neotericism in Mid-Sixteenth Century Medicine." McVaugh and Siraisi both in *Osiris* 6 (1990).

23. Karl Sudhoff, "Pestschriften aus den ersten 150 Jahren nach der Epidemie des 'Schwarzen Todes' (1348)," *Archiv für Geschichte der Medizin* (= SA) 4 (1911): 191–222, 389–424; 5 (1912): 36–87 and 332–96; 6 (1913): 313–79; 7 (1914): 57–114; 8 (1915): 175–215 and 236–89; 9 (1916): 53–78 and 117–67; 11 (1917): 44–92 and 121–76; 17 (1925): 12–139 and 241–91 (list, and editions of many texts). The content of a group of the earliest plague tractates is anlayzed in Campbell, *Black Death*, 34–92.

24. Some of these tracts are listed and their conclusions summarized in Thorndike, *History of Magic* 3: 289–92, 303–9, 326–37.

25. The explanations provided by Antonio Guaineri (d. after 1448), Michele Savonarola, and Jacques Despars (d. 1458) are analyzed in Danielle Jacquart, "Contradictory Tendencies in Fifteenth-Century Medicine," in *Osiris* 6 (1990). Understanding of the role of rats and fleas in transmitting bubonic plague followed the identification of the plague bacillus in the late nineteenth century.

26. Darrel W. Amundsen, "Medical Deontology and Pestilential Disease in the Late Middle Ages," JHM 32 (1977): 403–21.

27. Linda Deer Richardson, "The Generation of Disease: Occult Causes and Diseases of the Total Substance," in *The Medical Renaissance*, ed. Wear, French, and Lonie, 175–94. Vivian Nutton, "The Seeds of Disease: An Explanation of Contagion and Infection from the Greeks to the Renaissance," *Medical History* 27 (1983): 1–34. The problem of the origin of syphilis in Europe is discussed and recent research summarized in Mirko D. Grmek, *Diseases in the Ancient Greek World*, trans. Mireille Muellner and Leonard Muellner (Baltimore, 1989), 133–51.

28. Peter Richards, *The Medieval Leper and His Northern Heirs* (Cambridge, 1977). Grmek, *Diseases*, 152–76. Luke Demaitre, "The Description and Diagnosis of Leprosy by Fourteenth-Century Physicians," BHM 59 (1985): 327–44 (this article also includes bibliography of the controversy over whether references to sexual transmission in some of the *lepra* descriptions may imply the presence of syphilis in medieval Europe). For medieval moralizing about leprosy and the social and religious position of the leper, see Saul N. Brody, *The Disease of the Soul: Leprosy in Medieval Literature* (Ithaca, N.Y., 1974).

29. Pietro d'Abano, *Conciliator*, differentia 75, fol. 113ᵛ.

30. *De febrium differentiis*, ed. Kühn, 7:273–405.

31. Arnald of Villanova, *Tractatus de amore heroico*, ed. Michael R. McVaugh, in Arnald's *Opera medica*, vol. 3 (Barcelona, 1986), 43–54, provides a late-thirteenth-century medical summary of the subject of the lover's malady; a modern overview is contained in the editor's introduction, ibid. 11–39.

32. Rhazes, *Almansor*, Book 9, chap. 74, in Rhazes, *Opera*, 261.

33. Petrus Hispanus, *Thesaurus pauperum*, in his *Obras médicas*, 42, 58–63, 79.

34. The acceptance of sorcery as one of the causes of impotence by canon lawyers, and their discussions of whether this type of impotence was grounds for annulment

of marriage, are described in James A. Brundage, *Law, Sex, and Christian Society in Medieval Europe* (Chicago, 1987), 290–92, 376–78.

35. Mondino de' Liuzzi, *Mesue cum expositione Mondini super Canones universales* (Venice, 1508), fol. 38(37)$^{r-v}$, summarized in Siraisi, *Taddeo*, 68.

36. Malagola, *Statuti*, 264.

37. On ominous days in general, see Anthony Grafton and Noel M. Swerdlow, "Calendar Dates and Ominous Days in Ancient Historiography," *Journal of the Warburg and Courtauld Institutes* 51 (1988): 14–42. Galen's treatises are edited in his *Opera*, ed. Kühn, 9:550–941.

38. This explication of crisis and critical days follows Pietro d'Abano, *Conciliator*, differentia 104, fol. 154^{r-v}.

39. Galen, *De diebus decretoriis* 3.9, ed. Kühn, 9:928–33; for an example of uncritical use of the concept by a western medieval medical writer, see Siraisi, *Taddeo*, 186.

40. Pietro d'Abano, *Conciliator*, differentia 104, fols. 154^v–155^r. The preceding and the two following differentiae are also dedicated to crisis and critical days and the entire discussion extends from fol. 153^r to 157^v.

41. C. H. Talbot, *Medicine in Medieval England* (London, 1965), 125–27; and his "A Medieval Physician's Vade Mecum."

42. One who did suggest such modifications is described in Michael R. McVaugh, "The Two Faces of a Medical Career: Jordanus de Turre of Montpellier," in *Mathematics and Its Applications to Science and Natural Philosophy in the Middle Ages*, ed. Edward Grant and John E. Murdoch (Cambridge, Mass., 1987), 301–24.

43. The classification is, for example, used in Avicenna, *Canon*, Book 1, fen 4 (on types of therapy).

44. Pietro d'Abano, *Conciliator*, differentia 167, fol. 223^r.

45. Voigts and McVaugh, *A Latin Technical Phlebotomy*, 36, 53. The editors' introduction, 1–7, summarizes the development of phlebotomy in the Middle Ages.

46. John M. Riddle, "Folk Tradition and Folk Medicine: Recognition of Drugs in Classical Antiquity," in *Folklore and Folk Medicines*, ed. John Scarborough (Madison, Wisconsin, 1987), 33–61, lists substances mentioned as medicinal in the Hippocratic Corpus and shows that a number of the same plants still find a place in modern guides. The account of medieval and Renaissance medical botany given here draws in addition on Scarborough, "Botany, Pharmacy"; Jerry Stannard, "Medieval Italian Medical Botany," *Atti del XXI Congresso Internazionale di Storia della Medicina, Siena 22–28 Settembre 1968*, 2:1554–65; idem, "Medieval Herbals and Their Development, *Clio Medica* 9 (1974): 23–33; idem, "Magiferous Plants and Magic in Medieval Botany," *The Maryland Historian* 8 (1977): 33–45; and idem, "Natural History," in *Science in the Middle Ages*, ed. David C. Lindberg (Chicago, 1978), 443–49. Tony Hunt, *Popular Medicine in 13th-Century England* (Wolfeboro, N.H.: Boydell and Brewer, 1990) contains an edition and detailed analysis of six collections of Anglo-Norman medical prescriptions.

47. John M. Riddle, "Dioscorides," *CTC* 4 (1980): 6–8. Galen, *De simplicium medicamentorum temperamentis ac facultatibus*, ed. Kühn, 11:379–892; 12:1–377.

48. Max Meyerhof, "Esquisse d'histoire de la pharmacologie et botanique chez les Musulmans d'Espagne," in his *Studies in Medieval Arabic Medicine*, no. 10, 1–41.

49. Guy Beaujouan, "Fautes et obscurités dans les traductions médicales du Moyen Age," *Revue de synthèse*, 3d ser., 89 (1968): 145–52.

50. L. C. MacKinney, "Medieval Medical Dictionaries and Glossaries," in *Medieval*

and Historiographical Essays in Honor of James Westfall Thompson, ed. J. L. Cate and E. N. Anderson (Chicago, 1938), 240–68; Dietlinde Goltz, *Studien zur Geschichte der Mineralnamen in Pharmazie, Chemie und Medizin von den Angfängen bis Paracelsus*. SA, Beiheft 14 (Wiesbaden, 1972), 321–33.

51. Index entries under the general heading *quid pro quo* in Lynn Thorndike and Pearl Kibre, A *Catalogue of Incipits of Mediaeval Scientific Writings in Latin* (2d ed., Cambridge, Mass., 1963), provide examples. The example cited is at col. 1128.

52. Arnald of Villanova, *Aphorismi de gradibus*, ed. Michael R. McVaugh, in Arnald's *Opera medica*, vol. 2 (Granada-Barcelona, 1975), editor's introduction, 1–87; the mathematical principles of Arnald's system are explained and examples of his calculations analyzed on 86–87 and 253–58. Examples of Arnald's recommendations in his practice are edited in Michael R. McVaugh, "The *Experimenta* of Arnald of Villanova," *Journal of Medieval and Renaissance Studies* 1 (1971): 107–18. For the relation of Arnald's system to wider issues in the history of medieval science, see idem, "Arnald of Villanova and Bradwardine's Law," *Isis* 58 (1967): 56–64, and "Quantified Medical Theory and Practice at Fourteenth-Century Montpellier," *BHM* 43 (1969): 397–413.

53. Park, *Doctors*, 29–30; Richard Palmer, "Pharmacy in the Republic of Venice in the Sixteenth Century," in *The Medical Renaissance*, ed. Wear, French, and Lonie, 100–17.

54. Giambatista Da Monte, commentary on Avicenna, *Canon* 1.1 (Venice, 1554), fols. 228^r–229^r.

55. Campbell, *Black Death*, 67–68.

56. *Processi*, ed. Lugano, 261, 264, 282–83, 305–07.

57. *Die Areolae des Johannes de Sancto Amando (13. Jahrhundert)*, ed. Julius Leopold Pagel (Berlin, 1893).

58. Petrus Hispanus, *Thesaurus pauperum* 12.1, in his *Obras médicas*, 151; Siraisi, *Taddeo*, 300–301.

59. Stannard, "Magiferous Plants," 37–40.

60. Shatzmiller, "In Search of the Book of Figures."

61. Marsilio Ficino, *Three Books on Life*, ed. and trans. Carol V. Kaske and John R. Clark (Binghamton, N.Y., 1989). Giancarlo Zanier, *La medicina astrologica e la sua teoria: Marsilio Ficino e i suoi critici contemporanei* (Rome, 1977); idem, "Ricerche sull'occultismo a Padova nel secolo XV," in *Scienza e filosofia all'Università di Padova nel Quattrocento*, ed. Antonino Poppi (Padua, 1983), 345–72.

62. Based on a survey of the bio-bibliographical information in Pesenti, *Professori*.

CHAPTER SIX

1. Pietro d'Abano, *Conciliator*, differentia 3, fol. 7^r.

2. *Processo*, ed. Menestò, witnesses no. 43 and 45, pp. 264–65, 265–66. For other cases apparently of hernia (termed *ernia, ruptus, fractus* or *fractura*; in these cases the two last words are not being used of a broken bone but refer fairly plainly to hernia), mostly in boys, see witness 52, pp. 306–7; witness 86, pp. 367–68; witness 91, pp. 371–73; witness 109, pp. 385–86; witness 132, pp. 407–8; witness 142, pp. 417–18; witness 143, p. 418; witness 217, pp. 495–96; witness 225, p. 501; witness 232, pp. 507–8.

3. Pierre Huard and M. D.Grmek, *Mille ans de chirurgie en Occident: V^e–XVe siècles* (Paris, 1966), 33.

4. For a general assessment of the technical problems and accomplishments of premodern surgery, see Owen H. Wangensteen and Sarah D. Wangensteen, *The Rise of Surgery: From Empiric Craft to Scientific Discipline* (Minneapolis, 1978), 3–15.

5. Guy de Chauliac, *Cyrurgie*, ed. Ogden, 4–5; *Cyrurgia* (Venice, 1498), fol. 2^r.

6. Examples of lists of wounds that are usually fatal include: Hippocrates, *Aphorisms* 6.18, in *Hipporcrates* (LCL) 4:182; Avicenna, *Canon*, Book 4, fen 4, tractatus 1, chap. 2, fol. 445^r; Bruno Longoburgo, *Cyrurgia magna*, Book 1, chap. 6, printed with Guy de Chauliac, *Cyrurgia*, fol. 85 (84)^v; Teodorico Borgognoni, *Cyrurgia*, Book 1, chap. 21, fol. 112 (111)^{r–v}, in the same volume (modern English translation as *The Surgery of Theodoric, ca. A.D. 1267*, trans. Eldridge Campbell and James Colton [2 vols., New York, 1955, 1960], with the passage cited at 1:80–83). Examples of the description of malignant tumors: Guy de Chauliac, *Cyrurgia*, tractatus 2, supplementary chapter on cancerous apostemata, fol. 17(16)^r (*Cyrurgia*, ed. Ogden, 127–28), and Bruno Longoburgo, *Cyrurgia magna*, Book 1, chap. 16, fol. 89(88)^v–90(89)^r, in the same volume. On the need for caution in tooth extraction, see Albucasis, *On Surgery and Instruments*, Book 2, chap. 30, ed. and trans. M. S. Spink and G. L. Lewis (London, 1973), 276–78.

7. *An Arab-Syrian Gentleman and Warrior in the Period of the Crusades*, trans. P. K. Hitti (New York, 1929), 162. On amputation, see Wangensteen and Wangensteen, *Rise of Surgery*, 16–18; Huard and Grmek, *Mille ans de chirurgie*, 71.

8. V. L. Kennedy, "Robert Courson on Penance," *Mediaeval Studies* 7 (1945): 291–336 (includes edited text), at 322.

9. Dino del Garbo, *Dinus in Chirurgia* (Venice, 1536), fols. 136^v–39^r.

10. Guglielmo da Saliceto, *Summa conservationis et curationis*, (Venice, 1489), Book 1, chaps. 149 and 183. Guglielmo was doubtful about the value of this type of dental treatment.

11. *Dinus in Chirurgia*, fols. 136^v–39^r.

12. Guglielmo da Saliceto, *Cyrurgia*, printed with his *Summa conservationis et curationis* (Venice, 1489), Book 2, chap. 15, sig. x4^v.

13. See Gundolf Keil, "Mittelalterliche Chirurgie," AMHP 30 (1983–84): 45–64, at 45–49; Stanley Rubin, *Medieval English Medicine* (Newton Abbot, 1974), 35–40, 130–51; Augusto Beccaria, *I codici di medicina del periodo presalernitano (secoli IX, X e XI)* (Rome, 1956). To provide only one of many possible examples, several laws in the code issued by the Lombard king Rothair in A.D. 643, referring to medical practitioners who treat wounds and fractures for a fee, show the absence of any distinction between medicine and surgery; see Rothair's Edict in *The Lombard Laws*, trans. Katherine Fischer Drew, with introduction by Edward Peters (Philadelphia, 1973), 65–71, items 78, 82–84, 87, 89, 96, 103, 106–7, 110–112, 118, 128.

14. L. D. Reynolds, *Texts and Transmission: A Survey of the Latin Classics* (Oxford, 1983), 46–47 (Celsus); Pearl Kibre, *Hippocrates latinus* (New York, 1985), 93–94, 110, 124, 234 (the few fragments of Hippocratic surgery available in the Latin Middle Ages); Eugene F. Rice, "Paulus Aegineta," CTC 4 (1980): 150–67.

15. Ullmann, *Die Medizin im Islam*, 86–87, 141–42, 150. The remark quoted is from Rice, "Paulus Aegineta," 148.

16. On the Arabic manuscripts of Albucasis' work and their illustration, see Emilie

Savage Smith, "Some Sources and Procedures for Editing a Medieval Arabic Surgical Tract," *History of Science* 14 (1976): 245–64, an essay review of Albucasis, *On Surgery and Instruments*, ed. and trans. Spink and Lewis. For discussion and reproduction of numerous examples of the tradition of illustration in the Latin manuscripts of the same work, see Karl Sudhoff, *Beiträge zur Geschichte der Chirurgie im Mittelalter* 2:16–74, *Studien zur Geschichte der Medizin*, Heft 11 and 12 (Leipzig, 1914, 1918).

17. Books 3–6 of Galen's *Methodus medendi*, a work also known in the Middle Ages as *De ingenio sanitatis*, deal with wounds, ulcers, and fractures; surgical topics are also dealt with in Books 13 and 14. Regarding the separate circulation of these portions, see Richard J. Durling, "Corrigenda and Addenda to Diels' Galenica. I. Codices Vaticani," *Traditio* 23 (1967): 474; Thorndike and Kibre, *Catalogue of Incipits*, col. 1495.

18. It is probable that Book 9, the surgical section, was the only part of the second, practical, division of Haly Abbas' work translated by Constantinus himself, the *Pantegni* being completed by a pupil after his death (Constantinus was, of course, responsible for the version of the whole of the first, theoretical, division in the *Pantegni*); the evidence is set out in Constantinus Africanus, *Chirurgia*, ed. with Italian translation and commentary by Marco T. Malato and Luigi Loria in *Pagine di storia della scienza e della technica* 13 (1960): 61–211, at 61–68. George W. Corner, "On Early Salernitan Surgery and Especially the 'Bamberg Surgery'," *BHM* 5 (1937): 1–28.

19. Keil, "Mittelalterliche Chirurgie," 49–51. Roger's origins and career, and the sequence and provenance of the early glosses and additions to his work have been the subject of considerable controversy among historians of medicine. The history of the debate is summarized and the points at issue discussed in Mario Tabanelli, *La chirurgia italiana nell'alto medioevo* (2 vols., Florence, 1965) 1:5–14, and Wolfgang Löchel, *Die Zahnmedizin Rogers und der Rogerglosse: Ein Beitrag sur Geschichte der Zahnheilkunde im Hoch- und Spätmittelalter*, WMF, vol. 4 (Hanover, 1976), 12–35. The text of the version of Roger's surgery edited by Guido of Arezzo the younger is edited in Sudhoff, *Beiträge*, 2:156–236; Guido was described as "logice professionis ministro" (ibid., 153). The works of Guillaume de Congenis and his student are edited ibid., 311–84, with introductory material at 297–310.

20. Keil, "Mittelalterliche Chirurgie," 51. The complicated history of Roger's text (ultimately including translation back into Latin from a vernacular version) is traced in Gundolf Keil, "Gestaltwandel und Zersetzung—Roger-Urtext und Roger-Glosse vom 12. bis ins 16. Jahrhundert," in *Medizin im mittelalterlichen Abendland*, ed. Baader and Keil, 476–94.

21. The dates and what little is known of the biographies of these figures come mostly from the prefatory material and other remarks in their treatises. All available biographical information regarding Rolando da Parma, Teodorico Borgognoni, Guglielmo da Saliceto, and Lanfranco is collected, summarized, and exhaustively discussed in Tabanelli, *Chirurgia*. Teodorico Borgognoni, the pupil and almost certainly the son of the surgeon Ugo of Lucca, was a Dominican friar; it is possible too that he is also to be identified with a contemporary bishop of the same name. For differing views on this issue, see Huard and Grmek, *Mille ans de chirurgie*, 26–27; and Tabanelli, *Chirurgia*, 1:203–8.

22. Biographical material on Guy de Chauliac and Henri de Mondeville is collected in Wickersheimer, *Dictionnaire* 1:214–15 and 282–83, respectively.

23. Löchel, *Zahnmedizin*, provides details.

24. Richard J. Durling, *A Catalogue of Sixteenth Century Printed Books in the National Library of Medicine* (Bethesda, Maryland, 1967), 271–73, nos. 2233–51, lists nineteen complete or partial editions of Guy de Chauliac's work in various languages; this list does not, of course, represent all the editions printed.

25. *Processo*, ed. Menestò, witness 74, pp. 356–57; witness 81, pp. 361–62. Francesco Petrarca, *Letters on Familiar Matters: Rerum familiarum libri IX–XVI*, 11.1, trans. Aldo S. Bernardo (Baltimore and London, 1982), 85 (Latin text in *Epistole di Francesco Petrarca*, ed. Ugo Dotti [Turin, 1978], 294); the episode occurred in 1350, twenty-four years before Petrarch's death. Dino Compagni's *Chronicle of Florence*, trans. Daniel E. Bornstein (Philadelphia, 1986), 98–99. "Knee' in the Italian text; Bornstein has "nose."

26. Examples of parallel passages from the works of Bruno and Teodorico are printed in Tabanelli, *Chirurgia*, 1:485–89. Henri de Mondeville, *Chirurgie*, ed. Pagel, 11.

27. Margaret S. Ogden, "The Galenic Works Cited in Guy de Chauliac's *Chirurgia magna*," JHM 28 (1973): 24–33, esp. 26 and 33.

28. Proem to Bruno Longoburgo, *Cyrurgia magna*, printed with Guy de Chauliac, *Cyrurgia*, fol. 83 (82)^r; Lanfranco, *Ars completa totius cyrurgie*, tractatus 3, doctrina 1, chap. 6, fol. 182 (181)^v in the same volume (a Middle English translation of this work is edited under the title *Lanfrank's "Science of Cirurgie". Part I. Text*, ed. Robert v. Fleischhacker, EETS, no. 102 [Berlin, New York, and Philadelphia, 1894], with the passage cited at p. 193); Teodorico, *Cyrurgia*, printed with Guy de Chauliac, *Cyrurgia*, proem, fol. 106 (105)^r (*Surgery of Theodoric*, 1:4). For a summary of the career of Ugo of Lucca, see Siraisi, *Taddeo*, 14–15.

29. The most comprehensive study of western European medieval surgical illustration is still Sudhoff, *Beiträge*, 1 (entire) and 2:1–90, and accompanying plates; also valuable are Loren MacKinney, *Medical Illustrations in Medieval Manuscripts* (London, 1965), chap. 8, and plates, and Peter Murray Jones, *Medieval Medical Miniatures* (Austin, Texas, 1985), 96–118.

30. Guglielmo da Saliceto, *Cyrurgia*, printed with his *Summa conservationis*, Book 2, chap. 5, sig. x^r; chap. 7, sig. x^v.

31. Lanfranco, *Cyrurgia*, printed with Guy de Chauliac *Cyrurgia*, tractatus 2, chap. 1, fol. 176 (175)^r (*Science of Cirurgie*, ed., Fleischhacker, 127–29).

32. In the following discussion of this topic, I have benefited greatly from the advice of Robert J. T. Joy, M.D., and Dale C. Smith.

33. Henri de Mondeville, *Chirurgie*, ed. Pagel, tractatus 2, introductory notabilia 21, pp. 125–26. The passage, together with Mondeville's explanation of his method, is translated from a French version in Grant, *Source Book in Medieval Science*, 802–6.

34. Teodorico, *Cyrurgia* Book 1, chaps. 1, 11 and 12, printed with Guy de Chauliac, *Cyrurgia*, fols. 106(105)^v, 109(108)^v–110(109)^v (*Surgery of Theodoric*, 1:15–17, 48–49, 54). Guido Majno, *The Healing Hand: Man and Wound in the Ancient World* (Cambridge, Mass., 1975), 183–89, and Grmek, *Diseases*, 123–32, discuss ancient treatment of wounds and observations and ideas about pus. Huard and Grmek, *Mille ans de chirurgie*, 66.

35. Rolando, *Libellus de cyrurgia*, printed with Guy de Chauliac, *Cyrurgia*, Book 3, chap. 25, fol. 157 (156)^r; Teodorico, *Cyrurgia*, in the same volume, Book 2, chap. 17, fol. 117^v (*Surgery of Theodoric*, 1:149).

36. *Notulae* to the surgical tract of Guillaume de Congenis, ed. Sudhoff, *Beiträge*, 2:327, 370. Examples of treatises providing a recipe for a soporific sponge include the twelfth-century Salernitan compilation known as the Bamberg Surgery (Corner, "On

Early Salernitan Surgery," 12) and Teodorico, *Cyrurgia*, printed with Guy de Chauliac, *Cyrurgia*, Book 4, chap. 8, fol. 146ʳ (*Surgery of Theodoric*, 1:212–14). Marguerite L. Baur, "Recherches sur l'histoire de l'anesthésie avant 1846," *Janus* 31 (1927): 24–39, 63–90, 124–37, 170–82; Willem F. Daems, "Spongia somnifera: Philologische und pharmakologische Probleme," *Beiträge zur Geschichte der Pharmazie* 22 (1970): 25–26; MacKinney, *Medical Illustrations*, 8, 63, makes the point about miniatures. See also Huard and Grmek, *Mille ans de chirurgie*, 66–67.

37. Lanfranco, *Cyrurgia*, tractatus 1, doctrina 3, chap. 9, printed with Guy de Chauliac, *Cyrurgia*, fol. 172(171)ʳ (*Science of Cirurgie*, ed. Fleischhacker, 69–70).

38. Lanfranco, ibid., tractatus 2, chap. 1, fol. 177(176)ʳ (*Science of Cirurgie*, ed. Fleischhacker, 140); tractatus 3, doctrina 2, chap. 5, fol. 187(186) (*Science of Cirurgie*, ed. Fleischhacker, 220–21).

39. *Treatises of Fistula in Ano, Haemorrhoids, and Clysters by John Arderne from an Early Fifteenth-Century Manuscript Translation*, ed. D'Arcy Power. EETS, no. 139 (Oxford, 1910; repr. 1968), 1–3.

40. Guglielmo da Saliceto, *Chirurgia*, printed with his *Summa conservationis*, proem, sig. tᵛ.

41. Ibid., Book 1, chap. 1, sig. t2ᵛ.

42. Ibid., Book 2, chap. 5, sig. xʳ.

43. Avicenna, *Canon*, Book 4, fen 3, 4, and 5. Haly Abbas, *Liber regius*, Part 2 (Practice), Book 9 (Lyon, 1523), fols. 272ʳ–290ᵛ. This is the Stephen of Antioch version of Haly Abbas' work; for Constantinus Africanus' use of Book 9, see n. 18 in this chapter.

44. Surgical writers who made use of the idea of surgery as the third instrument of medicine included Rolando da Parma (*Libellus de Cyrurgia*, proem, fol. 147 [146]ʳ); Bruno Longoburgo (*Cyrurgia magna*, proem, fol. 83 [82]ʳ), and Henri de Mondeville (*Chirurgie*, ed. Pagel, tractatus 2, proem, p. 62).

45. Guglielmo da Saliceto, *Cyrurgia*, printed with his *Summa conservationis*, proem, sig. tᵛ. The preface to the *Summa conservationis* (sig. a2ʳ) contains citations of Aristotle's *Metaphysics*, *On Sense and Sensation*, and *On Sleep and Waking*. Guy de Chauliac, *Cyrurgia*, proem, fol. 2ʳ (*Cyrurgie*, ed. Ogden, 3).

46. Siraisi, *Taddeo*, 281, 289–90, 293, 296–98.

47. Guglielmo da Saliceto, *Summa conservationis*, proem, sig. a2ʳ⁻ᵛ; idem, *Cyrurgia*, introductory chapter, sig. t2ʳ.

48. *Processi*, ed. Lugano, 180.

49. *Notulae* on surgical treatise of Guillaume de Congenis, 3.12, ed. Sudhoff, *Beiträge*, 2:358.

50. Wolfram von Eschenbach, *Parzival* 10.506, 516, trans. Helen M. Mustard and Charles E. Passage (New York, 1961), 270–71, 275–76. The first passage is cited in Keil, "Mittelalterliche Chirurgie," 53. B. D. Haage, "Chirurgie nach Abū L-Qāsim im 'Parzival' Wolframs von Eschenbach," *Clio Medica* 19 (1984): 193–205, strongly maintains Wolfram's use of Albucasis.

51. *Notulae* on the surgical treatise of Guillaume de Congenis, 1.34, ed. Sudhoff, *Beiträge*, 2:331.

52. For example, for such legislation at Montpellier, see Louis Dulieu, *La chirurgie à Montpellier de ses origines au début du XIX siècle* (Avignon, 1975), 29.

53. Bruno Longoburgo, *Cyrurgia magna*, printed with Guy de Chauliac, *Cyrurgia*, fol. 83 (82)ʳ.

54. The decree is translated, with commentary, in Amundsen, "Medieval Canon Law on Medical and Surgical Practice by the Clergy," 40. For a recent evaluation of the impact of the prohibition, see André Goddu, "The Effect of Canonical Prohibitions on the Faculty of Medicine at the University of Paris in the Middle Ages," MJ 20 (1985): 342–62. Evidence regarding Teodorico is summarized in Siraisi, *Taddeo*, 16–17.

55. *Statuti*, ed. Malagola, 247–48.

56. *Dinus in Chirurgia*, fol. 1ʳ. Siraisi, *Taddeo*, 55–58, 109–10.

57. Park, *Doctors and Medicine*, 19–20, 62–66, 153, 167–70. Tiziana Pesenti Marangon, "'Professores chirurgie,' 'medici ciroici' e 'barbitonsores' a Padova nell'età di Leonardo Buffi da Bertipaglia (m. dopo il 1448)," *Quaderni per la storia dell'Università di Padova* 11 (1978): 1–38.

58. Keil, "Mittelalterliche Chirurgie," 53–54. Vern L. Bullough, "Training of the Nonuniversity-Educated Medical Practitioners in the Later Middle Ages," JHM 14 (1959): 446–58.

59. Henri de Mondeville, *Chirurgie*, ed. Pagel, Tractatus 2, introductory notabilia, pp. 79–80.

60. *Notulae* on the surgical treatise of Guillaume de Congenis 1.6, ed. Sudhoff, *Beiträge*, 2:317; discussed in Vern Bullough, "The Teaching of Surgery at the University of Montpellier in the Thirteenth Century," JHM 15 (1960): 202–4.

61. Dulieu, *Chirurgie à Montpellier*, 25–26, 30.

62. R. Theodore Beck, *The Cutting Edge: Early History of the Surgeons of London* (London, 1974), provides an account of these developments and of the early history of the London Barbers Company and Fellowship of Surgeons. See also note 10 to Chapter 3, and accompanying text.

63. Keil, "Mittelalterliche Chirurgie," 54; for Flanders and German regions in general, ibid., 54–55, 56–60.

64. Guy de Chauliac, *Cyrurgie*, ed. Ogden, v–vi.

65. Philippe Contamine, *War in the Middle Ages*, trans. Michael Jones (Oxford and New York, 1984), 258.

66. J. R. Hale, *War and Society in Renaissance Europe, 1450–1620* (New York, 1985), 46–74.

67. The provisions of the contract are summarized in Siraisi, *Taddeo*, 15.

68. In the passage referred to in n. 33 in this chapter.

69. George Gask, "The Medical Services of Henry the Fifth's Campaign on the Somme in 1415," *Essays in the History of Medicine* (London, 1950), 94–102. A translation of Morestede's petition is printed in C. T. Allmand, ed., *Society at War* (Edinburgh, 1973), 64–65. Getz, "Medicine at Medieval Oxford."

70. Arderne, *Treatises of Fistula in Ano*, 8–29. A. Neiger, *Atlas of Practical Proctology* (Bern, Stuttgart, Vienna, 1973), 47–52. James H. MacLeod, *A Method of Proctology* (Hagerstown, N.Y., 1979), 44–56. Wagensteen and Wagensteen, *Rise of Surgery*, 14–15.

71. Albucasis, *On Surgery and Instruments*, 3.80, 504–8; Arderne, *Treatises of Fistula in Ano*, ed. D'Arcy Power, notes the parallel passages, xvi–xvii; see also xvii–xviii and 112 for a critique of Arderne's procedure.

72. Teodorico, *Cyrurgia*, Book 2, chap. 3, printed with Guy de Chauliac, *Cyrurgia*, fol. 114(113)ᵛ (*Surgery of Theodoric*, 1:110).

EPILOGUE

1. Giovanni Manardo, *In Galeni doctrina et Arabum censura celeberrimi et optime meriti epistolarum medicinalium libri* XX (Basel, 1540), 1. For some of the sources of the brief sketch of sixteenth-century medicine in the epilogue, and for further information on these developments, see works listed in the Guide to Further Reading.

GUIDE TO FURTHER READING

The large secondary literature on early European medicine is of variable quality. The highly selective list of secondary works that follows has been drawn up with a view to introducing the reader to some examples of recent scholarship of merit on each of various aspects of the subject. The list of secondary works is confined to book-length studies and a few articles of broad scope. However, it is followed by a list of journals and bibliographies that provides a point of entry to the more specialized literature. No attempt has been made to provide a guide to manuscript materials. Only works in English are listed.

The reader should note that in a number of cases introductory material to translations of primary sources listed in the following section includes valuable historical and interpretative essays.

CHAPTER ONE

Amundsen, Darrel W. 1971. "Visigothic Medical Legislation." *Bulletin of the History of Medicine* 45:553–69.

———. 1982. "Medicine and Faith in Early Christianity." *Bulletin of the History of Medicine* 56:326–50.

D'Alverny, Marie-Thérèse. 1982. "Translators and Translations." In *Renaissance and Renewal in the Twelfth Century*, edited by Robert L. Benson and Giles Constable, 421–62. Cambridge, Mass.

De Lacey, Philip. 1972. "Galen's Platonism." *American Journal of Philology* 93:27–39.

Edelstein, E. J. and Edelstein, L. 1945. *Asclepius: A Collection and Interpretation of the Testimonies.* 2 vols. Baltimore.

Edelstein, L. 1967. *Ancient Medicine.* Edited by O. and C. L. Temkin. Baltimore.

Grmek, Mirko D. 1989. *Diseases in the Ancient Greek World.* Translated by Mireille Muellner and Leonard Muellner. Baltimore.

Harris, C. R. S. 1973. *The Heart and the Vascular System in Ancient Greek Medicine from Alcmaeon to Galen.* Oxford.

Lloyd, G. E. R. 1983. *Science, Folklore and Ideology: Studies in the Life Sciences in Ancient Greece.* Cambridge.

Longrigg, J. 1963. "Philosophy and Medicine, Some Early Interactions." *Harvard Studies in Classical Philology* 67:147–75.

Majno, Guido. 1975. *The Healing Hand: Man and Wound in the Ancient World.* Cambridge, Mass.

Meyerhof, Max. 1984. *Studies in Medieval Arabic Medicine: Theory and Practice.* Edited by Penelope Johnstone. London.

Nutton, Vivian. 1984. "From Galen to Alexander, Aspects of Medicine and Medical Practice in Late Antiquity." In *Symposium on Byzantine Medicine. Dumbarton Oaks Papers,* no. 38:1–14 (This and other articles by this author also in Nulton, *From Democedes to Harvey* [London, 1988]).

Phillips, E. D. 1987. *Aspects of Greek Medicine.* Philadelphia.

Riddle, John M. 1985. *Dioscorides on Pharmacy and Medicine.* Austin, Texas.

Rubin, Stanley. 1974. *Medieval English Medicine.* Newton Abbot. (Mostly on the Anglo-Saxon period.)

Scarborough, John. 1969. *Roman Medicine.* Ithaca, N.Y.

Smith, Wesley D. 1973. *The Hippocratic Tradition.* Ithaca, N.Y.

Temkin, Oswei. 1973. *Galenism: Rise and Decline of a Medical Philosophy.* Ithaca, N.Y. (Includes discussion of medieval and Renaissance Galenism.)

Ullmann, Manfred, 1978. *Islamic Medicine.* Edinburgh.

Von Staden, Heinrich, 1989. *Herophilus: The Art of Medicine in Early Alexandria.* Cambridge.

Voigts, Linda E. 1979. "Anglo-Saxon Plant Remedies and the Anglo-Saxons." *Isis* 70:250–68.

CHAPTER TWO

Amundsen, Darrel W. 1978. "Medieval Canon Law on Medical and Surgical Practice by the Clergy." *Bulletin of the History of Medicine* 52:39–56.

Benton, John. 1985. "Trotula, Women's Problems, and the Professionalization of Medicine in the Middle Ages." *Bulletin of the History of Medicine* 59:30–53.

Demaitre, Luke E. 1980. *Doctor Bernard de Gordon: Professor and Practitioner.* Toronto.

Friedenwald, Harry. 1944. *The Jews and Medicine. Essays.* 2 vols. Baltimore.

Garcia Ballester, Luis, Michael R. McVaugh, and Augustin Rubio Vela. *Medical Licensing and Learning in Fourteenth-Century Valencia. Transactions of the American Philosophical Society* (forthcoming).

Green, Monica H. 1989. "Women's Medical Practice and Medical Care in Medieval Europe." *Signs* 14:434–73.

Kealey, Edward J. 1981. *Medieval Medicus: A Social History of Anglo-Norman Medicine.* Baltimore.

Kibre, Pearl. 1953. "The Faculty of Medicine at Paris, Charlatanism and Unlicensed Medical Practice in the Late Middle Ages." *Bulletin of the History of Medicine* 27:1–20.

Lockwood, Dean Putnam. 1951. *Ugo Benzi, Medieval Philosopher and Physician, 1376–1439.* Chicago.

Nutton, Vivian. 1981. "Continuity or Rediscovery? The City Physician in Classical Antiquity and Medieval Italy." In *The Town and State Physician in Europe from the Middle Ages to the Enlightenment,* edited by Andrew W. Russell, 9–46. Wolfenbüttel.

Park, Katherine. 1985. *Doctors and Medicine in Early Renaissance Florence.* Princeton.

Pelling, Margaret. 1982. "Occupational Diversity: Barbersurgeons and the Trades of Norwich." *Bulletin of the History of Medicine* 56:484–511.

Rawcliffe, Carol. 1988. "The Profits of Practice: The Wealth and Status of Medical Men in Later Medieval England." *Social History of Medicine* 1:63–78.

Roth, Cecil. 1953. "The Qualification of Jewish Physicians in the Middle Ages." *Speculum* 28:834–43.

Shatzmiller, Joseph. 1983. "On Becoming a Jewish Doctor in the High Middle Ages." *Sefarad* 43:239–50.

Talbot, Charles H. 1967. *Medicine in Medieval England*. London.

Talbot, Charles H., and E. A. Hammond. 1965. *The Medical Practitioners of Medieval England: A Biographical Register*. London.

CHAPTER THREE

Bullough, Vern L. 1959. "Training of the Nonuniversity-Educated Medical Practitioners in the Later Middle Ages," *Journal of the History of Medicine and Allied Sciences* 14:446–58.

———. 1966. *The Development of Medicine as a Profession: The Contribution of the Medieval University to Modern Medicine*. New York.

Kristeller, Paul Oskar. 1956. "The School of Salerno: Its Development and Its Contribution to the History of Learning." In his *Studies in Renaissance Thought and Letters*, 495–551. Rome.

Ohl, Ronald. 1980. *The University of Padua 1405–1509. An International Community of Students and Professors*. Ph.D. dissertation. University of Pennsylvania.

Siraisi, Nancy G. 1981. *Taddeo Alderotti and His Pupils: Two Generations of Italian Medical Learning*. Princeton.

CHAPTER FOUR

Bullough, Vern. 1973. "Medieval Medical and Scientific Views of Women." *Viator: Medieval and Renaissance Studies* 4:485–501.

French, Roger. 1979a. "*De Juvamentis Membrorum* and the Reception of Galenic Physiological Anatomy." *Isis* 70:96–109.

———. 1979b. "A Note on the Anatomical Accessus of the Middle Ages." *Medical History* 23:461–68.

———. 1985. "Gentile da Foligno and the *via medicorum*." In *The Light of Nature: Essays in the History and Philosophy of Science Presented to A. C. Crombie*, edited by J. D. North and J. J. Roche, 21–34. Dordrecht, Boston, Lancaster.

Hall, Thomas H. 1971. "Life, Death and the Radical Moisture: A Study of Thematic Patterns in Medical Theory." *Clio Medica* 6:3–23.

Herrlinger, Robert. 1970. *A History of Medical Illustration from Antiquity to A.D. 1600*. London.

Hewson, M. Anthony. 1975. *Giles of Rome and the Medieval Theory of Conception*. London.

Jacquart, Danielle. 1988. "Aristotelian Thought in Salerno." In *A History of Twelfth-Century Western Philosophy*, edited by Peter Dronke, 407–28. Cambridge.

Jacquart, Danielle, and Claude Thomasset. 1988. *Sexuality and Medicine in the Middle Ages*. Princeton.

Keele, Kenneth D. 1983. *Leonardo da Vinci's Elements of the Science of Man*. New York.

Kibre, Pearl. 1945. "Hippocratic Writings in the Middle Ages." *Bulletin of the History of Medicine* 18:371–412.

Lawn, Brian. 1963. *The Salernitan Questions: An Introduction to the History of Medieval and Renaissance Problem Literature.* Oxford.

MacKinney, Loren C. 1965. *Medical Illustrations in Medieval Manuscripts.* London.

McVaugh, Michael R. 1974. "The 'humidum radicale' in Thirteenth-Century Medicine." *Traditio* 30:259–83.

Murray Jones, Peter. 1986. *Medieval Medical Miniatures.* Austin, Texas.

Nutton, Vivian. 1983. "The Seeds of Disease: An Explanation of Contagion and Infection from the Greeks to the Renaissance." *Medical History* 27:1–34.

O'Malley, Charles D., and J. B. de C. M. Saunders. 1952. *Leonardo da Vinci on the Human Body.* New York.

Siraisi. 1981. (see list for chap. 3).

Tester, S. J. 1987. *A History of Western Astrology.* Woodbridge.

CHAPTER FIVE

Arano, Luisa Cogliati. 1976. *The Medieval Health Handbook: Tacuinum sanitatis.* New York. (Reproductions of miniatures from medieval manuscripts, with art historical commentary.)

Arnaldi de Villanova opera medica omnia. 1975–. Edited by L. Garcia Ballester, J. A. Paniagua, and Michael R. McVaugh. Granada-Barcelona. (Contains modern scholarly editions of the Latin works of the leading medical author at medieval Montpellier; texts are in Latin, but vols. 2 [*Aphorismi de gradibus*, 1975], 3 [*De amore heroico, De dosi tyriacalium medicinarum*, 1985], and 16 [*Translatio libri Galieni de rigore et tremore et iectigatione et spasmo*, 1981] contain lengthy, scholarly, and informative introductions in English by Michael R. McVaugh on, respectively, pharmacology, the lover's malady and theriac, and concepts of rigor and spasm with attention to the elaboration of Latin technical medical vocabulary.)

Blunt, Wilfrid, and Sandra Raphael. 1979. *The Illustrated Herbal.* London.

Campbell, Anna M. 1931. *The Black Death and Men of Learning.* New York. (Facsimile reprint, 1966.)

Camporesi, Piero. 1988. *The Incorruptible Flesh. Bodily Mutation and Mortification in Religion and Folklore.* Translated by Tania Croft-Murray. Cambridge. (Mostly concerns popular religiosity in the early modern period, but includes much incidental information about late medieval and Renaissance medicaments, foodstuffs, parasites, and concepts regarding putrefaction.)

Carmichael, Ann G. 1986. *Plague and the Poor in Renaissance Florence.* Cambridge.

Jarcho, Saul. 1980. *The Concept of Heart Failure: From Avicenna to Albertini.* Cambridge, Mass.

Majno, Guido. 1975. (See list for chap. 1.)

Park, Katharine. 1985. "The Medieval Hospital." *FMR* 8:127–38.

Richards, Peter. 1977. *The Medieval Leper and His Northern Heirs.* Cambridge.

Riddle, John M. 1985. (See list for chap. 1.)

Stannard, Jerry. 1974. "Medieval Herbals and Their Development." *Clio Medica* 9:23–33.

Ziegler, Philip. 1969. *The Black Death.* New York.

CHAPTER SIX

Ackerknecht, Erwin. 1967. "Primitive Surgery." In *Diseases of Antiquity. A Survey of Diseases, Injuries and Surgery of Early Populations.* Edited by Don Brothwell and A. T. Sandison. Springfield, Illinois. (Deals with traditional surgery in the Third World, not early European surgery, but suggests interesting comparisons.)

Beck, R. Theodore. 1974. *The Cutting Edge: Early History of the Surgeons of London.* London.

Bullough, Vern L. 1959. (See list for chap. 3.)

MacKinney, Loren C. 1965. His chap. 8. (See list for chap. 4.)

Majno, Guido. 1975. (See list for chap. 1.)

Ogden, Margaret S. 1973. "The Galenic Works Cited in Guy de Chauliac's *Chirurgia Magna.*" *Journal of the History of Medicine and Allied Sciences* 28:24–33.

Rubin, Stanley. 1974. (See list for chap. 1.)

Smith, Emilie Savage. 1976. "Some Sources and Procedures for Editing A Medieval Arabic Surgical Tract." *History of Science* 14:245–64.

Wangensteen, Owen H., and Sarah D. Wangensteen. 1978. *The Rise of Surgery: From Empiric Craft to Scientific Discipline.* Minneapolis.

EPILOGUE

Arber, Agnes. 1986. *Herbals, Their Origin and Evolution. A Chapter in the History of Botany 1470–1670,* 3d Ed. Cambridge.

Bylebyl, Jerome J. 1985. "Medicine, Philosophy, and Humanism in Renaissance Italy." In *Science and the Arts in the Renaissance,* edited by John W. Shirley and F. David Hoeniger, 27–49. Washington, D.C.

Nutton, Vivian. 1987. *John Caius and the Manuscripts of Galen.* The Cambridge Philological Society. Supplementary volume no. 13. Cambridge.

O'Malley, Charles D. 1964. *Andreas Vesalius of Brussels 1514–1564.* Berkeley.

Pagel, Walter. 1958. *Paracelsus. An Introduction to Philosophical Medicine of the Era of the Renaissance.* Basel and New York.

Reeds, Karen. 1976. "Renaissance Humanism and Botany." *Annals of Science* 33:519–42.

Siraisi, Nancy G. 1987. *Avicenna in Renaissance Italy. The Canon and Medical Teaching in Italian Universities after 1500.* Princeton.

Wear, A., French, R. K., and Lonie, I. M., eds. 1985. *The Medical Renaissance of the Sixteenth Century.* Cambridge.

Webster, Charles, ed. 1979. *Health, Medicine and Mortality in the Sixteenth Century.* Cambridge.

SCHOLARLY JOURNALS AND REFERENCE TOOLS

Major English language journals of the history of medicine include the *Bulletin of the History of Medicine, Clio Medica,* the *Journal of the History of Medicine and Allied Sciences,* and *Medical History.* The principal bibliographical guides are the National Library of Medicine *Bibliography of the History of Medicine* (annual, cumulated every five years) and the

Wellcome Historical Medical Library *Subject Catalogue of the History of Medicine* (18 vols., Munich, 1980), updated in the quarterly *Current Work in the History of Medicine*. The *Isis Cumulative Bibliography* and *Isis* annual bibliographies of the history of science include history of medicine. Peter Murray Jones, "Medical Books Before the Invention of Printing," in *Thornton's Medical Books, Libraries, and Collectors* (ed. Alain Besson, 3rd rev. ed., Aldershot: Brookfield, Vermont, 1990), pp. 1–29, is a useful guide to specialized bibliographies and catalogues.

SELECTED PRIMARY SOURCES
AVAILABLE IN ENGLISH
TRANSLATION

Much ancient, medieval, and Renaissance medical writing has never been translated into any modern language; and many medieval and Renaissance works are available only in manuscript or in early printed editions. The following list of ancient, medieval, and Renaissance medical texts available in English translation makes no claims to completeness but indicates some of the sources in which readers who are confined to works available in English can study the content of early medicine at first hand. Readers should, however, be aware that modern translations of Greek and Arabic works into English are likely to have been made directly from the original languages, not from the Latin versions of the same texts in use in Europe during the Middle Ages and Renaissance.

Agnellus of Ravenna. 1981. *Lectures on Galen's De sectis*. Ed. and trans. Classics Seminar 609, State University of New York at Buffalo, Buffalo.

Albert the Great. 1987. *Man and the Beasts*. Trans. James J. Scanlon. Binghamton. (Includes short sections on human reproduction from Albertus Magnus' *De animalibus*.)

Albucasis. 1973. *On Surgery and Instruments*. Trans. M. S. Spink and G. L. Lewis. London.

Avicenna. 1966. *The General Principles of Avicenna's Canon of Medicine*. Trans. Mazhar H. Shah. Karachi. (Bk. 1, with summary of bks. 2–5.)

———. 1930. *Canon*, bk. 1. In R. Cameron Gruner. *A Treatise on the Canon of Medicine Incorporating a Translation of the First Book*. London.

Berengario da Carpi, 1990. *On Fracture of the Skull or Cranium*. Trans. L. R. Lind. *Transactions of the American Philosophical Society*. Vol. 80, pt. 4. Philadelphia.

Brain, Peter. 1986. *Galen on Bloodletting*. Cambridge. (Study including translated texts.)

Corner, George W. 1927. *Anatomical Texts of the Earlier Middle Ages*. Washington, D.C. (Includes the Salernitan manuals on anatomy.)

Ficino, Marsilio. 1989. *Three Books on Life*. Ed. and trans. Carol V. Kaske and John R. Clark, Binghamton. (Books 1 and 2 are on regimen in health; Book 3 is chiefly on astral magic.)

Galen. 1979. *On the Natural Faculties*. Trans. A. W. Brock. Loeb Classical Library. Cambridge and London. (Originally issued 1916.)

———. 1985. *Three Treatises on the Nature of Science. On the Sects for Beginners. An Outline of Empiricism. On Medical Experience*. Trans. R. Walzer and M. Frede. Indianapolis.

———. 1968. *On the Usefulness of the Parts of the Body*. Trans. Margaret T. May. 2 vols. Ithaca.

Grant, Edward, ed. 1974. *A Source Book in Medieval Science*. Pp. 700–807. Cambridge, Mass. (A well chosen and well organized set of excerpts from primary sources in English translation selected by Michael R. McVaugh. Among the major texts are portions of the *Isagoge* of Johannitius, the *Canon* of Avicenna, the *Anatomy* of Mondino de' Liuzzi, the gynecological treatise attributed to Trotula, and the *Surgery* of Henri de Mondeville, as well as samples of commentaries, *consilia*, works on diagnosis by pulse and urine, pharmacology, and other surgical treatises.)

Guy de Chauliac. 1971. *The Cyrurgie of Guy de Chauliac.* Ed. Margaret S. Ogden, Early English Text Society no. 265. Oxford. (Text in Middle English.)

Hippocrates, 6 vols., 1972–88. Trans. W. H. S. Jones et al. Loeb Classical Library. Cambridge and London. (Vols. 1 and 2 originally issued 1923; vol. 3, 1928; vol. 4, 1931).

[Johannes de Ketham]. 1925. *The Fasciculo di Medicina, Venice 1495.* Ed. Charles Singer. 2 vols. Florence. (A facsimile of an early printed collection of medical treatises in Italian, accompanied by modern scholarly apparatus. Includes an English translation of the *Anatomy* of Mondino de' Luzzi, or Liuzzi, 2:59–99. Unfortunately, the facsimile was printed in a small number of copies and is not widely available.)

John of Arderne. 1910. *Treatises of Fistula in Ano, Haemorrhoids, and Clysters by John Arderne from an Early Fifteenth-Century Manuscript Translation.* Ed. D'Arcy Power. Early English Text Society no. 139. Oxford. (Reprinted 1968.)

Leonard of Bertapaglia, 1989. *On Nerve Injuries and Skull Fractures.* Trans. Jules C. Ladenheim. Mount Kisco, New York.

Lind, R. L. 1975. *Studies in Pre-Vesalian Anatomy: Biography, Translations, Documents.* Philadelphia. (Includes the text of anatomical treatises by Alessandro Benedetti [1497], Niccolo Massa [1559], Andreas de Laguna [1535], Johannes Dryander [1535] and a commentary on the *Anatomy* of Mundinus [Mondino] by Berengario da Carpi [1521].)

Lloyd, G. E. R., ed. 1978. *Hippocratic Writings.* Harmondsworth.

Maimonides, 1984. *Medical Writings.* Trans. Fred Rosner, M.D. Haifa.

Rowland, Beryl, ed. and trans. 1981. *Medieval Woman's Guide to Health.* Kent, Ohio. (A gynecological treatise.)

Saffron, Morris H., ed. and trans. 1972. *Maurus of Salerno Twelfth Century "Optimus Physicus" with His Commentary on the Prognostics of Hippocrates. Transactions of the American Philosophical Society.* Vol. 62, pt. 1. Philadelphia.

Sharpe, William D., ed. and trans. 1964. *Isidore of Seville: The Medical Writings. Transactions of the American Philosophical Society.* Vol. 54, pt. 2. Philadelphia.

Teodorico Borgognoni (Theodoric of Lucca). 1955–60. *The Surgery of Theodoric.* Trans. Eldridge Campbell and James Colton. 2 vols. New York.

Voigts, Linda E., and Michael R. McVaugh, eds. 1984. *A Latin Technical Phlebotomy and Its Middle English Translation. Transactions of the American Philosophical Society.* Vol. 74, pt. 2. Philadelphia.

Wallner, Björn, ed. 1969. *The Middle English Translation of Guy de Chauliac's Treatise on Fractures and Dislocations. Book 5 of the Great Surgery.* Lund. (Other sections of Guy de Chauliac's work have also been translated by Wallner in the same series.)

BIBLIOGRAPHY

Only works cited in the notes are included in the bibliography. Well-known works on nonmedical subjects that have been cited for one brief passage or reference (e.g., Augustine of Hippo, De civitate Dei) are not included. The list of abbreviations used is to be found at the head of the notes.

Acta graduum academicorum gymnasii patavini ab anno 1406 ad annum 1450. Edited by G. Zonta and G. Brotto. 1970. 2 vols. 2d ed. Padua.

Agnellus of Ravenna. 1981. *Lectures on Galen's De sectis.* Edited and translated by Seminar Classics 609, State University of New York at Buffalo. Buffalo.

Agrimi, Jole, and Chiara Crisciani. 1978. *Medicina del corpo e medicina dell'anima: Note sul sapere del medico fino all'inizio del secolo XIII. Episteme.* Milan.

———. 1988. *Edocere medicos: Medicina scolastica nei secoli XIII–XV.* Naples.

Albucasis. 1973. *On Surgery and Instruments.* Edited and translated by M. S. Spink and G. L. Lewis. London.

Amundsen, Darrel W. 1971. "Visigothic Medical Legislation." BHM 45:553–69.

———. 1977. "Medical Deontology and Pestilential Disease in the Late Middle Ages." JHM 32:403–21.

———. 1978. "Medieval Canon Law on Medical and Surgical Practice by the Clergy." BHM 52:39–56.

———. 1981. "Casuistry and Professional Obligations: The Regulation of Physicians by the Court of Conscience in the Late Middle Ages." *Transactions & Studies of The College of Physicians of Philadelphia* 3:21–39, 93–112.

———. 1982. "Medicine and Faith in Early Christianity." *Bulletin of the History of Medicine* 56:326–50.

———. 1986. "The Medieval Catholic Tradition." In *Caring and Curing: Health and Medicine in the Western Religious Traditions,* edited by Ronald L. Numbers and Darrel W. Amundsen, 65–107. New York and London.

Arano, Luisa Cogliati. 1976. *The Medieval Health Handbook: Tacuinum sanitatis.* New York.

Arbesmann, Rudolph. 1954. "The Concept of 'Christus medicus' in St. Augustine." *Traditio* 10:1–28.

Aristotle. 1984. *The Complete Works,* edited by Jonathan Barnes. 2 vols. Princeton.

Arnaldi de Villanova opera medica omnia. 1975–. Edited by L. Garcia Ballester, J. A. Paniagua, and M. R. McVaugh. Granada-Barcelona.

Arnald of Villanova. 1975. *Aphorismi de gradibus.* Edited by Michael R. McVaugh. In Arnald's *Opera medica omnia,* vol. 2. Granada-Barcelona.

————. 1981. *Translatio libri Galieni De rigore et tremore et iectigatione et spasmo.* Edited by Michael R. McVaugh. In Arnald's *Opera medica omnia,* vol. 16. Barcelona.

————. 1985a. *Doctrina Galieni De interioribus.* Edited by Richard J. Durling. In Arnald's *Opera medica omnia,* vol. 15. Barcelona.

————. 1985b. *Tractatus de amore heroico. Epistola de dosi tyriacalium medicinarum.* Edited by Michael R. McVaugh. In Arnald's *Opera medica omnia,* vol. 3. Barcelona.

Averroes. 1562. *Colliget libri VII.* In vol. 10 of *Opera* of Aristotle and Averroes. Venice.

Avicenna. 1507. *Liber Canonis.* Venice. Facsimile, Hildesheim, 1964.

Baader, Gerhard. 1968. "Zur anatomie in Paris im 13. und 14. Jahrhundert." MJ 3:40–53.

————. 1974. "Die Entwicklung der medizinischen Fachsprache im hohen und späten Mittelalter." In *Fachprosaforschung,* edited by G. Keil and P. Assion, 88–123. Berlin.

————. 1981. "Galen in mittelalterlichen Abendland." In *Galen: Problems and Prospects,* edited by Vivian Nutton, 213–28. London.

Baader, Gerhard, and Gundolf Keil, eds. 1982. *Medizin im mittelalterlichen Abendland.* Darmstadt.

Baur, Marguerite L. 1927. "Recherches sur l'histoire de l'anesthésie avant 1846." *Janus* 31:24–39, 63–90, 124–37, 170–82.

Beaujouan, Guy. 1962. *Manuscrits scientifiques médiévaux de l'université de Salamanque et de ses "Colegios Mayores."* Bibliothèque de l'Ecole des Hautes Etudes Hispaniques, Fasc. 32. Bordeaux.

————. 1968. "Fautes et obscurités dans les traductions médicales du Moyen Age." *Revue de synthèse,* 3d series, 89:145–52.

Beccaria, Augusto. 1956. *I codici di medicina del periodo presalernitano (secoli IX, X e XI).* Rome.

————. 1959, 1961, 1971. "Sulle tracce di un antico canone latino di Ippocrate e di Galeno." *Italia Medioevale e Umanistica* 2:1–56; 4:1–75; 14:1–23.

Beck, R. Theodore. 1974. *The Cutting Edge: Early History of the Surgeons of London.* London.

Bellomo, Manlio. 1979. *Saggio sull'università nell'età del diritto comune.* Catania.

Beltran de Heredia, Vicente, O.P. 1970–73. *Cartulario de la Universidad de Salamanca.* 6 vols. Salamanca.

Benton, John. 1985. "Trotula, Women's Problems, and the Professionalization of Medicine in the Middle Ages." BHM 59:30–53.

Birkenmajer, Aleksander. 1970. "Le rôle joué par les médecins et les naturalistes dans la réception d'Aristote au XIIe et XIIIe siècles." In his *Etudes d'histoire des sciences et de la philosophie du Moyen Age,* 73–87. Studia Copernicana, vol. 1. Wroclaw, Warsaw, Cracow. (Originally published 1930.)

Borgognoni, Teodorico. 1498. *Cyrurgia.* Printed with Guy de Chauliac, *Cyrurgia.* Venice.

————. 1955–60. *The Surgery of Theodoric.* Translated by Eldridge Campbell and James Colton. 2 vols. New York.

Bornstein, Daniel E., trans. 1986. *Dino Compagni's Chronicle of Florence.* Philadelphia.

Brain, Peter. 1986. *Galen on Bloodletting.* Cambridge.

Brody, Saul N. 1974. *The Disease of the Soul: Leprosy in Medieval Literature.* Ithaca.

Brown, Elizabeth A. R. 1981. "Death and the Human Body in the Later Middle Ages: The Legislation of Boniface VIII on the Division of the Corpse." *Viator: Medieval and Renaissance Studies* 12:221–70.

Brown, Peter. 1981. *The Cult of the Saints: Its Rise and Function in Latin Christianity.* Chicago.

Bullough, Vern L. 1959. "Training of the Nonuniversity-Educated Medical Practitioners in the Later Middle Ages," JHM 14:446–58.

———. 1960. "The Teaching of Surgery at the University of Montpellier in the Thirteenth Century." JHM 15:202–4.

———. 1966. *The Development of Medicine as a Profession: The Contribution of the Medieval University to Modern Medicine.* New York.

———. 1973. "Medieval Medical and Scientific Views of Women." *Viator: Medieval and Renaissance Studies* 4:485–501.

Bylebyl, Jerome J. 1971. "Galen on the Non-Natural Causes of Variation in the Pulse." BHM 45:482–85.

Bynum, Caroline Walker. 1987. *Holy Feast and Holy Fast: The Religious Significance of Food to Medieval Women.* Berkeley.

Campbell, Anna M. 1966. *The Black Death and Men of Learning.* New York. (Originally published 1931.)

Camporesi, Piero. 1988. *The Incorruptible Flesh. Bodily Mutation and Mortification in Religion and Folklore.* Translated by Tania Croft-Murray. Cambridge. (Originally published in Italian as *La carne impassibile*, Milan, 1983.)

Carmichael, Ann G. 1986. *Plague and the Poor in Renaissance Florence.* Cambridge.

Cartulaire de l'Université de Montpellier . . . Tome 1 (1181–1400). 1890. Montpellier.

Chartularium universitatis Parisiensis. Edited by H. Denifle and E. Chatelain. 1889. Vol. 1. Paris.

Chartularium universitatis portugalensis (1288–1537). Edited by A. Moreira de Sá. 1966–81. Vols. 1–8. Lisbon.

Clagett, Marshall. 1941. *Giovanni Marliani and Late Medieval Physics.* New York.

Constable, Giles, ed. 1967. *The Letters of Peter the Venerable.* 2 vols. Cambridge, Mass. (Letters 158a and b and appendices.)

Constantinus Africanus. 1960. *Chirurgia.* Edited by Marco T. Malato and Luigi Loria. In *Pagine di storia della scienza e della tecnica* 13:61–211.

Corner, George W. 1927. *Anatomical Texts of the Earlier Middle Ages.* Washington, D.C.

———. 1937. "On Early Salernitan Surgery and Especially the 'Bamberg Surgery'." BHM 5:1–28.

Corsini, A. 1925. "Nuovo contributo di notizie intorno alla vita di maestro Tommaso del Garbo." *Rivista di storia delle scienze mediche e naturali* 16:268–78.

Cosman, Madeleine Pelner. 1973. "Medieval Malpractice: The Dicta and the Dockets." *Bulletin of the New York Academy of Medicine* 49:22–47.

Daems, Willem F. 1970. "Spongia somnifera: Philologische und pharmakologische Probleme." *Beiträge zur Geschichte der Pharmazie* 22:25–26.

D'Alverny, Marie-Thérèse. 1982. "Translators and Translations." In *Renaissance and Renewal in the Twelfth Century,* edited by Robert L. Benson and Giles Constable, 421–62. Cambridge, Mass.

De Laccy, Philip. 1972. "Galen's Platonism." *American Journal of Philology* 93:27–39.

Del Garbo, Dino, 1514. *Dyni florentini super quarta fen primi Avicenne preclarissima commentaria que Dilucidatorium totius practice generalis medicinalis scientie nuncupatur.* Venice.

———. 1536. *Dinus in Chirurgia.* Venice.

Demaitre, Luke. 1976. "Nature and the Art of Medicine in the Later Middle Ages." *Medievalia* 2:23–47.

———. 1980. *Doctor Bernard de Gordon: Professor and Practitioner.* Toronto.

———. 1985. "The Description and Diagnosis of Leprosy by Fourteenth-Century Physicians." BHM 59:327–44.

De Renzi, Salvatore. 1845–48. *Storia della Medicina in Italia*. 5 vols. Naples.

Dronke, Peter, 1984. *Women Writers of the Middle Ages*. Cambridge.

Dulieu, Louis. 1975. *La chirurgie à Montpellier de ses origines au début du XIX siècle*. Avignon.

———. 1976[?] *La médicine à Montpellier*. Vol. 1: *Le Moyen Age*. n.p., n.d.

Durling, Richard J. 1967a. *A Catalogue of Sixteenth Century Printed Books in the National Library of Medicine*. Bethesda, Md.

———. 1967b, 1981. "Corrigenda and Addenda to Diels' Galenica. I. Codices Vaticani,"; "II. Codices miscellanei." *Traditio* 23:461–76; 37:373–81.

———, ed. 1976. *Burgundio of Pisa's Translation of Galen's Peri Kraseon "De complexionibus." Galenus latinus*, vol. 1. Berlin and New York.

Eamon, William, and Gundolf Keil. 1987. "'Plebs amat empirica': Nicholas of Poland and His Critique of the Medieval Medical Establishment," SA 71:180–196.

Edelstein, E. J., and Edelstein, L. 1945. *Asclepius: A Collection and Interpretation of the Testimonies*. 2 vols. Baltimore.

Edelstein, Ludwig. 1967. *Ancient Medicine*. Edited by Owsei and C. Lilian Temkin. Baltimore.

Favreau, Robert. 1978. "L'université de Poitiers et la société poitevine à la fin du Moyen Age." In *Les universités à la fin du Moyen Age*, edited by Jacques Paquet and Jozef Ijsewijn, 549–83. Louvain.

Fazio, Bartolomeo. 1745. *De viribus illustribus liber*, edited by L. Mehus. Florence.

Fichtner, Gerhard. 1972–73. "Padova e Tübingen: La formazione medica nei secoli XVI e XVII." AMHP 19:43–62.

———. 1982. "Christus als Arzt. Ursprünge und Wirkungen eines Motivs," *Frühmittelalterliche Studien: Jahrbuch des Instituts für Frühmittelalterforschung der Universität Münster* 16:1–17.

Ficino, Marsilio. 1989. *Three Books on Life*. Edited and translated by Carol V. Kaske and John R. Clark. Binghamton, N.Y.

Finucane, Ronald C. 1977. *Miracles and Pilgrims: Popular Beliefs in Medieval England*. Totowa, N.J.

Fleischhacker, Robert v., ed. 1894. *Lanfrank's "Science of Cirurgie."* Part 1. Text. EETS no. 102. Berlin, New York, and Philadelphia.

French, Roger. 1979a. "*De Juvamentis Membrorum* and the Reception of Galenic Physiological Anatomy." *Isis* 70:96–109.

———. 1979b. "A Note on the Anatomical Accessus of the Middle Ages." *Medical History* 23:461–68.

———. 1983. "Medical Teaching in Aberdeen: From the Foundation of the University to the Middle of the Seventeenth Century." *History of Universities* 3:127–28.

———. 1984. "An Origin for the Bone Text of the 'Five-Figure Series.'" SA 68:143–56.

———. 1985. "Gentile da Foligno and the *via medicorum*." In *The Light of Nature: Essays in the History and Philosophy of Science Presented to A. C. Crombie*, edited by J. D. North and J. J. Roche, 21–34. Dordrecht, Boston, Lancaster.

Friedenwald, Harry. 1944. *The Jews and Medicine. Essays*. 2 vols. Baltimore.

Fuiano, Michele. 1973. *Maestri di medicina e filosofia a Napoli nel Quattrocento*. Naples.

Galen, *De diebus decretoriis*, Kühn, 9:928–33.

———. *De febrium differentiis*, Kühn 7:273–405.

———. *De locis affectis*, Kühn, 8:1–452.

———. *De simplicium medicamentorum temperamentis ac facultatibus*, Kühn, 11:379–892.

———. *Methodus medendi*, Kühn, vol. 10.

———. 1968. *On the Usefulness of the Parts of the Body.* Translated by Margaret T. May. 2 vols. Ithaca.

———. 1979. *On the Natural Faculties.* Edited and translated by A. W. Brock. LCL. Cambridge and London. (Originally issued 1916.)

———. 1985. *Three Treatises On the Nature of Science. On the Sects for Beginners. An Outline of Empiricism. On Medical Experience.* Translated by Richard Walzer and Michael Frede. Indianapolis.

Garcia Ballester, Luis. 1982. "Arnau de Vilanova (c. 1240–1311) y la reforma de los estudios médicos en Montpellier (1309): El Hipócrates latino y la introducción del nuevo Galeno." *Dynamis* 2:97–158.

———. 1984. *Los Moriscos y la medicina: Un capítulo de la medicina y la ciencia marginadas en la España del siglo XVI.* Barcelona.

———. 1987. "Medical Science in Thirteenth-Century Castile: Problems and Prospects." BHM 61:183–202.

Garcia Ballester, Luis, Michael R. McVaugh, and Agustin Rubio Vela, 1989. *Medical Licensing and Learning in Fourteenth-Century Valencia. Transactions of the American Philosophical Society.* Vol. 79, pt. 6. Philadelphia.

Garcia Ballester, Luis, Michael R. McVaugh, and Agustin Rubio Vela. *Medical Licensing and Learning in Fourteenth-Century Valencia. Transactions of the American Philosophical Society* (forthcoming).

Gask, George E. 1950. "The Medical Services of Henry the Fifth's Campaign on the Somme in 1415." In his *Essays in the History of Medicine*, 94–102. London.

Gentile da Foligno. 1520. *Questiones et tractatus extravagantes.* Venice.

Getz, Faye M. "Medicine at Medieval Oxford." Forthcoming in *History of the University of Oxford*, Vol. 2, *Late Medieval Oxford*, edited by J. I. Catto.

Goddu, André. 1985. "The Effect of Canonical Prohibitions on the Faculty of Medicine at the University of Paris in the Middle Ages," MJ 20:342–62.

Goehl, Konrad. 1984. *Guido d'Arezzo der Jüngere und sein "Liber mitis."* WMF, vol. 32. Hanover.

Goehl, Konrad, and Gundolf Keil. 1987. "Eine Salzburger spätmittelhochdeutsche Stuhlschau." SA 71:113–15.

Goerke, Heinz. 1972. "Die medizinische Fakultät von 1472 bis zur Gegenwart." In *Die Ludwig-Maximilians-Universität in ihren Fakultäten*, vol. 1, edited by Laetitia Boehm and Johannes Spörl. Berlin.

Goltz, Dietlinde. 1972. *Studien zur Geschichte der Mineralnamen in Pharmazie, Chemie und Medizin von den Angfängen bis Paracelsus.* SA. Beiheft 14. Wiesbaden.

Gottfried, Robert A. 1984. "English Medical Practitioners, 1340–1530." BHM 58: 164–82.

Grafton, Anthony, and Noel M. Swerdlow. 1988. "Calendar Dates and Ominous Days in Ancient Historiography." *Journal of the Warburg and Courtauld Institutes* 51:14–42.

Grant, Edward, ed. 1974. *A Source Book in Medieval Science*, 700–808 ("Medicine"). Cambridge, Mass.

Green, Monica H. 1985. "The Transmission of Ancient Theories of Female Physiology and Disease Through the Early Middle Ages." Ph.D. dissertation, Princeton University.

———. 1987. "The *De genecia* Attributed to Constantinus Africanus." *Speculum* 62:299–323.

———. 1989. "Women's Medical Practice and Medical Care in Medieval Europe." *Signs* 14:434–73.

Grmek, Mirko D. 1989. *Diseases in the Ancient Greek World.* Translated by Mireille Muellner and Leonard Muellner. Baltimore.

Guglielmo da Saliceto. 1489a. *Cyrurgia.* Printed with his *Summa conservationis et curationis.* Venice.

———. 1489b. *Summa conservationis et curationis.* Venice.

Guillaume de Conches. 1974. *Philosophia mundi.* Edited by Gregor Maurach. Pretoria.

Guy de Chauliac. 1498. *Cyrurgia Guidonis de Cauliaco. Et Cyrurgia Bruni Theodorici Rogerii Rolandi Bertapalie Lanfranci.* Venice.

———. 1971. *The Cyrurgie of Guy de Chauliac.* Vol. 1. *Text.* Edited by Margaret S. Ogden. EETS no. 265. Oxford.

Haage, B. D. 1984. "Chirurgie nach Abū L-Qāsim im 'Parzival' Wolframs von Eschenbach." *Clio Medica* 19: 193–205.

Hall, Thomas H. 1971. "Life, Death and the Radical Moisture: A Study of Thematic Patterns in Medical Theory." *Clio Medica* 6:3–23.

Haly Abbas. 1523. *Liber totius medicine.* [Lyon?]

Harris, C. R. S. 1973. *The Heart and the Vascular System in Ancient Greek Medicine from Alcmaeon to Galen.* Oxford.

Haskins, Charles Homer. 1927. "A List of Text-Books From the Close of the Twelfth Century." In his *Studies in the History of Mediaeval Science,* 2d Ed., 356–76. Cambridge, Mass.

Henri de Mondeville. 1892. *Die Chirurgie des Heinrich von Mondeville (Hermondaville).* Edited by Julius Leopold Pagel. Berlin.

Herrlinger, Robert. 1970. *A History of Medical Illustration from Antiquity to A.D. 1600.* New York.

Hewson, M. Anthony. 1975. *Giles of Rome and the Medieval Theory of Conception.* London.

Hippocrates. 1972–88. 6 vols. Edited and translated by W. H. S. Jones et al. LCL. (Vols. 1 and 2 originally issued 1923; vol. 3, 1928; vol. 4, 1931.)

Holste, Thomas. 1976. *Der Theriakkrämer. Ein Beitrag zur Frühgeschichte der Arzneimittelwerbung.* WMF, vol. 5. Hanover.

Huard, Pierre, and Mirko Drazen Grmek. 1966. *Mille ans de chirurgie en Occident: V^e-XVe siècles.* Paris.

Humphreys, K. W. 1954. "The Medical Books of the Medieval Friars." *Libri: International Library Review* 3:95–103.

Hunt, R. W. 1984. *The Schools and the Cloister: The Life and Writings of Alexander Nequam (1157–1217).* Edited and revised by Margaret Gibson. Oxford.

Hunt, Tony. 1985. "Recettes médicales en vers français d'apres le manuscrit 0.8.27 de Trinity College, Cambridge." *Romania* 106:57–83.

———, 1990. *Popular Medicine in Thirteenth-Century England.* Woodbridge, Suffolk.

Iohannis Alexandrini commentaria in librum De sectis Galeni. 1982. Edited by C. D. Pritchet. Leiden.

Iohannis Alexandrini commentaria in librum De sectis Galeni. 1982. Edited by C. D. Pritchet. Leiden.

Jacquart, Danielle. 1979. See under Wickersheimer. 1936.

———. 1980. "Le regard d'un médecin sur son temps: Jacques Despars (1380?–1458)." *Bibliothèque de l'Ecole des Chartes* 138:35–86.

———. 1981. *Le milieu médical en France du XIIe au XV siècle. En annexe 2e supplément au "Dictionnaire" d'Ernest Wickersheimer.* Geneva.

———. 1984. "De *crasis* à *complexio:* Note sur le vocabulaire du tempérament en Latin médiéval." In *Textes médicaux latins antiques,* edited by G. Sabbah, 71–76. Centre Jean Palerne, *Mémoires,* vol. 5. Saint-Etienne.

———. 1985. "La réception du *Canon* d'Avicenne: Comparaison entre Montpellier et Paris au XIIIᵉ et XIVᵉ siècles." *Histoire de l'école médicale de Montpellier, Colloque. Actes du 110ᵉ Congrès National des Sociétés Savantes (Montpellier, 1985)* 2:69–77. Paris.

———. 1986. "A l'aube de la Renaissance médicale des XIᵉ–XII siècles: L'Isagoge Johannitii' et son traducteur." *Bibliothèque de l'Ecole des Chartes* 144:209–40.

———. 1988. "Aristotelian Thought in Salerno." In *A History of Twelfth-Century Western Philosophy,* edited by Peter Dronke, 407–28. Cambridge.

Jacquart, Danielle, and Claude Thomasset. 1988. *Sexuality and Medicine in the Middle Ages.* Princeton.

James, M. R. 1903. *The Ancient Libraries of Canterbury and Dover.* Cambridge.

Jarcho, Saul. 1980. *The Concept of Heart Failure: From Avicenna to Albertini.* Cambridge, Mass.

[Johannes de Ketham]. 1925. *Fasciculo di medicina.* Edited by Charles Singer. 2 vols. Florence.

John of Arderne. 1910. *Treatises of Fistula in Ano, Haemorrhoids, and Clysters by John Arderne from an Early Fifteenth-Century Manuscript Translation.* Edited by D'Arcy Power. EETS, no. 139. Oxford. (Reprinted 1968.)

Jordan, Mark D. 1977. "Medicine and Natural Philosophy in Aquinas." In *Thomas von Aquin,* edited by Albert Zimmerman. *Miscellanea Mediaevalia,* vol. 19. Berlin and New York.

Kealey, Edward J. 1981. *Medieval Medicus: A Social History of Anglo-Norman Medicine.* Baltimore.

Keele, Kenneth D. 1983. *Leonardo da Vinci's Elements of the Science of Man.* New York.

Keil, Gundolf. 1959. "Das Arzneibuch Ortolfs von Baierland: Sein Umfang und sein Einfluss auf die 'Cirurgia magistri Petri de Ulma'." SA 43:20–60.

———. 1982. "Gestaltwandel und Zersetzung—Roger-Urtext und Roger-Glosse vom 12. bis ins 16. Jahrhundert. In *Medizin im mittelalterlichen Abendland,* edited by Gerhard Baader and Gundolf Keil. Darmstadt.

———. 1983–84. "Mittelalterliche Chirurgie." AMHP 30:45–64.

Kennedy, V. L. 1945. "Robert Courson on Penance." *Mediaeval Studies* 7:291–336.

Kibre, Pearl. 1945. "Hippocratic Writings in the Middle Ages." BHM 18:371–412.

———. 1953. "The Faculty of Medicine at Paris, Charlatanism and Unlicensed Medical Practice in the Later Middle Ages." BHM 27:1–20.

———. 1985. *Hippocrates latinus: Repertorium of Hippocratic Writings in the Middle Ages.* New York.

Kleineidam, Erich. 1964, 1969. *Universitas Studii Erffordensis.* 2 vols. Leipzig.

Kristeller, Paul Oskar. 1956. "The School of Salerno: Its Development and Its Contribution to the History of Learning." In his *Studies in Renaissance Thought and Letters,* 495–551. Rome.

———. 1986. *Studi sulla scuola medica salernitana.* Naples.

Krist, Rüdiger. 1987. *Berthold Blumentrosts "Quaestiones disputatae circa tractatum Avicennae de generatione embryonis et librum meteorum Aristotelis": Ein Beitrag zur Wissenschaftsgeschichte des mittelalterlichen Würzburgs.* WMF, vol. 43. Hanover.

Kudlien, Fridolf. "Mondinos Standort innerhalb der Entwicklung der Anatomie." In *Frühe Anatomie,* edited by Robert Herrlinger and Fridolf Kudlien, 1–14. Stuttgart.

Kuhn, Werner. 1971. *Die Studenten der Universität Tübingen zwischen 1477 und 1534. Ihr Studium und ihre späterer Lebenstellung.* 2 vols. Goppingen.

Lanfranco. 1498. *Ars completa totius cyrurgie.* Printed with Guy de Chauliac, *Cyrurgia*. Venice.

Lawn, Brian. 1963. *The Salernitan Questions: An Introduction to the History of Medieval and Renaissance Problem Literature.* Oxford.

————, ed. 1979. *The Prose Salernitan Questions.* London.

Lenhardt, Friedrich. 1986 [1982]. *Blutschau: Untersuchungen zur Entwicklung der Hämatskopie.* WMF, vol. 22. Hanover.

Lind, R. L. 1975. *Studies in Pre-Vesalian Anatomy: Biography, Translations, Documents.* Philadelphia.

Liuzzi, Mondino de'. 1508. *Mesue cum expositione Mondini super Canones universales.* Venice.

Lloyd, G. E. R. 1983. *Science, Folklore and Ideology: Studies in the Life Sciences in Ancient Greece.* Cambridge.

Lockwood, Dean Putnam. 1951. *Ugo Benzi, Medieval Philosopher and Physician, 1376–1439.* Chicago.

Löchel, Wolfgang. 1975. *Die Zahnmedizin Rogers und der Rogerglosse: Ein Beitrag sur Geschichte der Zahnheilkunde im Hoch- und Spätmittelalter.* WMF, vol. 4. Hanover.

Longoburgo, Bruno. 1498. *Cyrurgia magna.* Printed with Guy de Chauliac, *Cyrurgia*. Venice.

Longrigg, J. 1963. "Philosophy and Medicine, Some Early Interactions." *Harvard Studies in Classical Philology* 67:147–75.

López de Meneses, Amada. 1952. "Documentos culturales de Pedro el Ceremonioso." *Estudios de Edad Media de la Corona de Aragon* 5:669–737.

Lugano, Placido Tommaso, O.S.B., ed. 1945. *I processi inediti per Francesca Bussa dei Ponziani (Santa Francesca Romana) 1440–1453.* Vatican City.

Macdonald, Michael. 1981. *Mystical Bedlam.* Cambridge.

MacKinney, Loren C. 1938. "Medieval Medical Dictionaries and Glossaries." In *Medieval and Historiographical Essays in Honor of James Westfall Thompson*, edited by J. L. Cate and E. N. Anderson, 240–68. Chicago.

————. 1962. "The Beginnings of Western Scientific Anatomy: New Evidence and A Revision in Interpretation of Mondeville's Role." *Mdical History* 6:233–39.

————. 1965. *Medical Illustrations in Medieval Manuscripts.* London.

Maclean, Ian. 1980. *The Renaissance Notion of Woman: A Study in the Fortunes of Scholasticism and Medical Science in European Intellectual Life.* Cambridge.

Maimonides. 1984. *Medical Writings.* Translated by Fred Rosner, M.D. Haifa.

Majno, Guido. 1975. *The Healing Hand: Man and Wound in the Ancient World.* Cambridge, Mass.

Marangon, Paolo. 1977. *Alle origini dell'Aristotelismo padovano (sec. XII-XIII).* Padua.

————. 1978. "Il rapporto culturale tra università e ordini mendicanti nella Padova del Duecento." *Il Santo* 18:129–32.

Martines, Lauro. 1968. *Lawyers and Statecraft in Renaissance Florence.* Princeton.

McVaugh, Michael R. 1967. "Arnald of Villanova and Bradwardine's Law," *Isis* 58:56–64.

————. 1970. "The *Experimenta* of Arnald of Villanova." *The Journal of Medieval and Renaissance Studies* 1:107–18.

————. 1972. "Theriac at Montpellier, 1285–1325." *SA* 56:113–44.

————. 1974. "The 'humidum radicale' in Thirteenth-Century Medicine." *Traditio* 30:259–83.

————. 1975. "An Early Discussion of Medicinal Degrees at Montpellier by Henry of Winchester." BHM 49:57–71.

————. 1987. "The Two Faces of a Medical Career: Jordanus de Turre of Montpellier." In *Mathematics and Its Applications to Science and Natural Philosophy in the Middle Ages*, edited by Edward Grant and John E. Murdoch, 301–24. Cambridge, Mass.

McVaugh, Michael R., and Nancy G. Siraisi, guest editor, 1990. *Renaissance Medical Learning: Evolution of a Tradition. Osiris 6.*

Menestò, Ernesto, ed. 1984. *Il processo di canonizzazione di Chiara da Montefalco.* Perugia.

Meyerhof, Max. 1984. *Studies in Medieval Arabic Medicine: Theory and Practice.* Edited by Penelope Johnstone. London.

Michler, Markwart. 1967. "Guy de Chauliac als Anatom." In *Frühe Anatomie*, edited by Robert Herrlinger and Fridolf Kudlien, 15–32. Stuttgart.

Montero Cartelle, Enrique, ed. 1983. *Constantini liber de coitu: El tratado de andrología de Constantino el Africano.* Santiago de Compostela.

Münster, Ladislao. 1954. "Alcuni episodi sconosciuti o poco noti sulla vita e sull'-attività di Bartolomeo da Varignana." *Castalia: Rivista di storia della medicina* 10: 207–15.

————. 1955. "La medicina legale in Bologna dai suoi albori fino alla fine del secolo XIV." *Bollettino dell'Accademia Medica Pistoiese Filippo Pacini* 26:257–71.

Murdoch, John E. 1984. *Album of Science: Antiquity and the Middle Ages.* New York.

Murray Jones, Peter. 1985. *Medieval Medical Miniatures.* Austin, Texas.

Naso, Irma. 1982. *Medici e strutture sanitarie nella società tardo-medievale: Il Piemonte dei secoli XIV e XV.* Milan.

Niederhellman, Annette. 1983. *Arzt und Heilkunde in der Frühmittelalterlichen leges.* Berlin and New York.

Nutton, Vivian. 1981. "Continuity or Rediscovery? The City Physician in Classical Antiquity and Medieval Italy." In *The Town and State Physician in Europe from the Middle Ages to the Enlightenment*, edited by Andrew W. Russell, 9–46. Wolfenbüttel (also in Nutton, 1988).

————. 1983. "The Seeds of Disease: An Explanation of Contagion and Infection from the Greeks to the Renaissance." *Medical History* 27:1–34 (also in Nutton, 1988).

————. 1984. "From Galen to Alexander, Aspects of Medicine and Medical Practice in Late Antiquity." In *Symposium on Byzantine Medicine. Dumbarton Oaks Papers.* no. 38:1–14 (also in Nutton, 1988).

————. 1985. "Murders and Miracles: Lay Attitudes to Medicine in Classical Antiquity." In *Patients and Practitioners*, edited by Roy Porter, 23–53. Cambridge. (also in Nutton, 1988).

————. 1988. *From Democedes to Harvey.* London.

Ogden, Margaret S. 1973. "The Galenic Works Cited in Guy de Chauliac's *Chirurgia Magna*." JHM 28:24–33.

Ohl, Ronald. 1980. *The University of Padua 1405–1509. An International Community of Students and Professors.* Ph.D. dissertation, University of Pennsylvania.

O'Malley, Charles D., and J. B. de C. M. Saunders. 1952. *Leonardo da Vinci on the Human Body.* New York.

O'Neill, Ynez Violé. 1969. "The Fünfbilderserie Reconsidered." BHM 43:236–45.

Ongaro, Giuseppe. 1981. "La medicina nello Studio di Padova e nel Veneto." In *Storia della cultura veneta*, edited by G. Arnaldi and M. Pastore. Vol. 3, pt. 3. Vicenza.

Ottosson, Per-Gunnar. 1984. *Scholastic Medicine and Philosophy: A Study of Commentaries on Galen's Tegni (ca. 1300–1450)*. Naples.

Overfield, James H. 1984. "University Studies and the Clergy in Pre-Reformation Germany." In *Rebirth, Reform and Resilience: Universities in Transition 1300–1700*, edited by James M. Kittelson and Pamela J. Transue. Columbus, Ohio.

Pagel, Julius Leopold, ed. 1893. *Die Areolae des Johannes de Sancto Amando (13. Jahrhundert)*. Berlin.

Palmer, Richard. 1981. "Physicians and the State in Post-Medieval Italy." In *The Town and State Physician in Europe from the Middle Ages to the Enlightenment*, edited by Andrew W. Russell. Wolfenbüttel.

————. 1983. *The Studio of Venice and Its Graduates in the Sixteenth Century*. Padua and Trieste.

————. 1985. "Pharmacy in the Republic of Venice in the Sixteenth Century." In *The Medical Renaissance of the Sixteenth Century*, 100–117. Edited by A. Wear, R. French, and I. M. Lonie. Cambridge.

Pantaleoni, Marina. 1965. "La spongia somnifera al vaglio della critica moderna." *Atti del XXI Congresso Nazionale di Storia della Medicina, Perugia 11–12 Settembre, 1965* 2: 485–90.

Pardi, Giuseppe. 1903. *Lo studio di Ferrara nei secoli XVᵉ e XVIᵉ*. Ferrara.

Park, Katharine. 1985a. "The Medieval Hospital." FMR 8:127–38.

————. 1985b. *Doctors and Medicine in Early Renaissance Florence*. Princeton.

————. "Medicine and Society in Medieval Europe." Forthcoming in *History of Medicine in Society*, edited by Andrew Wear. Cambridge.

Paschetto, Eugenia. 1984. *Pietro d'Abano, medico e filosofo*. Florence.

Pelling, Margaret. 1982. Occupational Diversity: Barbersurgeons and the Trades of Norwich." BHM 56:484–511.

Pelling, Margaret, and Charles Webster. 1979. "Medical Practitioners." In *Health, Medicine and Mortality in the Sixteenth Century*, edited by Charles Webster. Cambridge.

Perarnau i Espelt, Josep. 1982. "Activitats i fórmules supersticioses de guarició a Catalunya en la primera meitat del segle XIV." *Arxiu de Textos Catalans Antics* 1:47–78.

Pesenti Marangon, Tiziana. 1978a. "La miscellanea astrologica del prototipografo padovano Bartolomeo Valdizocco e la diffusione dei testi astrologici e medici fra i lettori padovani del '400," *Quaderni per la Storia dell'Università di Padova* 11:87–106.

————. 1978b. "'Professores chirurgie,' 'medici ciroici' e 'barbitonsores' a Padova nell'età di Leonardo Buffi da Bertipaglia (m. dopo il 1448)." *Quaderni per la storia dell'Università di Padova* 11:1–38.

Pesenti, Tiziana. 1983. "Generi e pubblico della letteratura medica padovana nel Tre- e Quattrocento." In *Università e società nei secoli XII-XVI. Atti del nono Convegno Internazionale di studio tenuto a Pistoia nei giorni 20–25 settembre 1979*, 523–45. Bologna.

————. 1984. *Professori e promotori di medicina nello studio di Padova dal 1405 al 1509: Repertorio bio-bibliografico*. Padua and Trieste.

Petrarca (Petrarch), F. 1554. *Rerum senilium libri*. Book 12. In his *Opera*. Basel (facsimile reprint, Ridgewood, N.J., 1965).

————. 1978a. *Invectiva contra medicum: Testo latino e volgarizzamento di Ser Domenico Silvestri*. Edited by Pier Giorgio Ricci and Bortolo Martinelli. Revised edition. Rome.

————. 1978b. *Rerum familiarum libri* 11.1 (Latin text). In *Epistole di Francesco Petrarca*. Edited by Ugo Dotti. Turin.

————. 1982. *Rerum familiarum libri* 11.1. In *Letters on Familiar Matters: Rerum familiarum libri IX–XVI*. Translated by Aldo S. Bernardo. Baltimore and London.

Petrus Hispanus. 1973. *Thesaurus pauperum*. In his *Obras médicas*, edited by Maria Helena da Rocha Pereira. Coimbra.

Phares, Symon de. 1929. *Recueil des plus célèbres astrologues et quelques hommes doctes*. Edited by Ernest Wickersheimer. Paris.

Phillips, E. D. 1987. *Aspects of Greek Medicine*. Philadelphia.

Piana, Celestino, O. F. M. 1966. "Lauree in arti e medicina conferite a Bologna negli anni 1419–1434." In his *Nuove ricerche su le Università di Bologna e di Parma*, 110–74. Florence.

Pietro d'Abano. 1565. *Conciliator*. Venice. Facsimile, Padua, 1985.

Pouchelle, Marie-Christine. 1990. *The Body and Surgery in the Middle Ages*. Translated by Rosemary Morris. New Brunswick: Rutgers University Press. (French edition published 1983.)

Powell, James M., trans. 1971. *The Liber Augustalis or Constitutions of Melfi Promulgated by the Emperor Frederick II for the Kingdom of Sicily in 1231*. Title XLIV (1) and Title LXV (23)(1), pp. 130–31. Syracuse, N.Y.

Préaud, Maxime. 1984. *Les astrologues à la fin du Moyen Age*. Paris.

Ptolemy. *Tetrabiblos*. Edited and translated by F. E. Robbins. In *Manetho. Ptolemy, Tetrabiblos*. LCL. 1964. London and Cambridge, Mass. (Originally issued 1940.)

Rashdall, F. H. 1936. *The Universities of Europe in the Middle Ages*. Edited by F. M. Powicke and A. B. Emden. 3 vols. Oxford. (Reissued 1988.)

Rawcliffe, Carol. 1988. "The Profits of Practice: The Wealth and Status of Medical Men in Later Medieval England." *Social History of Medicine* 1:63–78.

Raymond of Capua. 1866. *Vita Sanctae Caterinae*. *Acta Sanctorum* April, 3:898–903. Paris and Rome.

————. 1960. *The Life of St. Catherine of Siena*. Translated by George Lamb. New York.

Reisert, Robert. 1986. *Der siebenkammerige Uterus: Studien zur mittelalterlichen Wirkungsgeschichte und Entfaltung eines embryologischen Gebärmuttermodells*. WMF, vol. 39. Hanover.

Renardy, Christine. 1979. *Le monde des maîtres universitaires du diocèse de Liège 1140–1350*. Paris.

Reynolds, L. D. 1983. *Texts and Transmission: A Survey of the Latin Classics*. 46–47 (Celsus). Oxford.

Rhazes. 1544. *Almansor*. In his *Opera*. Basel. (Facsimile reprint, Brussels, 1973.)

Rhazes. 1544. *Aphorismorum libri 2*. In his *Opera*. Basel. (Facsimile reprint, Brussels, 1973.)

Rice, Eugene F. 1980. "Paulus Aegineta." In CTC, vol. 4. Washington, D.C.

Richards, Peter. 1977. *The Medieval Leper and His Northern Heirs*. Cambridge.

Richardson, Linda Deer. 1985. "The Generation of Disease: Occult Causes and Diseases of the Total Substance." In *The Medical Renaissance of the Sixteenth Century*, edited by A. Wear, R. French, and I. M. Lonie, 175–94. Cambridge.

Richler, Benjamin. 1982. "Manuscripts of Avicenna's Kanon in Hebrew Translation: A Revised and Up-to-date List," *Koroth* 8:145*–68*.

Riddle, John M. 1980. "Dioscorides." In CTC, vol. 4. Washington, D.C.

————. 1985. *Dioscorides on Pharmacy and Medicine*. Austin, Texas.

————. 1987. "Folk Tradition and Folk Medicine: Recognition of Drugs in Classical Antiquity." In *Folklore and Folk Medicines*, edited by John Scarborough, 33–61. Madison, Wisconsin.

Rolando. 1498. *Libellus de cyrurgia*. Printed with Guy de Chauliac, *Cyrurgia*. Venice.

Roth, Cecil. 1953. "The Qualification of Jewish Physicians in the Middle Ages." *Speculum* 28:834–43.

Rowland, Beryl, ed. and trans. 1981. *Medieval Woman's Guide to Health*. Kent, Ohio.

Rubin, Stanley. 1974. *Medieval English Medicine*. Newton Abbot.

Russell, Andrew W., ed. 1981. *The Town and State Physician from Antiquity to the Enlightenment*. Wolfenbüttel.

Saffron, Morris H., ed. and trans. 1972. *Maurus of Salerno, Twelfth Century "Optimus Physicus," With His Commentary on the Prognostics of Hippocrates. Transactions of the American Philosophical Society*. Vol. 62, pt. 1. Philadelphia.

Sarti, Mauro, and Mauro Fattorini. 1888, 1896. *De claris archigymnasii bononiensis professoribus*. Edited by Carlo Malagola. 2 vols. Bologna.

Savonarola, Michele. 1952. *Ad mulieres ferrarienses de regimine pregnantium et noviter natorum usque ad septennium*. Edited by Luigi Belloni. Milan.

———. 1982. *Libreto de tute le cosse che se manzano: Un libro di dietetica di Michele Savonarola, medico padovano del secolo XV*. Edited by Jane Nystedt. Stockholm.

Scarborough, John. 1969. *Roman Medicine*. Ithaca, N.Y.

———. 1987. "Botany, Pharmacy, and the Culinary Arts." In *The Rational Arts of Living*, edited by A. C. Crombie and Nancy Siraisi, 161–202. Smith College Studies in History, vol. 50. Northampton, Mass.

Schipperges, Heinrich. 1964. *Die Assimilation der arabischen Medizin durch das lateinische Mittelalter. SA. Beiheft* 3. Wiesbaden.

Schmitt, Charles B. 1985. "Aristotle Among the Physicians." In *The Medical Renaissance of the Sixteenth Century*, edited by A. Wear, R. K. French, and I. M. Lonie, 1–15. Cambridge.

Schultz, John B. 1985. *Art and Anatomy in Renaissance Italy*. Ann Arbor.

Schwinges, Rainer Christoph. 1986. *Deutsche Universitätbesucher im 14. und 15. Jahrhundert: Studien zur Sozialgeschichte des alten Reiches*. Stuttgart.

Sears, Elizabeth. 1986. *The Ages of Man*. Princeton.

Sezgin, Fuat. 1970. *Geschichte des arabischen Schrifttums*, vol. 3. Leiden.

Sharpe, William D., ed. and trans. 1964. *Isidore of Seville: The Medical Writings. Transactions of the American Philosophical Society*. Vol. 54, pt. 2. Philadelphia.

Shatzmiller, Joseph. 1980. "Livres médicaux et éducation médicale: à propos d'un contrat de Marseille en 1316," *Mediaeval Studies* 42:463–70.

———. 1982–83. "In Search of the 'Book of Figures': Medicine and Astrology in Montpellier at the Turn of the Fourteenth Century." *AJSreview* 7–8:383–407.

———. 1983. "On Becoming a Jewish Doctor in the High Middle Ages." *Sefarad* 43:239–50.

Siraisi, Nancy G. 1973. *Arts and Sciences at Padua*. Toronto.

———. 1980. "The Medical Learning of Albertus Magnus." In *Albertus Magnus and the Sciences*, edited by James A. Weisheipl, O.P. Toronto.

———. 1981. *Taddeo Alderotti and His Pupils: Two Generations of Italian Medical Learning*. Princeton.

———. 1987a. *Avicenna in Renaissance Italy. The Canon and Medical Teaching in Italian Universities after 1500*. Princeton.

———. 1987b. "The Physician's Task: Medical Reputations in Humanist Collective Biographies." In *The Rational Arts of Living*, edited by A. C. Crombie and Nancy Siraisi, 105–33. Smith College Studies in History, vol. 50. Northampton, Mass.

Smith, Emilie Savage. 1976. "Some Sources and Procedures for Editing A Medieval Arabic Surgical Tract." *History of Science* 14:245–64.

Smith, Wesley D. 1973. *The Hippocratic Tradition*. Ithaca, N.Y.

Stannard, Jerry. 1968. Jerry Stannard, "Medieval Italian Medical Botany." *Atti del XXI Congresso Internazionale di Storia della Medicina, Siena 22–28 Settembre 1968* 2: 1554–65.

———. 1974. "Medieval Herbals and Their Development." *Clio Medica* 9:23–33.

———. 1977. "Magiferous Plants and Magic in Medieval Medical Botany." *The Maryland Historian* 8:33–45.

———. 1978. "Natural History." In *Science in the Middle Ages*, edited by David C. Lindberg, 429–60. Chicago.

Statuti delle Università e dei Collegi dello Studio bolognese, edited by Carlo Malagola. 1888. Bologna.

Sudhoff, Karl. 1914, 1918. *Beiträge zur Geschichte der Chirurgie im Mittelalter*. 2 vols. *Studien zur Geschichte der Medizin*, vol. 11 and 12. Leipzig.

———. "Pestschriften aus den ersten 150 Jahren nach der Epidemie des Schwarzen Todes (1348)." *Archiv für Geschichte der Medizin*. (= SA) 4 (1911): 191–222, 389–424; 5 (1912): 36–87, 332–96; 6 (1913): 313–79; 7 (1914): 57–114; 8 (1915): 175–215 236–89; 9 (1916): 53–78 117–67; 11 (1917): 44–92 121–76: 17 (1925): 12–139 241–91.

Tabanelli, Mario. 1965. *La chirurgia italiana nell'alto medioevo*. 2 vols. Florence.

Talbot, C. H. 1961. "A Medieval Physician's Vade Mecum." JHM 16:213–33.

———. 1967. *Medicine in Medieval England*. London.

Talbot, C. H., and E. A. Hammond. 1965. *The Medical Practitioners in Medieval England: A Biographical Register*. London.

Temkin, Owsei. 1973. *Galenism: Rise and Decline of a Medical Philosophy*. Ithaca, N.Y.

Tester, S. J. 1987. *A History of Western Astrology*. Woodbridge.

Thorndike, Lynn, 1923, 1934. *History of Magic and Experimental Science*. Vols. 1–3. New York.

———. ed. 1949. *The Sphere of Sacrobosco and Its Commentators*. Chicago.

Thorndike, Lynn, and Pearl Kibre. 1963. *A Catalogue of Incipits of Mediaeval Scientific Writings in Latin*, 2d Ed. Cambridge, Mass.

Ullmann, Manfred. 1970. *Die Medizin im Islam*. Leiden.

———. 1978. *Islamic Medicine*. Edinburgh.

Villani, Filippo. 1847. *Liber de civitatis Florentiae famosis civibus*. Edited by G. C. Galletti. Florence.

Voigts, Linda E. 1979. "Anglo-Saxon Plant Remedies and the Anglo-Saxons." Isis 70:250–68.

———. 1982. "Editing Middle English Medical Texts: Needs and Issues." In *Editing Texts in the History of Science and Medicine*, edited by Trevor H. Levere, 39–66. New York and London.

———. 1988. "Report and Reviews: Old and Middle English Medicine." *Society for Ancient Medicine and Pharmacy Newsletter*, no. 16 (October, 1988): 31–36.

———. 1989. "Scientific and Medical Books." In *Book Production and Publishing in Britain, 1375–1475*, edited by Jeremy Griffiths and Derek Pearsall. 345–402. Cambridge.

Voigts, Linda E., and Michael R. McVaugh, eds. 1984. *A Latin Technical Phlebotomy and Its Middle English Translation. Transactions of the American Philosophical Society*. Vol. 74, pt. 2. Philadelphia.

Wallner, Björn, ed. 1969. *The Middle English Translation of Guy de Chauliac's Treatise on Fractures and Dislocations. Book V of the Great Surgery.* Lund.

Wangensteen, Owen H., and Sarah D. Wangensteen. 1978. *The Rise of Surgery: From Empiric Craft to Scientific Discipline.* Minneapolis.

Wear, A., French, R. K., and Lonie, I. M., eds. 1985. *The Medical Renaissance of the Sixteenth Century.* Cambridge.

Whitteridge, Gweneth. 1977. "Some Italian Precursors of the Royal College of Physicians." *Journal of the Royal College of Physicians* 12:67–80.

Wicher, Helen Brown. 1986. "Nemesius Emesenus." In CTC, vol. 6. Washington, D.C.

Wickersheimer, Ernest. 1936. *Dictionnaire biographique des médicins en France au moyen âge.* 2 vols. Paris. With *Supplément*, edited by Danielle Jacquart. Geneva, 1979.

William of Conches. 1567. *Dragmaticon (De substantiis physicis)*, bk. 6. Strasburg. (Facsimile Frankfurt/Main 1967.)

Zanier, Giancarlo. 1977. *La medicina astrologica e la sua teoria: Marsilio Ficino e i suoi critici contemporanei.* Rome.

———. 1983. "Ricerche sull'occultismo a Padova nel sec. XV." In *Scienza e filosofia all'Università di Padova nel Quattrocento*, edited by Antonino Poppi, 345–72.

INDEX

Frequently occurring names (e.g. Galen, Avicenna) are indexed selectively; some names referred to only incidentally are not indexed. Bibliographic citations in the notes are not indexed. References to figures are to the content of the captions. *Parts of the body, medicines and medicinal ingredients,* and *surgical procedures* are grouped as subentries under those headings. As far as possible, the subentries grouped under the headings *diseases and afflictions* and *physiology* use the concepts and terminology of the medical system described in this book.

London: College of Physicians, 18, 190; conjoint college of physicians and surgeons, 56, 180; medical and surgical practitioners in, 20, 56–57, 180

Longoburgo, Bruno, of Calabria, 164, 167, 177

Lucretius, 130

Magic and magical remedies, 11, 34, 35, 46, 132, 149, 152

Maimonides, 29

Manardo, Giovanni, 190

Marliani, Giovanni, 124

Materia medica. See Medicines and medicinal ingredients

Maurus of Salerno, 124

Medical and surgical practitioners, vii, 5, 6, 10–11, 13–14; attitudes toward patients, 40, 116, 124, 172, 175–76; biographies, 47; distribution (see names of cities and geographic regions); hierarchy of categories, 20; income, 21–22 (see also Salaries and fees); non-medical activities, 26, 36; numbers, 23–25; practice of astrology, 36; relations among categories, 34–35, 172, 177–80, 188; status, economic and social, 20, 21, 26; titles and terms for, 20–21; trade secrets of, 185; varieties of medical employment, 21, 36–39. See also Clergy, practice of medicine by; Jewish medicine and medical practitioners; Moriscos; Surgeons; Surgery; University faculties of medicine (university-educated practitioners); Women and medicine

Medicine, personification of, fig. 1

Medicines and medicinal ingredients, 3, 126, 141, 172, figs. 30, 31, 33; alcohol, 148, 185; from animals, 148; compounds, 146; dosage, 146; emetics and laxatives, 148; exotica, 143, 146, 147; herbs and vegetable substances, 116, 121, 141–43, 147–49; means of application (internal, external, by inhalation, fumigation, as ointments, pills, powders, liquids), 116, 129, 147, 169, 170; methods of preparation, 148; mineral, 147, 193; nomenclature and identification, 143; pharmacological theory, 141, 144–46, 191; simples, 145; social factors in prescription, 147;

substitutions, 143; theriac, 32–33, 118–19, 146; wine, 148, 170, 185. See also Herbals; Magic and magical remedies; Recipes and remedy collections

Mercato of Gubbio, medical practitioner, 39

Merovingian Gaul, 10

Merton College, Oxford, 56

Methodists. See Sects, medical, ancient

Milan, 100

Military medicine, 35, 176–77, 181–83, 192

Milk, 105, 111

Monasteries and nunneries, employment of medical practitioners by, 9, 14, 38–39, 115–18

Monastic medicine, 7, 9, 10, 25, 50. See also Clergy, practice of medicine by

Mondeville, Henri de, 85, 90, 96, 166, 179–80, 180, 182

Monte Cassino, 14, 58

Montpellier, 14, 32, 34, 55, 62, 85, 119, 141, 152, 153, 166; surgery at, 180

Montpellier, University of, 63, 64, 66, 69, 71, 72, 80, 84; dissection at, 86; origins and development of medical faculty, 58–59

Morestede, Thomas, 182

Moriscos, 23, 29

Music of pulse, 127

Muslim world, medicine in, ix, 11–13, 58, 188

Naples, 86; medical practitioners in, 27

Natural philosophy, 3, 12, 15, 21, 32, 41, 52, 58, 60, 107; relation with medicine, 2–3, 12, 67, 79, 80, 84–85, 100, 146, 191. See also Reconciliation of Aristotle and Galen

Naturals, things natural, 101

Nequam, Alexander, 59

Neutral state (between health and sickness), 119, 123, 137

New diseases, recognition of, 129, 191

New Testament, miracles of healing in, 8–9

Niccolo, medical practitioner of Spoleto, 40

Nicholas of Poland, OP, 32–33

Non-naturals, 101, 120, 123

North Africa (Roman), 6